Understanding
Chronic Illness

Understanding Chronic Illness

The Medical and Psychosocial
Dimensions of Nine Diseases

Toba Schwaber Kerson, D.S.W.
with
Lawrence A. Kerson, M.D.

FP

THE FREE PRESS
A Division of Macmillan, Inc.
NEW YORK

Collier Macmillan Publishers
LONDON

The Free Press
A Division of Macmillan, Inc.
866 Third Avenue, New York, N. Y. 10022

Collier Macmillan Canada, Inc.

Printed in the United States of America

printing number

3 4 5 6 7 8 9 10

Library of Congress Cataloging in Publication Data

Kerson, Toba Schwaber.
 Understanding chronic illness.

 Bibliography: p.
 Includes index.
 1. Chronic diseases—Psychological aspects. 2. Chronic
diseases—Social aspects. I. Kerson, Lawrence A.
II. Title. [DNLM: 1. Chronic Disease. 2. Chronic
Disease—psychology.   WT 500 K41u]
 RC108.K465 1985   616   84-28622
 ISBN 0-02-918200-X

This book is in memory of **Joseph Schwaber Jr.,** who fought the good fight with great dignity and with trust in God and his doctors; and for **Jennie Kerson,** who still believes that Daddy, the doctor, can heal any hurt.

Contents

Acknowledgments

Several hundred people were interviewed in the course of gathering information for this book. Many more read drafts of various chapters or helped with the collection of data.

At the risk of offending those whom I neglect to mention, I would like to thank Susan Dawson, Renee Weisman, Judy Regeuiro, Judy Gross, Rosemary Boyle, Sue Davis, Marian Frank, Doris Schwartz, Loretta Dugan, Leslie and John Alexander, Carolyn McGrory, Gary Gordon, Faye Soffen, Carleton Dallery, June Axinn, Elihu Goren, Roberta Gonzalez, Julina Gylfe, Sheldon Lisker, Nancy Interante, Richard Katz, Jonathan Satinsky, Sherri Alper, Linda Smith, Cynthia Shockley, Camille DiSilvestro, Marianne Sachs, Maryann De Dominic, Eliza Wingate, and Lorraine Wright.

Laura Wolff, editor at The Free Press, made only thoughtful suggestions and urged me toward clarity and depth of content. A special thank you to Betsy Blades for her contribution to the data collection and writing in the respiratory disease chapter.

In addition, I would like to thank the National Epilepsy Foundation, American Diabetes Association, Juvenile Diabetes Foundation, Al-Anon, American Cancer Society, American Lung Association, American Heart Association, Alzheimer's Disease and Related Disorders Association, Progressive Epilepsy Network, Alcoholics

Anonymous, and the National Arthritis Foundation and representatives of many governmental agencies for their help.

I extend grateful acknowledgment to Bryn Mawr College's
Rosalyn R. Schwartz Fund and to Richard Gaskins of the Graduate
School of Social Work and Social Research for their support.

Finally, I am grateful to Lawrence A. Kerson, medical and
grammatical consultant, who made the writing of this book a
priority because it was important to me.

Understanding
Chronic Illness

1

Introduction

CHRONIC DISEASES ARE long-lasting; they affect and even disrupt the lives of the ill individual and those around her.* The word "chronic" has nothing but negative connotations. People are described not as chronically happy or healthy but as chronically depressed or ill. Caused by nonreversible pathological alterations in the body, chronic diseases generally require long periods of supervision, observation, care, and rehabilitation. Most are characterized by periods of recurrence and remission. Because there are rarely cures, the goal of treatment for these illnesses becomes control of the progression of the disease, which means its tendency to involve and damage increasing amounts of body tissue. Chronic illness is often marked by a loss of physical or mental ability, which curtails a person's capacity to look after her needs. Each disease disables differently, so much of the impact a chronic illness has on the life of an individual and her family members is inextricably bound to the facts of the particular disease.

Understanding Chronic Illness is written for people who face decisions affecting others who are chronically ill: those dispensing medical care, those in positions of authority in the community, and those who seek to be better informed in their relationship with the chronically ill. A social worker who has to decide whether a child can continue to live with her grandmother who has had a stroke; a manager who must decide whether

*Because no single word exists for he/she or her/his, and the use of those solutions seems heavy-handed, I will generally alternate, using "her" and "she" as representative of both sexes in some chapters and "he" and "him" in others. This introduction will use "her" and "she" as the general terms. The pronoun used has no bearing on the incidence of the disease discussed among males or females.

to permit someone who has cancer or heart disease to return to work; a teacher who must decide how to explain a student's seizures to the rest of the class; or a minister who must counsel a despondent congregant about her husband's emphysema are examples of readers who should find help here.

The book describes the medical, social, and psychological aspects of nine chronic diseases: arthritis, cancer, dementia, diabetes, epilepsy, heart disease, respiratory illness, stroke, and substance abuse. These illnesses were chosen because they are among the most devastating of the chronic diseases with greatest prevalence. Each affects several million people in the United States. Sinusitis, the chronic condition with the greatest prevalence in the United States (about 31 million), is not usually devastating, so it was not included. Multiple sclerosis can be devastating, but the Multiple Sclerosis Society estimates its prevalence at less than 250,000, and the National Center for Health Statistics at less than 100,000, so it also is not included. End stage renal disease (about 60,000) and sickle cell anemia (about 50,000) are not included for the same reason.

Some of the included diseases rank high among causes of death in the United States. In 1982 the National Center for Health Statistics reported the ten leading causes of death as heart diseases, 38.2 percent; malignant neoplasms (cancer), 21.9 percent; cerebrovascular diseases (stroke), 8 percent; accidents, 4.8 percent; chronic obstructive pulmonary diseases and allied conditions (respiratory illness), 3 percent; pneumonia and influenza, 2.5 percent; diabetes mellitus, 1.7 percent; suicide, 1.4 percent; chronic liver disease and cirrhosis, 1.4 percent; and arteriosclerosis, 1.3 percent. Although some of the diseases included in this book are not on this list, suffering from one of them can place a person at greater risk for these high-mortality diseases. Diabetes puts one at greater risk for heart disease and stroke, for example, and alcoholism increases the risk for several of these illnesses, including liver disease. In March 1983 the Department of Health and Human Services announced that Alzheimer's disease and its complications cause 100,000 deaths a year. Although the mortality statistics for such illnesses as epilepsy and arthritis are not high, the degree of disability and the impact on the life of an affected individual are great.

Framework for Understanding Chronic Disease

Each chapter loosely follows the following outline as a guide for presenting information on the medical, social, and psychological aspects of a chronic illness:

    I. Medical Information
       A. Description of the disease
         1. Definition

2. Classification
3. Etiology
4. Prevalence and incidence
5. Populations at risk for the illness
6. Association with other diseases
7. Prognosis
   B. Natural history
   1. Stages
   2. Symptoms
   C. Diagnostic procedures
   1. History
   2. Physical examination
   3. Laboratory tests
   D. Treatment
   1. Drugs
   2. Surgery
   3. Radiography
   4. Other
   E. Anticipated course of the treated disease
II. Psychosocial Information
   A. Modifications in life-style
   1. Diet
   2. Exercise
   3. Restraint from activity
   4. Restriction from activity
   5. Sleep or rest patterns
   6. Relaxation techniques
   7. Daily schedule
   8. Other
   B. Impact of the disease on social life
   1. Legal aspects
      a. Restrictions
         (1) Driving
         (2) Marriage
         (3) Training or work
         (4) Other
      b. Protection
         (1) Right to work
         (2) Right to retraining
         (3) Guardianship
   2. Social aspects
      a. Insurance
         (1) Medical
         (2) Life
         (3) Automobile
         (4) Social Security disability
      b. Relationships with others
         (1) Family members

           (2) Strangers
           (3) Increased dependence
           (4) Increased confinement
           (5) Isolation
      c. Work
      d. Diet
      e. Recreational activity
      f. Daily schedule
   3. Psychological aspects
      a. Self-concept
      b. Particular psychological responses
      c. Stages of psychological response
      d. Sexual response
      e. Changes in appearance
      f. Changes in mood and affect
      g. Other
  III. How to Be Helpful to Someone Who Has the Illness

The first part of each chapter presents medical information, with an emphasis on clarifying the decision-making processes of the medical team. The disease is defined, and information about mortality, progression, and predictability is presented. The classification involves a breakdown of the broad term into specific types. For example, diabetes can be classified as insulin-dependent or non-insulin-dependent, and cancer can be assorted into more than one hundred categories based on anatomic site and type of tumor. Both prognosis and treatment plan depend on classification.

Etiology or cause of the disease is discussed, although often little is understood about causation. The prevalence and incidence of each disease and its main categories are also described. Prevalence means the number of people who have the particular disease or type at a specified time, and incidence refers to the number of new cases of a disease in a given year. Unless otherwise stated, reported statistics are for the United States, and the source for almost all of them is the National Center for Health Statistics. Particular populations who are at risk for contracting the disease are described as well. For example, women whose mothers or sisters have a history of breast cancer have a greater chance of contracting breast cancer than women without a family history. Smokers have a far greater chance of contracting lung cancer than nonsmokers, and people with uncontrolled hypertension are at greater risk of a stroke than those with normal blood pressure. Next, the prognosis or forecast of the probable course of the disease is presented.

The natural history, the course the disease would take if left untreated, is described in terms of stages and symptoms. Particularly addressed are the frequency and duration of pain, sensory loss, inability to control bodily functions, behavioral changes, mood changes, changes in thought processes, fatigue, and weakness.

The means used to arrive at a diagnosis are described: the symptoms the physician looks for in history-taking, the particular findings the physician looks for in the physical examination, and the tests used to support or rule out the diagnosis. Possible complications resulting from tests are also noted.

The discussion of treatment touches on measures directed at both decreasing the likelihood of a recurrence or progress of the disease and preventing or controlling symptoms. Drug, surgical, and radiographic therapies relevant to specific diseases are discussed. The means presented for diagnosis and treatment represent the standard of medical practice in relation to each illness. The final topic of the medical section is the anticipated course of the treated disease.

The second section of each chapter discusses the social and psychological aspects of the disease. First addressed are the kinds of changes one must make in life-style to adapt to the illness. Diet, exercise, climate change, restraint from or restriction of certain activities, sleep or rest patterns, recreational activities, and daily schedule are among the areas where changes may occur. Examples of life-style changes are the special attention to diet demanded by diabetes and the importance of a specific kind of exercise program for someone with rheumatoid arthritis.

Federal legislation affects the rights and entitlements of many people who are chronically ill. Especially important are the several titles of the Social Security Act relating to aid for the chronically ill such as Medicare (for those over sixty-five), Medicaid (for the indigent), Crippled Children's Programs (for certain handicapping conditions), and Disability Insurance (for those whose severely disabling conditions prevent them from working). Although most individuals are covered by health insurance through the workplace until retirement, the likelihood of contracting one or more chronic diseases rises with age, so many of the chronically ill, being elderly, are insured through Medicare. Medicaid covers the poorest segments of society, especially impoverished dependent children and those (most often elderly people) needing custodial care. Medicare, Medicaid, Crippled Children's Programs, and Social Security Disability Insurance will now be explained briefly in general terms.

Federal Medical Insurance Programs

In 1966 Congress passed Titles 18 and 19 of the Social Security Act. Title 18 called for the establishment of Medicare, and Title 19 the establishment of Medicaid. The Health Care Financing Administration, under the Department of the Health and Human Services, is responsible for the Medicare program, federal participation in the Medicaid program, and other health care programs. Both Medicare and Medicaid are important for those who are chronically ill, Medicare because the likelihood of chronic illness increases with age, and Medicaid because it is for the poor. It is not uncommon for a person who has become severely disabled as a result of a chronic illness to become poor because of the expense of her care, her inability to earn income, and sometimes her caretaker's loss of income.

Medicare

Medicare is a federally administered health insurance program in which money from trust funds pays medical bills for insured people who are sixty-five or older and for some disabled people under sixty-five. Almost every citizen of the United States who is sixty-five or over is eligible for Medicare. Those who have sufficient work credits under Social Security automatically have hospital insurance when they reach sixty-five. They may purchase medical insurance by signing up during the three months immediately before or after they reach sixty-five or during the first three months of any year thereafter. The medical insurance part of Medicare requires a monthly payment, which is increased by a percentage for every year in which one could have been but was not enrolled. People who have received Social Security Disability benefits for two years or who have chronic renal disease requiring dialysis or transplant are also eligible for Medicare. Total Medicare expenditures were more than $35.7 billion in 1980. In July 1981, 29 million aged or disabled people were enrolled in the Medicare program.

Medicare has two parts: hospital insurance and medical insurance. Both parts will pay only for services specifically covered, and both require some degree of co-payment or deductible, so that the ill person is sharing the expenses. Hospital insurance helps pay for inpatient hospital care and for posthospital care in a skilled nursing facility or at home. In regard to inpatient hospital care, it covers room and board in a semiprivate room in an approved hospital for the first sixty-day period except for a substantial deductible, and for the next thirty days in each benefit period except for a per diem co-payment. Sixty additional lifetime "reserve days" can be used in case hospitalization extends beyond ninety days in a benefit period. The "reserve days" pay all covered expenses except a per diem co-payment and are not replaced once they are used.

Also covered are laboratory and x-ray services, regular hospital nursing services, drugs used in inpatient treatment, blood and packed red blood cells after the third pint in a calendar year (the first three pints must be bought or replaced through donation), use of operating room and recovery room, intensive care and coronary care units, medical supplies such as surgical dressings or casts, use of appliances such as stretchers or wheelchairs, and rehabilitation services such as physical, speech, and occupational therapy. Services specifically not covered are the extra cost of a private room unless it is required for medical reasons, private duty nursing, items like telephone and TV that are requested by the patient for personal convenience, physicians' services except at some teaching hospitals (these may be covered under medical insurance), and room and board in a psychiatric hospital beyond a lifetime total of 190 days.

Inpatient care in a skilled nursing facility is also covered for up to one hundred days per benefit period following a hospital stay of at least three days within the last thirty days. To be eligible for a skilled nursing facility, the patient must require skilled nursing or skilled rehabilitation services. Patients who require custodial care but not skilled nursing or rehabilitation services are ineligible for this coverage.

Home health care pays for prescribed part-time skilled nursing care, physical therapy, and speech therapy if one is confined to her home. The home treatment plan must be set up within fourteen days of the patient's discharge from a hospital or skilled nursing facility. Drugs, full-time nursing, and care that is mainly custodial are not covered.

Medical insurance helps pay for doctors' services, outpatient hospital services, and some other services and supplies not covered under hospital insurance. Specifically, it covers physicians' medical and surgical services, including those in the hospital, the physician's office, the patient's home, or anywhere in the United States. Also covered are dentists' services when they are of the kind covered when furnished by physicians; supplies and services relating to diagnosis or treatment such as x-rays and electrocardiograms; and prosthetic devices such as artificial limbs. Medicare will pay for the rental of durable medical equipment for home use such as hospital beds and oxygen; outpatient physical and speech therapy when prescribed by a physician; rehabilitation services from an approved center; ambulance service to the nearest appropriate facility when other modes of transportation would be unsafe; blood and packed blood beginning with the fourth pint in a calendar year; and home health visits by an approved agency. Not covered are routine physical examinations, cosmetic surgery unless needed to correct malfunction or because of injury, optometrists' services except for prosthetic lenses, podiatrist's services for routine foot care, payments for mental illness in excess of $250 annually, most immunizations, false teeth, eyeglasses except for prosthetic use, hearing aids, orthopedic shoes, drugs, and full-time nursing and custodial care.

Recently legislation was enacted in response to the explosive costs of Medicare, which have created a crisis for reimbursement. The crisis has occurred primarily for two reasons: The number of elderly has grown more rapidly than the rest of the population, and changes in per capita health expenditures have been greater for those over sixty-five years old than for others. Since the enactment of Medicare, life expectancy at age sixty-five has jumped from 14.6 to 16.4. Expenditures rise generally with age, not because of age *per se*, but because the proportion of people near death increases with age. Expenditures are particularly large in the last year of life. In 1976 the average Medicare reimbursement for those in the last year of life was 6.6 times as high as for those who survived. The United States is spending about 1 percent of its GNP on health care for the elderly in the last year of life. In 1982 Medicare accounted for 7 percent of all federal outlays. That is the crisis to which the legislation was a response.

TEFRA (TAX EQUITY AND FISCAL RESPONSIBILITY ACT)

The first piece of legislation is the Tax Equity and Fiscal Responsibility Act of 1982 (TEFRA). TEFRA changed Medicare's hospital reimbursement methods in several ways. It made the basis for reimbursement the case (the disease category of the patient) rather than the cost to the hospital or providing daily care for the patient. It incorporated case-mix, that is, the kinds of patients in that particular hospital in the payment system, and it limited the rate at which the costs could be increased per case. In addition TEFRA mandated that the Secretary of Health and Human Services develop a prospective payment plan.

MEDICARE PROSPECTIVE PAYMENT SYSTEM

The Medicare Prospective Payment system established a patient classification system of 468 diagnosis-related groups (DRGs). Hospitals are no longer reimbursed according to a per diem figure based on what it costs them to take care of the patient. Rather, they are now paid according to the diagnosis of the patient. Payments per DRG are to be a function of urban or rural location, area wages, and the number of full-time interns and residents on the staff of the particular hospital. Capital costs and direct education are to be separate from DRGs for the present. The three-year phase-in period for the program is to be completed by 1987.

One concern about the prospective payment system is whether it accounts sufficiently for severity of illness. For example, people who are admitted to the hospital for cataract surgery will usually be discharged very quickly. The course in hospital for those admitted because of the progression of a systemic illness such as cancer or diabetes will often be less predictable. Acute episodes of chronic illnesses are of special concern.

HOSPICE

Section 122 of TEFRA is the Hospice Bill. In effect in November 1983, the bill extended Medicare coverage of both inpatient and home care to Medicare-eligible patients with a six-months-or-less terminal diagnosis. It is thought that the bill was passed because the Congressional Budget Office reported that the hospice legislation would save Medicare $109 million in the first five years after passage, or $1,100 during the last forty-five days of each hospice patient's life. Medicare-reimbursed hospice programs must provide assurances to the federal government that 80 percent of the days in which their total patient population was enrolled in its program were home days and not inpatient days. The aggregate reimbursement limit (per hospice) is $7,600. Thus, the success and, in fact, the survival of the hospice program as a federally reimbursed service is dependent on its adherence to those fiscal guidelines. To date, relatively few of the hospice programs have joined the Medicare program, because it is felt that the fiscal constraints would, in fact, bankrupt the hospices.

Although hospices could be a useful approach for people dying as a result of many causes, it is estimated that more than 90 percent of hospice patients have cancer. The National Hospice Organization has included questions about population diagnoses in the survey it will conduct of the more than 2,000 hospice programs in the United States.

Central to the hospice concept is the management of the illness in ways that allow patients to be alert and free of pain, and to live with their families as much as possible, and that allow the families to grieve in a healthy manner and live without guilt after the patient dies. The goal is to keep life comfortable and meaningful for all concerned. In addition to symptom relief and emotional support, hospice programs also provide respite for exhausted family members by having volunteers spend time with the ill person at home or by briefly admitting the ill person to an inpatient facility. Hospice programs are usually interdisciplinary and physician-directed, either based in a hospital or a visiting nurse or home-care program or coordinated by a community group. The hospice is a fashionable concept but a very old one. Continuing to care and be supportive when one can no longer hope to cure is a value in nursing, social work, gerontology, and the ministry as well as in medicine. The institutionalization of such care, it is to be hoped, will make its watchwords of sensitivity and support the rule and not the exception.

Medicaid

Medicaid is an assistance program in which states design their own programs within federal guidelines to pay medical bills for specific categories of needy and low-income people. It is a vendor payment program, which means that payments are made directly to providers of care, who must accept the Medicaid reimbursement as full payment. All states except Arizona have Medicaid programs. As of November 1981 Arizona established the Health Care Cost Containment System, a demonstration program supported by the Health Care Financing Administration that provides health care to the poor based on a prepaid, capitation basis.

Federal law governs certain aspects of Medicaid. For example, it mandates coverage for two low-income groups: single-parent families and some two-parent families with one unemployed parent that are part of the Aid to Families with Dependent Children Program (AFDC), and disabled people who are part of the Supplemental Security Income program (SSI).

Medicaid varies from state to state. The federal government requires states to provide a basic set of services to people eligible for Medicaid. However, since states establish eligibility for AFDC and the federal government mandates Medicaid coverage for all AFDC recipients, the states in fact determine Medicaid eligibility by determining AFDC eligibility. Some states also include other needy and low-income people.

Medicaid pays for at least the following services: inpatient hospital care, outpatient hospital services, laboratory and x-ray services, skilled nursing facility services, physicians' services, screening, diagnosis and treatment of children under twenty-one, home health care services, family planning services, and rural health clinic services. In many states Medicaid also pays for some dental care; prescribed drugs; eyeglasses; clinic services; specified diagnostic, screening, preventive, and rehabilitative services; and intermediate care facility services. In 1980 there were approximately 28.6 million Medicaid recipients. The state and federal Medicaid expenditures for that year were more than $23 billion. Forty-two percent of the expenditures were for nursing home care, 28 percent for inpatient hospital care, and 30 percent primarily for physicians' services, outpatient hospital care, and medications. Medicaid is the primary source of payment for more than half of all nursing home patients. In long-term care institutions, individuals must turn over income in excess of the maintenance needs of themselves and their spouses to help pay for their care. Also, most states have buy-in agreements with Medicare under which Medicaid pays the Part B Medicare premiums and cost sharing for people covered under both programs.

State Medicaid programs provide many services for the chronically ill that Medicare does not cover, such as skilled nursing home facility care beyond the hundred-day posthospital coverage provided by Medicare, long-term care in intermediate care facilities, prescription drugs, eyeglasses, and hearing aids. However, eligibility for these benefits is based on a very low income and is generally related to the level of payment in Aid to Families with Dependent Children. The AFDC benefit rate now ranges nationwide from $96 to $130 per month.

Crippled Children's Program

The Crippled Children's Program was one of two child health programs created by the Social Security Act of 1935 giving federal grants-in-aid to the states to provide preventive services to children through early detection of handicapping conditions in the total child population. States usually set eligibility requirements, the diagnostic categories accepted for care, and sliding scales to determine payment. The focus of Crippled Children's Programs remains the prevention, detection, and treatment of handicapping conditions. However, money is now distributed to the states through block grants, which means that state Crippled Children's Programs must compete with many other programs for funds. As a result of block grant funding, most state Crippled Children's Programs are now less well funded. Those state programs which have maintained or raised funding or have succeeded in having special funds made available to them through new state legislation have done so through lobbying efforts of interest groups such as self-help organizations. Thus, state health departments continue to serve chronically ill children, but disease categories, eligibility, services, and now funding are determined by each state.

Social Security Disability Insurance

The last type of aid, Social Security Disability Insurance, began in 1956 to provide benefits to those who were too disabled to continue working. Criteria for receiving payments are strict. A person must have a physical or mental disability that lasts at least one year or results in death. The individual must be unable to do any substantial gainful work. Specific evidence of disability must be furnished by the claimant to substantiate her claim. Such evidence would include relevant medical history and objective evidence such as laboratory test results. The evaluators look for inability to perform significant functions required to work such as sitting, standing, grasping, traveling, hearing, speaking, and handling objects. Disability benefits are based on the individual's earning history. As of August 1983 there were about 4 million people collecting disability payments; 2.7 million were disabled workers and the rest were dependents. In 1980 the Social Security Disability Amendments (PL 96–265) allowed the deduction of some nonvocational expenses in calculating income benefits and extended the trial period for the disabled to work.

Other Federal Programs

Several other pieces of legislation have special relevance to the chronically ill. The Rehabilitation Act of 1973 (PL 93–112) authorizes a variety of research, training, and civil rights programs for disabled people. It prohibits discrimination against otherwise qualified handicapped individuals under any program or activity receiving federal financial assistance. It gives the more severely disabled priority in receiving services. In 1978 the act was amended (PL 95–602) to provide funding for independent living centers and to make independent living a priority for state vocational rehabilitation programs.

The Architectural Barriers Act of 1968 (PL 90–480) states that buildings with federal funds or leased by the federal government must be made accessible to persons with disabilities. The Developmental Disabilities Services Facilities and Construction Act of 1970 (PL 91–517) expanded the responsibility of the states in planning and implementing comprehensive services for the developmentally disabled. In 1975 the Developmental Disabilities Assistance and Bill of Rights Act (PL 94–103) established advocacy and protection services for the developmentally disabled.

Some of those laws affect each chronically ill individual; most, however, affect people according to the kind of disease they have and the degree of disability they experience.

Other Psychosocial Issues

For a chronically ill person, social issues can range from her ability to obtain medical, life, and automobile insurance, through her relationships with others, to her ability to work. Relationships with family members and strangers are affected by illness, as are the degree of dependence, confinement, and isolation the ill person experiences.

The section on psychological impact addresses issues of self-concept, mood, and affect, as well as the impact of a particular disease on developmental stage, appearance, and sexual response. It also describes a person's psychological response to her illness as well as the specific stages of psychological response through which she may pass. For example, people who have had strokes have a predictable pattern of despair and hope throughout their rehabilitation process.

The final section of each chapter discusses very generally the relationship of the reader to someone with this particular disease. Of course, each relationship has its own history and set of expectations, but each disease also evokes certain responses that tend to reinforce the isolation that a chronically ill person already feels. Thus, this final portion offers advice on "how to be helpful." The book concludes with a directory of self-help groups and government organizations dealing with chronic diseases, a glossary, and a bibliography, each divided into sections corresponding to the chapters.

Sources of Data

Multiple sources of data include a review of the available research and literature in the fields of medicine, nursing, social work, gerontology, rehabilitation, physical therapy, occupational therapy, and pastoral counseling relevant to the general subject of chronic disease as well as to the specific illnesses addressed. Extensive interviews were conducted with individuals who have the illnesses and family members (cited in the text as "informant"), as well as physicians, social workers, nurses, physical therapists, occupational therapists, rehabilitation counselors, representatives of societies and foundations devoted to helping people with specific diseases, members of self-help groups, lawyers, insurance experts, and representatives of government agencies. The anthropological term informant is used often in the text because it depicts the stance used to gather data. People were asked to describe their relationship to a particular illness— what they knew, how it felt, what it meant to them. People who have a chronic disease are referred to in that way even though it would have been easier to call them patients, epileptics, diabetics, or sufferers, because a purpose of this book is to see their illness as part of their identity but not all, or even most. The standard of practice for care of each particular disease is described. Obviously, not all medical personnel, ill people, or family members are good, kind, trustworthy, or even competent. However, the professionals consulted for this book were chosen because they are considered to be excellent.

Purposes

Understanding Chronic Illness has several agendas. First, it is meant to provide very specific medical and psychosocial information about diseases that afflict great numbers of people and are potentially devastating. Second, through providing information about general as well as disease-specific resources, self-help groups, and readings, it offers ways for the reader to extend her knowledge of each and to become intelligently involved in research, treatment, support, and advocacy activities. Third, the framework used as a guide for each chapter is meant to provide a handy way for the reader to find the kind of information she needs on the disease in which she is primarily interested and to compare it with similar data for other diseases. Last, by stringing together these thousands of bits of information, the book attempts to address the meaning of illness—the ways it touches the life of the ill individual and her circle and the ways people find to manage disease.

2

Arthritis

ARTHRITIS MEANS inflammation of the joints. It causes limitation of function, pain, and fatigue, symptoms that characterize the disease. Arthritis can be mild, resulting in one painful finger joint or an occasionally stiff knee, or it can be severe, affecting many joints, to the point of disfigurement and debilitation. It is said that everyone who is past the age of sixty has a bit of arthritis, but this chapter will focus primarily on rheumatoid arthritis, the kind that is in many instances the most disabling.

The pain of arthritis has been likened to a headache or a toothache: throbbing, sometimes distracting, and periodically unbearable. Generally one can manage the pain, but extraordinary discomfort is a signal that prompt medical intervention is necessary. Because fatigue is also an important symptom, people with arthritis learn to schedule times each day to rest and conserve their joints. While medication, rest, and physical therapy can address the symptoms and sometimes bring arthritis into remission, the disease may progress, attacking joints that were previously healthy and further affecting already diseased joints.

Medical Information

The term "arthritis" represents more than one hundred conditions that cause pain and aching in joints and connective tissue throughout the body. Some of these conditions are rare and some are common. Some are trivial, requiring little intervention, and some are serious, requiring a monitored medical regimen. The disease is not fatal in itself and is often progressive. Neither its course nor its crises is predictable.

The Arthritis Foundation estimates that there are 31,600,000 people with arthritis in the United States. Of this total number it estimates that 6,500,000 have rheumatoid arthritis, 250,000 children have some form of arthritis, and 16 million people have osteoarthritis serious enough to cause them problems. The National Center for Health Statistics reported 27,238,293 people with arthritis in 1981. The Health Interview Survey of the National Center for Health Statistics reported in 1976 that 7,300,000 people with arthritis were disabled at any one time, there were 525 million days of restricted activity annually as a result of arthritis, and there were 26,600,000 days lost from work at a regular job annually.

The Arthritis Foundation also reports that in 1980 the annual cost of arthritis in medical care bills and lost wages was $13 billion, with more than $4.5 billion spent in direct costs for medical care.

Classification

Arthritis is classified by cause or by the part of the joint structure it affects. The Arthritis Foundation's *Primer on the Rheumatic Diseases* lists thirteen categories: "Polyarthritises of Unknown Origin," "Connective Tissue Disorders," "Rheumatic Fever," "Degenerative Joint Disease," "Nonarticular Rheumatism," "Diseases with Which Arthritis is Frequently Associated," "Associated with Known Infectious Agents," "Traumatic and/or Neurogenic Disorders," "Associated with Biochemical or Endocrine Abnormalities," "Neoplasms," "Allergy or Drug Reactions," "Inherited and Congenital Factors," and "Miscellaneous Disorders." The six commonly known kinds of arthritis are classified within four of these categories.

POLYARTHRITISES OF UNKNOWN ORIGIN

Rheumatoid arthritis, juvenile rheumatoid arthritis, and ankylosing spondylitis are polyarthritises of unknown origin in which there is inflammation of several joints at one time.

Rheumatoid arthritis (RA). Rheumatoid arthritis affects three times as many women as men and usually begins in middle age. The term "rheum" refers to the aching and fatigue that are part of the disease. Here joints become inflamed, the cells in the membrane divide, and other inflamed cells enter the joint from other parts of the body. Because of the inflammation, the joints look swollen and feel warm. As part of the disease process, enzymes are released into the joint space, causing increased pain. If the process continues for years, the enzymes can gradually break down the bone and cartilage of the joint. This is generally a symmetrical condition, affecting both sides of the body similarly.

Rheumatoid arthritis almost always affects the wrists and the knuckles and often involves the knees and joints of the foot, the hips, spine, and other joints. It is the most destructive kind of arthritis; bone erosion, ruptured tendons, and slipped joints are all possible. Most people with rheumatoid arthritis do not develop all these problems, and many do not develop deformities.

The course of the disease can follow one of three patterns: monocyclic, polycyclic, and chronic. The monocyclic course is a brief illness lasting a few months at most and leaving no impairment. The polycyclic course usually does not result in much disability but includes several flareups of the illness followed by remissions. The chronic course lasts for a longer period and sometimes for life. Here the chance of crippling increases, but serious crippling is unusual. During periods of remission the disease is less violent and stiffness and fatigue might decrease, but old destruction cannot be corrected. Thus it is critical that the disease be treated correctly in its early stages so that the person will be left with maximum mobility when the illness activity subsides.

Juvenile Rheumatoid Arthritis (JRA).   Juvenile rheumatoid arthritis is usually seen before a person is sixteen years old. There are three forms, each of which has a different pattern of onset and different symptoms. Pauciarticular JRA begins by affecting only a few large joints and rarely affects the same joint of both sides of the body. Boys tend to have low back and hip stiffness in the early part of the disease, while girls may develop iridocyclitis, an inflammation of the iris and ciliary body of the eye. Polyarticular JRA begins in many joints. It usually affects the small joints of the hands and fingers and sometimes the weight-bearing joints. This type is often symmetrical and is found more frequently in girls than boys. The onset of systemic JRA (Still's disease) is marked by a high fever, chills, shaking, and a rash. The arthritis generally affects many joints, and there can be recurrent episodes over a number of years. Other problems can include inflammation of the lining of the lungs (pleuritis) and of the outer lining of the heart (pericarditis), severe anemia, a high level of white cells in the blood, and abdominal pain.

Many children who have JRA, especially the first two types, will have no problems with arthritis as adults. Many more will have long periods of remission. Again, early treatment is important to prevent permanent disability that would continue even in long periods of remission.

Ankylosing Spondylitis.   Ankylosing spondylitis is an inflammatory disease of the spine in which hereditary disposition plays an important role. It is thought that more men contract the disease than women. In ankylosing spondylitis, ligaments of the spine and the sacroiliac joints (those near the base of the spine) are usually affected first. Thus, pain in the lower back and legs is often an early symptom. It is most frequently a mild condition, but in some instances intact bones fuse together and stiffness of the spine can progress until it is completely rigid. At that point there is immobility and no pain. The term "poker spine" has been used to describe the symptom.

Age of onset seems to be around twenty, but the diagnosis is rarely made until the mid-thirties, because symptoms before that time have not been significant. Good medical treatment, physical therapy, and postural routine prevent much discomfort and deformity. The disease is usually self-limiting after several years. Most people have a normal life span, and death due to the disease is highly unusual. Many patients lead vigorous, active lives not limited by the disease.

CONNECTIVE TISSUE DISORDERS (ACQUIRED)

Within the category called connective tissue disorders (acquired) are systemic lupus erythematosus and scleroderma. Connective tissue diseases are also called autoimmune or collagen-vascular diseases.

Systemic Lupus Erythematosus (SLE).   Systemic lupus erythematosus, also called SLE or lupus, is a rheumatic disease that affects not only joints but organs, the nervous system, and particularly the immune system. It is chronic, systemic, and inflammatory. There are two common forms: discoid and systemic. Discoid lupus is a mild form that usually involves only a rash but sometimes develops into systemic lupus. Systemic lupus is the form in which many parts of the body may be affected.

Scleroderma.   Scleroderma is a relatively uncommon disease of the connective tissue, with accompanying symptoms of arthritis. It causes a hardening and thickening of the skin and of the connective tissue in many parts of the body, including the blood vessels, joints, the esophagus, the kidneys, lungs, and bowel. Because of impaired circulation through the small blood vessels, it can eventually lead to scarring, tightening, and stiffness of the skin. Joint inflammation is usually mild and overshadowed by skin and soft tissue involvement. However, it can lead to deformities that are like those associated with rheumatoid arthritis. It affects more women than men and often begins in middle age. Sometimes it progresses rapidly, with severe kidney and lung involvement, and sometimes it follows a course of flareups and remissions. It is a difficult illness to treat, but it is often reponsive to medication, specific exercises, and joint and skin protection.

DEGENERATIVE JOINT DISEASE

Degenerative joint disease includes primary and secondary osteoarthritis and osteoarthrosis. In this category, the cartilage that absorbs the shock of joint motion wears out, leaving the two surfaces of the bone in contact with each other. Inflammation is less significant than in rheumatoid arthritis but can still be a problem. The most common form of arthritis in this and all categories is osteoarthritis.

Osteoarthritis.   Nearly everyone gets some osteoarthritis if he or she lives long enough. Although it typically occurs in old people, it can be seen in younger people after trauma. It is generally mild and attacks individual joints. Most often it affects the weight-bearing joints of hips and knees and the vertebrae. It involves some joint pain, stiffness, immobility, and muscle weakness. When bone changes have taken place in people with advanced disease, joints begin to look knobby. If the knees or hips are badly affected, joint replacement might be indicated.

Osteoarthritis affects both sexes, and age of onset is usually between forty-five and ninety. The progress of the disease is slow, crippling is relatively rare, and most people with osteoarthritis often have pain-free periods. Weight control, joint protection, drugs, rest, special exercises, and heat help in the relief of symptoms.

ASSOCIATED WITH BIOCHEMICAL OR ENDOCRINE ABNORMALITIES

Gout.   Gout is the best-known or prototypical disease in this category. With gout, a high buildup of uric acid creates crystals, which are deposited in a joint. The needlelike crystals irritate the lining of the joint, causing it to be inflamed and very painful. Most commonly gout occurs in the base of the big toe, but it is also found in the knee, the ankle, the instep of the foot, fingers, elbows, wrists, and knees. Gout is rare in women and children. It generally affects men between the ages of forty and fifty, but it can occur at any age and does affect some postmenopausal women.

Gout often results from an inherited defect in body chemistry, but it can occur after the use of diuretics to rid the body of excess fluid or to lower blood pressure. Attacks of gout are sudden and extremely painful. The affected joint is swollen and warm and often looks red or purple and shiny.

Gout can be controlled by reducing the uric acid in a person's system to tolerable levels. A group of drugs called uricosuric agents enable the body to increase its discharge of uric acid. An example is probenecid (Benemid). A drug called allopurinol (Zyloprim) helps reduce the body's production of uric acid. Medication controls but does not cure the illness. Thus, medication to control the amount of uric acid in the body may have to be taken for life.

Etiology

The exact cause of most types of arthritis is unknown, but there has been a great deal of discussion about factors contributing to an arthritic condition. They include aging, stress, bacteria, virus, and predisposition. For example, the cause of a localized arthritis like tennis elbow is clear in that there is an abnormal physical stress causing injury to the joint.

Also, it has been established that in the process of aging joint wear eventually causes some degree of osteoarthritis. Osteoarthritis is likely to develop in any joint that has taken a lot of abuse. For example, an overweight person puts additional stress on her hips and knees; particular sports put extraordinary stress on certain joints; specific kinds of work stress certain joints; and joints can become injured in accidents. Thus a joint subject to unusual stress is likely to operate imperfectly and is more susceptible to osteoarthritis.

In joint infection, acute or chronic arthritis can be caused by various kinds of bacteria invading the joints. There is now speculation that rheumatoid arthritis, like a number of other diseases, might be caused by a latent virus, which may lie dormant in the body for years and then become active, causing illness. Also, in many kinds of arthritis, there is an inherited predisposition toward contracting the disease. This is true, for example, of gout, rheumatoid arthritis, and ankylosing spondylitis.

Finally, emotional stress is thought to contribute to some kinds of arthritis. Symptoms sometimes appear after a crisis, and in patients who already have some form of the disease symptoms are often worse during time of emotional stress.

In the past there has been great speculation about a premorbid rheumatoid personality, but there is no convincing evidence that it exists. (See, especially, Zeitlin, 1977, in the bibliography.) It was supposed to have comprised the following traits: overreaction to illness, masochism, self-sacrifice, rigidity, moralism, conformity, inhibition, perfectionism, and difficulty in dealing with aggression. Research has demonstrated that these traits are common to people who have many different chronic illnesses, apparently consequent rather than antecedent to coping with debilitation. The current thinking favors a predispositional matrix of genetic, autoimmune, infectious, and psychosocial factors, which can be triggered to produce rheumatoid arthritis.

Populations at Risk for the Illness

Besides what has already been noted on this subject in the earlier sections on classification and etiology, it is important to point out that people who have a family history of one of these illnesses or who are involved in work or recreational activities that stress joints excessively should take extra care to protect their joints and to maintain a reasonable body weight. Women are most prone to some types of arthritis, like systemic lupus erythematosus, and men are more prone to gout and to ankylosing spondylitis. Osteoarthritis is generally a disease of the elderly.

Association with Other Diseases

Diseases with which rheumatoid arthritis is frequently associated are sarcoidosis, ulcerative colitis, relapsing polychondritis, regional enteritis, and several others. Sarcoidosis is a granulomatous disease that can affect any area of the body but most often affects the skin, lungs, lymphatic glands, or bones of the hand. Relapsing polychondritis is a recurring inflammation of the cartilage in many sites in the body. Henoch Schonlein's purpura is bleeding into and from the wall of the intestines. Ulcerative colitis is an inflammatory and ulcerative condition of the colon. Regional enteritis is an inflammatory and ulcerative condition of the ileum in which there are clear demarcations between healthy and affected portions of the bowel. Whipple's disease, characterized by diarrhea, weight loss, anemia, and increased pigmentation; Sjogren's syndrome, in which deficient secretion from salivary and other glands leads to a dry tongue and hoarse voice; and familial Mediterranean fever are also associated with rheumatoid arthritis but are rare.

Prognosis

All arthritic illnesses are chronic, even when they are in remission. A good prognosis for each depends on early intervention and continued attention to drug management, prescribed exercise, sufficient rest, and joint protection. In some kinds of arthritis, gout for example, symptoms can be controlled through medication, and the prognosis for managing the illness is excellent. In others, rheumatoid arthritis for example, the prognosis is uncertain, but the best possible prognosis again depends on intervention and attentiveness.

Natural History

If left untreated, each of these diseases would progress until, unpredictably, it would go into remission. Even the most violent forms of arthritis have some inactive periods. If the diseases were not treated during active periods, many people would find their mobility severely limited and their pain sometimes unbearable.

If rheumatoid inflammation is not treated, it can cause progressive damage in the joint. Inflammation begins in the synovial membrane, the lining of the joint capsule that secretes the fluid which lubricates the joint, swelling the membrane and spreading to other parts of the joint system. Inflammation can lead to distortion of the joints affecting the bones of the hand, particularly, so that fingers are pulled sideways and backward, becoming difficult to use. Outgrowths of the inflamed tissue invade the cartilage surrounding the bone ends and eventually destroy it. Then scar tissue can form between the ends of the bones, fusing and immobilizing the affected joint. Treated or untreated, the disease process remains unpredictable. Untreated, the disease might well result in increasing disability, crippling, and eventual immobility and dependence.

Diagnostic Procedures

Because the symptoms of many forms of arthritis seem to evolve slowly and because aches and pains in and around the joints can mean different things, many people do not consult a physician for several years after the onset of the illness. Therefore, the Arthritis Foundation has published arthritis warning signs designed to encourage people with the symptoms of arthritis to seek early intervention. The warning signs are:

- Persistent pain and stiffness on arising
- Pain, tenderness, or swelling in one or more joints
- Recurrence of these symptoms, especially when they involve more than one joint
- Recurrent or persistent pain and stiffness in the neck, lower back, knees, and other joints

Correct diagnosis is essential because, although all the arthritises share some common symptoms, each is treated very differently. For example, a joint infection is treated with antibiotics, which will cure the problem. On the other hand, rheumatoid arthritis is treated with an elaborate regimen designed to control the symptoms.

The diagnosis is made on the basis of a history, physical examination, laboratory tests, and x-rays. The process may be lengthy. First, the physician reviews the person's past and present symptoms and asks specifically about joint injury. The physician will also review the medical histories of family members. Next, the physician will examine the person, giving special attention to the joints, especially noting inflammation, loss of flexibility or range of motion, and any other joint abnormality.

In rheumatoid arthritis the physician looks for weakness, fatigue, joint swelling and stiffness, sweaty hands and feet, weight loss, and loss of appetite. Often joints on both sides of the person's body will be involved; for example, both hands, or both knees. In addition, people may have nodules under the skin, anemia, inflammation of the membrane covering the surface of the lung, or inflammation of the eyes. Continued observation over a long period may be necessary for diagnosis.

X-rays are used to determine the condition of bones and joints. Blood tests contribute to the diagnosis of bacterial infection and anemia. One group of tests for rheumatoid factor, a complex protein circulating in the blood of many persons with rheumatoid arthritis, may not be conclusive but may help to confirm a diagnosis. Another test measures sedimentation rate, the speed at which red blood cells settle to the bottom of a glass tube. The cells settle more rapidly than normal when there is chronic inflammation. Urine tests detect the presence of crystals or a high level of uric acid indicative of gout, and renal disease, which may be an indication of a collagen vascular disease like systemic lupus erythematosus.

The periodic analysis of joint fluid may help to make a diagnosis. The fluid is removed through a needle. Sometimes a biopsy will be performed in which a small piece of tissue is removed and examined under a microscope. Arthroscopy, a surgical procedure in which a fiberoptic instrument is inserted into a joint allowing a physician to see the interior of a joint, is sometimes used to examine or to excise a piece of tissue for diagnosis.

Therapies

The purpose of therapy is to control symptoms, to maximize joint protection and flexibility, and to minimize pain. Therapies include medication, physical therapy, an exercise program to maintain the best possible range of motion for the affected joints, rest, stress reduction, techniques used to distract a person from his pain, and the surgical replacement of severely diseased joints.

DRUGS

No drug for rheumatoid arthritis actually stops the disease process, but several reduce pain and inflammation. Because people vary in their reaction to drugs and because there is so much variation in the disease process itself, the physician has to design and monitor an individual regimen for each person. Drugs have different degrees of effectiveness at different times for different people. The Arthritis Foundation refers to a pyramid of drugs, with the least toxic and most often prescribed at the bottom and the most toxic, experimental drugs, which are used least often, at the top. Most prescribed are the anti-inflammatory drugs, which reduce inflammation, pain, and swelling. Aspirin is the most frequently prescribed, and it is taken regularly in large doses, even in periods of remission. Because people vary in their tolerance for aspirin, and prolonged use of aspirin can cause dangerous side effects, its use must be monitored by a physician. Ringing in the ears or stomach irritation means that the dose must be adjusted.

Also in the anti-inflammatory category are the nonsteroidal anti-inflammatory drugs (NSAID) which work like aspirin, are much more expensive, but sometimes have fewer side effects. Some drugs in that category are Clinoril (sulindac), Motrin (ibuprophin), Feldene (piroxicam), Nalfon (fenoprofen), Tolectin (tolmetin), Indocin (indomethacin), Meclomen (meclofenamate), Butazolidin (phenylbutazone), and Naprosyn (naproxen).

Gold salts have been found useful in the treatment of rheumatoid arthritis. On injection, they can reduce inflammation for 65 percent of rheumatoid patients and may reverse some of the bone erosion. The use of gold salts can have some side effects, including skin, blood cell, and kidney involvement, but most side effects are reversible if the treatment is discontinued. At a later point gold salts can be used again with no side effects. Thus monitoring is critical. This treatment is very expensive, costing about eight hundred dollars for the initial twenty-week course. Because the use of gold salts can result in remission, however, it is a valuable approach.

Penicillamine works similarly to gold salts. It, too, is used for people with rheumatoid arthritis whose disease has not responded well to other treatment. Side effects are much the same as they are for gold salts except that additionally the connective tissue may be weakened. The healing of a cut may be delayed, making surgery more difficult for a person with whom this drug is being used. Antimalarial drugs are also used to reduce inflammation, but here, too, the use of the drug must be monitored for possible side effects.

The next group of drugs, corticosteroids, are the most potent anti-inflammatory drugs available and often bring about sensational reduction of inflammation and pain in a few hours. Steroids are occasionally injected into a particular joint to provide temporary relief. They may have serious side effects, especially if taken systemically in large doses over a long period. Taken in high doses for one week to one month, steroids can cause risk for psychotic, depressed, or euphoric mental states, ulcers, acne, and other kinds of infection, since it reduces the body's immune response. High doses taken for one month to one year can cause fat in the central part of the body with wasting of the arms and legs and a buffalo hump at the base of the neck, the growth of facial hair, and skin bruises. Over a long period the loss of calcium makes bones fragile and more likely to break. Cataracts may develop; there is a danger of adrenal crisis in which adrenalin and cortisone are no longer produced; blood pressure can drop; there can be an inability to react to physical stress; sodium can be lost and potassium retained; and the person can go into shock and die.

A new group of drugs, cytotoxic agents, can suppress the immune system. They are being used at present for cancer chemotherapy and in organ transplantation to prevent rejection of the new organ. These drugs are highly toxic and used only in severe rheumatoid arthritis when no other therapy is effective. Some of these drugs have been approved by the Food and Drug Administration for use with arthritis, but they are still used with great caution.

SURGERY

Surgery is carried out to relieve pain and to restore function. Best results are achieved when the problem is localized in the large joints like the hip or the knee. The decision to do the procedure is based on the degree and type of pain as well as an evaluation of the person's motivation and life requirements. In a surgical procedure the diseased or inflamed tissue is removed or the joint is removed and replaced. Specific operations are synovectomy, resections, back surgery, fusions, neurological operations, and joint replacement.

Synovectomy is removal of inflamed synovial membrane, the lining of the joint capsule, with the hope that reduction of that tissue will result in less damage to the joint. Joint stiffness is a frequent side effect, and the inflamed tissue often grows back. Whether synovectomy should be carried out early or late in the disease process is a matter of debate. It has been suggested that criteria include the worsening of a single joint when disease in other joints is inactive or the attempt to avoid the use of a drug that may be dangerous to the individual.

Resections are procedures for cutting away bone, for example, the bone on the outside of the wrist, bunions, or the metatarsal heads in the forefoot. Fusions, which unite two bones in order to stabilize joints, are meant to provide a platform for movement and to prevent pain in the fused area. However, flexibility is lost, additional strain may be placed on nearby joints, and fusion is not always successful. Although occasionally useful, such surgery has many drawbacks. Back surgery is not indicated unless there is demonstrable pressure on the nerve roots. Neurological operations are carried out in order to remove the structures that are pressing on the nerves or to remove the area that is sending abnormal signals.

In joint replacement, the joint is removed and replaced with a manmade joint composed of vitallium, stainless steel, and high-density plastics. A new biological cement that causes very little reaction and allows the prosthesis to be more strongly connected to the bone ends has been developed. The hip joint, first to be replaced, now has a success rate of about 98 percent. The present artificial hip lasts at least ten to fifteen years, greatly improves function, and relieves pain. The ball and socket joint of the hip is far easier to construct than the knee joint, which requires sideways stability in addition to sufficient flexibility, but knee replacements today are also generally successful. Joints in the wrists and elbows can also be replaced, but ankle and shoulder replacements remain experimental.

Operations on the small bones of the hands and feet are quite common. Such operations sometimes improve the appearance of a hand but do not improve its function. It may look normal but lacks strength and dexterity. In operations a simple silicone rubber implant is placed within and between two bones. During the healing process live, fibrous tissue forms around the implant, holding it into position. Muscles and tendons around the replaced joints must be retrained postoperatively. For people with systemic disease many joints may have deteriorated, and priorities must be established for the sequence of reconstructive procedures. It is thought that a person's chief complaint should be given highest priority, because she will be highly motivated for success, and success in the first replacement procedure will inspire confidence in the sequence. Some procedures, such as those on the hand and the knee, or the hand and the foot, can be combined. Age is no contraindication to surgery, and complications are rare.

Anticipated Course of the Treated Disease

Some forms of arthritis, like those resulting from bacterial infection, can be cured. Others, like gout, can reach a very high degree of symptom control. Still others, like rheumatoid arthritis, remain unpredictable. With early and continued treatment, and with good self-care, the maximum range of motion that the disease will allow can be maintained, and the inflammation can be treated to minimize joint and bone damage.

Psychosocial Information

People who have rheumatoid arthritis say the loss of spontaneous mobility is the worst aspect of the illness. Before undertaking almost any kind of physical activity, whether going to the store for a couple of items, to the beach for the day, or a vacation for a week, she must mentally preview the entire process to be sure she will be able to manage and that she will not be doing anything that could damage joints. The question is not just, "Do I have the energy to begin?" or "Can I carry out all parts of the activity?" but "Will I have the strength and flexibility to finish the activity?"

Modifications in Life-Style

EXERCISE

Exercise, sufficiently gentle to avoid undue stress on joints, is critical for maintaining the maximum range of motion in each joint. The great stress placed on joints by certain sports is harmful for people with arthritis and may even cause osteoarthritis. Range-of-motion exercises taught by physical therapists as part of rehabilitation services follow the principle of isometrics, in which muscle tone is maintained by pitting one part or muscle of the body against another or against an immovable object with a strong but motionless effort. (For a more extensive description, see the section on exercise in Chapter 7, "Heart Disease.")

DRIVING

If someone is unable to look over her shoulder or use side mirrors, her driving will be impeded. Hip, knee, ankle, or foot involvement may impair her ability to brake, and hand and wrist involvement may slow her steering. There is no specific legal restriction on driving. If someone with arthritis becomes a rehabilitation patient, a goal may be for her to pass her state driving examination again.

The alternatives to driving are worse. Walking long distances is difficult. Waiting on cold corners for long periods for buses that probably cannot "kneel" (entrance platforms of kneeling buses descend for passengers who cannot climb high steps) is difficult. Taxis are expensive and sometimes hard to find, and depending on friends or family for rides means loss of autonomy. People with arthritis therefore continue to drive as long as they are able to get into the car and turn on the ignition.

Parking a car can also become a problem. State departments of transportation now mandate that certain spaces in public parking lots be reserved for the handicapped. Any car with a handicapped license plate may park in those spaces. Ordinarily someone who lives in a city may have to park several blocks from home. However, on residential streets many state departments of transportation will mark the space in front of a handicapped person's home as reserved for handicapped. Those who park a vehicle without a handicapped license in a specially marked space can be ticketed.

DIET

The only exception is gout, in which certain foods containing the chemical purine, which can cause uric acid levels to rise, should be avoided. With one exception, diet has never been proved to be directly related to any form of arthritis. Still, diet is one area where quackery abounds, with promoters of exotic diets promising tremendous relief. Research has demonstrated that the promises are false. Weight control, on the other hand, is highly important for someone with arthritis. Excess weight places undue stress on the weight-bearing joints of hips and knees. Sound nutrition is also important for maintaining energy and staying as healthy as possible.

CLIMATE CHANGE

One popular but often ill-founded solution to the problems of arthritis is a move to a warm, dry climate, as in Arizona or New Mexico. The Arthritis Foundation and rheumatologists caution, however, that the small relief found through the climate change must be balanced against the effort of moving and especially the loss of long-established relationships and of social and emotional supports. Although rainy weather makes many people feel less well, and icy, snowy conditions do increase one's chances of falling, the joint discomfort for those with arthritis comes mainly with a change in barometric pressure rather than absolute weather conditions such as snow or rain. Spring, with its capricious weather, is thus an especially difficult time of the year.

SLEEP

In an acute phase arthritis makes sleep difficult. Joints are painful, and some people must wear splints to keep the joints of their hands or lower arms in a nonstressed position throughout the night. Arthritis patients say that splints feel strange at first, but they quickly get used to them and find that the joints protected by the splint feel better in the morning than they do without splinting.

For those with rheumatoid arthritis, the most difficult part of the day is often the beginning. Joints are generally stiff in the morning. They seem to jell while one is asleep. Getting up and getting going takes time. One does not bounce out of bed.

REST PATTERNS

Rest is a key issue in arthritis. Because the disease process is tiring, it is important to pace oneself and to schedule rest periods. Patients report that one day with no rest would result in at least one day of not feeling well and having to rest more later.

STRESS MANAGEMENT

Not only joint stress but emotional stress can exacerbate arthritic episodes. One informant described her life at the onset of an arthritic episode. A program she had developed and administered, and with which she was very closely identified, was threatened with discontinuance, as was the department where she taught. Already working fourteen-hour days and wearing three or four hats, she felt she was embroiled in a fight for her own survival. Although both program and department continued after all, she found that she had won a battle only to lose the war. Soon after the administrative questions were settled, rheumatoid arthritis, affecting her thumbs, her knees, and her feet, forced her into early retirement. She says she thinks it was not the stresses but the ways she managed them that created the problem. Little evidence has been gathered for the psychogenic onset of most arthritic disease. Coping with disease, disability, and pain is itself a source of tension, depression, and fatigue. Additional worries or crises cause muscle tension and exhaustion. Both can be alleviated through relaxation techniques.

Self-Help Aids

Many of the wide variety of aids available to people with arthritis are described in the *Self-Help Manual for Patients with Arthritis,* published by the Arthritis Foundation. Most of the aids address the activities of daily living: bed transfer, toilet aids, and help in walking, dressing and grooming, cooking, cleaning, and needlework. Practical examples include a plastic holder with a handle for a milk carton; a key ring that conserves wrist action in opening a door; elastic shoelaces; velcro fasteners; and orthopedic shoes that act as splints for the feet, giving them external support. These simple aids enable someone with severe arthritis to manage self-care. Without such aids she would have to have someone else pour her milk, unlock her door, or fasten her clothes. Simple activities of that kind are often the key to independence. Occupational and physical therapists are knowledgeable about such aids and qualified to teach correct use. They are able to survey someone's home to suggest adaptations like push-up boards on walls next to the toilet, a high stool with a foot rest and swivel seat in the kitchen, or a bed caddy to hold things one might need at night.

More elaborate aids are available too. Replacing stairs with ramps or installing elevators increase mobility and independence. Speaker phones and touch-tone or touch-a-matic dialing make telephoning easier. Electric typewriters with large carriage knobs, word processors, and electric calculators help those for whom writing is difficult.

Automobile aids and adapted vehicles ease driving and dealing with specific emergency situations, such as a flat tire (an aerosol can that can temporarily repair and inflate a tire quickly without the use of a jack) or signaling distress (a rotating reflector which suctions to a car roof). For those who rely on public transportation, some "kneeling" buses are available in most metropolitan areas.

Distractions from Pain

In order not to be disabled by the discomfort arthritis brings, it is important for people to distract themselves from the pain. Meaningful activity—

going to work and being involved with other people—is the most helpful distraction. One informant whose hands were affected chose to continue work as a typist, even though she often cried as she typed. Her physician said that the activity would not affect the disease process, and she valued her work and her colleagues enough to stay.

An engrossing hobby can be a powerful distraction. Even gardening, which one might think of as harmful because of the conditions under which most people garden, can be made easier through the use of trellises, dwarf fruit trees, containers, or window greenhouses.

Impact of the Disease on Social Life

INSURANCE

It is difficult for people with rheumatoid arthritis to find medical insurance if they were not previously insured. Generally they have to join a group plan through their work or wait until the particular time of the year when insurance companies have to offer coverage to anyone who applies. Life insurance is also difficult to obtain. The life span for people with rheumatoid arthritis is shortened, partly because their resistance to infection is lowered and they are more susceptible to pneumonia than the average person. The immobility caused by very severe arthritis causes additional health problems. Automobile insurance, however, is not difficult to obtain.

SOCIAL SECURITY DISABILITY

For someone with rheumatoid arthritis to obtain disability payments, signs of joint inflammation must persist or recur despite three months of medical treatment; the joint inflammation must result in significant restriction of function of the affected joints; and clinical activity of the disease must be expected to last for at least twelve months. The diagnosis must be corroborated through a specified series of laboratory tests. One such test is a biopsy of the affected joint tissue that shows changes characteristic of rheumatoid arthritis (synovial biopsy). Thus, a person must be severely disabled for many months without remission before Social Security will consider such a claim. The impairment must be severe enough to prevent a person from carrying on gainful activity.

Relationships with Others

Many people with rheumatoid arthritis try to act as if a limited range of motion, pain, and fatigue do not interfere with normal activity. Often they are faced with a reduction in mobility, in dexterity and strength, and in overall energy. To appear normal, people become skillful in planning ahead, scheduling rest times, and hiding how they feel. One patient recounted the following example to demonstrate the ways in which arthritis had made dating difficult. A man whom she liked a lot asked her to play tennis. She promptly bought herself a lightweight racket, found she could not swing it, and chose to break the date rather than explain why they would have to change the activity.

A psychologist who has rheumatoid arthritis said that arthritis is boring to people who don't have it: It is dull, aching pain with restricted mobility, and it is forever. It lacks drama. The way to keep up a normal life is to assume your mornings are stiff and slow, do what you can without overtaxing yourself, and, for goodness sake, keep quiet about how you feel.

Normalizing enhances some areas of relationship and confounds others. Acting as if one is normal helps colleagues, family, and friends to minimize the effects of the illness but can cause misjudgments of capacity. People with arthritis worry about becoming a burden to their family and adversely affecting the family with the amount of care they require.

Studies have shown that most women feel their husbands understand the disease, but they themselves have difficulty dealing with their husbands' anxiety. Generally those whose disease developed before marriage dealt with the arthritis better in their marriages than those whose arthritis developed after they were married. A primary problem is a spouse's inability to judge the limitations of the person with arthritis. Thus, a husband is either overprotective because he thinks his wife is able to do very little, or he is too demanding and does not believe that his wife is weak or in pain or tires quickly because she has arthritis. Because they are unable to understand limitations, family members may accuse the person with arthritis of malingering and may become angry. Continued dependence leads to resentment and fear on the part of everyone involved. Thus it is best if maximum independence for everyone is maintained.

When one person in the family is disabled, others also have to change roles. If it is a man with arthritis, his wife may have to assume a larger portion of the earning role. If it is the woman, as is generally the case, the man and the children have to assume more of the homemaking roles. This is especially difficult when young children require help with many activities. Adults in this situation have to avoid asking children to assume adult responsibilities. Helping Mom to take the top off of a bottle or to tie shoes or cut up her food is probably useful to the whole family, but no one benefits when the child assumes the responsibility for mothering.

SEXUAL ACTIVITY

The sexual parts of the body are rarely affected by arthritis, but the disease can indirectly affect sexual activity. Changes in appearance can affect self-concept, making one feel less desirable. A partner, too, may be put off by some disfigurement or afraid that he will worsen the ill person's pain or discomfort. Arthritis can also make a person, stiff, tired, and thus less desirous of sexual activity. The first step is the couple's acceptance of the changes wrought by the arthritis. That and a willingness to talk openly with each other and to learn to adapt sexual activity to the limitations imposed by the arthritis are critical to a rich sexual life.

A pamphlet called *Living and Loving: Information About Sex* (1982), available through The Arthritis Foundation, lists some general suggestions in planning for better sex. A person with arthritis should plan for sex at a time of the day when she generally feels best. The individual should time taking medication for the relief of pain so that its effects will not decrease libido during intercourse. Pacing daily activities will help one avoid extreme fatigue. Range-of-motion exercises will help reflex joints. A warm bath or shower before sex will be relaxing. Finally, supporting affected joints with pillows and finding the most comfortable positions for intercourse are helpful. The booklet provides drawings of seven positions for intercourse and describes the advantages of each position for people with different kinds of joint involvement. It suggests using vibrators and oral or manual stimulation when intercourse is not possible. Throughout, the emphasis is on the couple's awareness of their sexual desires, communicating them and working together on ways to satisfy themselves and each other.

STRANGERS

The prime factor in relationships with strangers is the invisibility of the disease. Even when someone with arthritis has some deformity, a stranger who looks at her cannot predict her limitations. Thus, strangers constantly underestimate or overestimate the capabilities of someone with arthritis. Problems arise because people with arthritis often need the kind of help from strangers that they might consider "child's play": opening doors, bending over to pick something up, zipping, or buttoning.

DEPENDENCE, CONFINEMENT, AND ISOLATION

For many people with arthritis the greatest dread is to end up wheelchair-bound, crippled, totally dependent, confined to a nursing home, and isolated from the community. Generally the fear is dealt with through the individual's rejection of the idea that it could happen to her, through maintaining maximum independence, and, when the disease is active, often through depression and despair. It is important to remember that there is almost always remission, and most people with arthritis do not become severely disabled. Only a small number of patients become wheelchair-bound, and that number is decreasing as technology advances. Still,

the response to discomfort, limitation, and fatigue can easily become isolation and confinement. People with arthritis and their friends and family
must work to avoid isolation. More time alone means less distraction from
pain and makes all aspects of the person's life less bearable. Although social activity, even if it requires some assistance, takes more effort than it
did before the onset of the illness, it is part of the treatment for the relief
from pain.

ABILITY TO WORK

The ability of a person with arthritis to continue working depends on
her occupation and her degree of disability. A seamstress whose hands are
badly deformed and painful may not be able to continue that work. If a
football player whose arthritic involvement is in his knees continues to
play with "pain killers" and great determination, he will increasingly
damage his knees until he is no longer able to play. Particular work situations can place great pressure on vulnerable joints. For example, a man
who played first clarinet in a major symphony orchestra retired early as
a result of arthritis in the joints of his thumbs. Although he could still play
extremely well and could endure the pain of supporting his instrument
with arthritic thumbs, his arthritis took away some of his former facility.
Rather than lose face through his inevitable replacement as first clarinet,
he chose to leave the orchestra.

A college professor with badly affected knee joints, who had refused
to carry a cane or tolerate any assistance as she worked, finally accepted
help from her students when she could no longer stand the looks on their
faces as they watched her get out of her chair to write on the chalkboard.
By accepting some assistance, she was able to continue to work.

One woman chose work as a rehabilitation counselor because of an
obvious interest in the field, but also because the work required little physical mobility and the schedule was flexible, allowing her to work harder
when she felt good and less hard when her disease was active. The kind
and amount of work someone with arthritis can do depends on the joint
stress in a particular occupation and some job flexibility, as well as the
extent of the individual's disability. Occupations that can damage affected
joints are to be avoided.

Psychological Aspects

SELF-CONCEPT

In our society the ability to be spontaneous, to have boundless energy,
to look perpetually eighteen years old, to jog, to dash here and there is
the ideal. The image of someone with rheumatoid arthritis has to be read-

justed—slowed down, more compulsive, more inner-directed. An additional problem in self-concept comes from the effects of arthritis on the body. One's body image is changed when hands, feet, shoulders, or knees are deformed.

A central theme in dealing with arthritis is the uncertainty generated by the disease process itself. The hope for relief or remission is juxtaposed with the progression of the disease. Coupled with uncertainty is the inability to predict the performance of the affected joints. At one point in the day someone can pick up a coffee pot with little difficulty; later the same day she may find it slipping out of her hand. One informant told of her embarrassment one day when she thought she could pour her own tea at a meeting and dropped the teapot, splashing tea all over herself, the table, and several women standing nearby. There is always the question of whether you will be able to get through the next activity, lift this, or tie that. In addition to this uncertainty, there is the dread of dependency. There is also a danger of withdrawal—deciding no longer to take the risks of occasionally embarrassing moments or of appearing dependent when asking for help.

STAGES OF PSYCHOLOGICAL RESPONSE

The degree and duration of incapacity influence people's reaction to their initial diagnosis, the first stage of psychological response. If the attack is frightening and powerful, they may be relieved to find out what is actually the matter. People almost always ask why it has happened to them and cite reasons often related to stress, injury, or punishment.

Certain anxieties about the disease process relate to role fulfillment. A young woman may worry about how the illness will affect her ability to have children, a wage-earner will worry about whether he can continue to do his job, and a child may worry about whether he will be able to play sports.

The second stage is often one of denial, especially when the disease is in remission. When the arthritis is stabilized, people often sound resigned and accepting. When the disease is exacerbated, anxiety, anger, sadness, and vulnerability may come to the fore. One informant said she is always depressed when her disease is active, because she is sure she will continue to get worse and worse until she is totally crippled and dependent. Her depression is worse when the disease attacks a new joint than when the disease in an already affected joint is reactivated. The length of each psychological stage seems to be tied to the disease process. The stages repeat themselves as the disease becomes active and abates, as new joints are involved, as treatment is effective, or as joints are replaced. Uncertainty about the course of the disease and about one's daily abilities remains throughout.

How to Be Helpful to Someone with Arthritis

As in other illnesses, the degree to which arthritis affects one's life depends on the severity of the illness, the person's psychological response to the illness, and her social supports. You cannot understand the limitations of a person with arthritis by looking at her. You have to ask her what she can or cannot do and what she would like you to do for her. Unless, after a long period, you decide that the person can really do more or less than she is telling you (and one of those alternatives is certainly as bad as the other), assume that you should follow her indications.

Some rules of social behavior have to be altered. For example, one often begins a relationship or seals a bargain with a firm handshake. For someone with arthritis, a handshake may be very painful. If the disease has affected her weight-bearing joints, prolonged standing can be extremely uncomfortable. It is considerate to offer someone with arthritis a chair that isn't very deep or very low, so that it will be easier for her to rise by herself. The person also needs enough room while sitting to straighten her knees. Some movie houses and charter airplane flights are impossible. When planning an excursion or an activity with someone who has arthritis, remember that rest is often a necessary part of the day and that wherever you go, you also have to get back. Early morning is difficult for people with arthritis. It takes a while to get stiff joints moving. The other difficult time of the day is late afternoon, when fatigue sets in.

Give the person room to be depressed when she needs to be. The disease itself is fraught with ups and downs, and there are many times when a person feels awful physically and psychologically. When she feels better physically, her depression will probably lift.

To understand pain in arthritis, one must be aware of the amount, the means a person uses to reduce the stress that may exacerbate it, and the methods she employs to distract herself from it. Uncertainty, limited mobility, fatigue, and pain remain important in the life of a person with arthritis. People seem to live best when they protect their joints, use self-help aids cleverly, and find ways to distract themselves from pain.

3

Cancer

CANCER MEANS the uncontrolled growth of cells. Among its definitions dictionaries include a malignant growth of tissue or a malignant evil that corrodes slowly and fatally. Like yesterday's tuberculosis, the word itself has become a metaphor for harmful and distressing aspects of society. It is used to describe our political enemies, the blight of our cities, or even what hatred can do to the psyche. Of all of the chronic diseases, it is the one met with greatest dread and ignorance.

At times people refer to their illness as a growth or a tumor rather than as cancer. When one hears that somebody is very sick but the illness is not specified, it is often assumed that the person has cancer. Many people mistakenly think that cancer is contagious. People who have been successfully treated often do not tell others that they have had cancer. For several reasons such fears are justified. We do not understand the processes of cancer. As with many other illnesses, genetic and environmental factors outside of one's control are thought to be related to etiology. The treatments for cancer sometimes seem to be as devastating to the body and psyche as the disease itself. The incidence of certain malignancies seems to be increasing. Finally, in their terminal phases certain kinds of cancer leave people looking gaunt and wasted, like the terrifying images of death one acquires in childhood.

However, it is a grave mistake to assume that all of the causes of cancer are outside of one's control or that cancer in all its forms is fatal. Many factors within one's control, including smoking and diet, affect the incidence of cancer. Many cancers are curable. Several others can have long remissions, and remissions are lengthening in many instances. Great strides are being made in research regarding the basic processes of cancer and in identifying specific risk factors for the disease. The outlook for understanding and treating cancer, therefore, is not only improving but hopeful.

Medical Information

Cancer is actually a group of diseases that share the common characteristic of the uncontrolled growth of abnormal cells. The basic difference between normal cells and cancer cells is the way they grow. The growth of normal body cells is controlled and coordinated to manage necessary functions of the body. For example, in pregnancy, natural blood replacement, or tissue repair, specific growth patterns are triggered to meet the required function. Once the goal has been attained and the baby is born, the blood restored, or the tissue repaired, the growth pattern returns to normal.

Malignant cells act differently from normal tissue. They continue to multiply, outstripping the body's ability to remove them. Such a mass can compress, become invasive, and destroy normal tissue. In the process abnormal cells lose their resemblance to normal cells in terms of both function and appearance. If they are not eliminated, after they reach a certain size, tumors shed cells, which can enter the bloodstream and/or drain into the lymph nodes. Traveling through the blood and lymphatic systems, they enter other organs and tissue. The process of spreading is called metastasis.

At the points where the abnormal cells have been carried, metastases or secondary cancerous deposits can develop, which again invade and destroy the normal tissue around them. A growth of new cells that proliferate without control and serve no useful function in the body is called a tumor. Since it is a new growth, it is also called a neoplasm. Some neoplasms remain at their original site and are benign. An example of a benign tumor is a fatty tumor or lipoma. Others are malignant or cancerous and spread or metastasize to other parts of the body. Although all cancers begin at the cellular level, many types of cancer can eventually affect the entire body.

Neither the course taken by nor the response to treatment for a particular type of cancer is truly predictable. Physicians tend to talk among themselves and to their patients in terms of odds. If a person with a metastatic colon cancer takes a particular chemotherapy regimen, the chances may be that three times in ten the therapy will be successful. These odds are based on previous experience with the drugs. Although sweeping statements are often made about kinds of cancer, however, the course followed by individuals is difficult to predict.

Today many types of cancer are curable. Hodgkin's disease, childhood leukemia and certain other childhood cancers, testicular tumors, and choriocarcinomas (placental tumors of pregnancy) are potentially curable even when they are widespread. In many other forms of cancer, when the disease has spread the aim or treatment becomes a matter of controlling the disease process rather than curing the disease. Control depends on the stage, location, and most importantly the type of cancer. For example, localized lymphoma can be managed more succesfully than metastatic lung cancer.

When the cancer is considered to be under control, it is said to be in remission. A partial remission means that the tumor shrinks or stops growing for a certain period. A complete remission implies that all indications of the disease disappear. The length of a remission is variable. If the signs of the disease process reappear, the person is said to have had a relapse or recurrence. At that point a new treatment plan is formulated in order to try to bring the disease back under control.

Classification

Cancer is classified by type of tissue (histology) and by anatomic site. Cancer cells are categorized as well-differentiated or anaplastic. Well-differentiated cells retain identifiable characteristics relating to their tissue of origin, while anaplastic cells lose their normal characteristics. These types are determined through microscopic examination of the malignant tissue.

Five prevalent histologic types are carcinoma, melanoma, sarcoma, lymphoma, and leukemia. Carcinoma is cancer arising from the epithelial cells, the surface layer of cells. Examples of such tissues are the skin, glandular tissue such as breast and prostate, and cellular linings of body organs and body cavities. A melanoma is a form of carcinoma that arises from the melanin-producing cells, which are responsible for pigment in the skin and hair. Sarcoma is cancer arising from the connective and supporting tissues, such as bone, cartilage, and fat. Lymphoma is cancer originating in, and characterized by the enlargement of, the lymph nodes. Examples of malignant lymphoma are Hodgkin's disease and non-Hodgkin's lymphoma. Leukemias are malignant transformations of the white blood cells (either the leukocytes or lymphocytes), which penetrate the bone marrow and other tissues like the lymph nodes or spleen and then circulate throughout the body in the blood. The leukemias are either acute or chronic. Acute leukemia occurs primarily in the young and is characterized by the presence of immature, very bizarre cells. The chronic type is somewhat less virulent and usually occurs at a later age.

The second aspect of classification, anatomic site, refers to the place in the body in which the malignant growth began. The principal sites are the lung, colon-rectum, breast, uterus, urinary system, oral cavity, pancreas, bone marrow, ovary, skin, lymphatic system, and brain. Each type has its own natural history and prognosis. The five most prevalent primary sites of cancer are lung, colon-rectum, breast, prostate, and uterus.

LUNG CANCER

Lung cancer accounts for the greatest number of new cases each year. It is also the greatest cancer killer of men and the second greatest cancer killer of women. The death rate of lung cancer among men has stayed stable for about twenty-five years. In that same period the rate has increased 200 percent in women.

Approximately 80 percent of lung cancer is caused by cigarette smoking. In 1983 more than 93,000 deaths could have been prevented by not smoking cigarettes. An additional 10 percent of lung cancer occurs in nonsmokers, some of whom have been exposed to toxic substances through their work. Occupations involving radioactive dust, inhalation of wood dust, beryllium dust, coal tar fumes and fogs, and nickel and chromium compounds are at increased risk. People who work with asbestos fibers who also smoke increase their risk. In addition, there is thought to be a genetic component to lung cancer.

The latent period for lung cancer, the period between exposure and symptoms, is between fifteen and thirty years. The disease is difficult to diagnose at an early stage. Early symptoms can include a persistent cough, increased sputum (the material brought up from the lungs), and shortness of breath. The spells of coughing grow more persistent and longer. Symptoms in later stages include chest pain and blood in the sputum (hemoptysis).

In designing a treatment plan for lung cancer, it is important to know the stage of the cancer as well as what kind of tumor is present. Four principal types of tumors account for more than 90 percent of all lung cancers: epidermoid or squamous cell, adenocarcinoma, large cell, and small or oat cell carcinoma. The type is identified through the microscopic examination of tumor cells. Sometimes a biopsy can be carried out by examining cells from the phlegm coughed up by the ill person, but usually either a bronchoscopic examination or a surgical procedure is required. A bronchoscopy allows the physician to look directly into the bronchi, the two tubes into which the lower end of the trachea (windpipe) divides, and to obtain a tissue specimen. Additional tests include a chest x-ray, CT scan of the chest and mediasternum, and aspiration needle biopsy. Sometimes a mediastinoscopy is carried out. Here, a small incision in the neck allows the physician to pass an instrument into the area between the lungs and behind the breastbone in order to obtain tissue from nearby lymph nodes. In that way the physician can determine whether there is any cancer in the lymph nodes. If it is determined that the person has a lung cancer that is potentially curable, a thoracotomy or surgical exploration of the lungs is carried out. In this procedure the chest is opened and the lungs and chest cavity are examined. In order to determine the stage of the cancer, the liver, spleen, bone, lung, and sometimes the brain are scanned. Bone marrow and lymph node aspiration biopsy may also be required.

Lung cancer is generally treated with a combination of surgery, radiation, and chemotherapy. If the cancer is thought to be contained in one lung or one part of one lung, the diseased lobe or lung is removed surgically. Generally only those cancers that can be removed surgically are potentially curable. Because it is so difficult to detect lung cancer in its early stages, it has usually spread beyond a local lesion before the ill person seeks medical treatment. It is thought that the cancer spreads so quickly because of the rich supply of lymphatic channels and blood vessels in the lungs.

In many cases surgery is not a solution. Sometimes the cancer has spread; at other times the existence of cardiac or respiratory problems makes surgical intervention impossible or tumors involving major blood vessels or areas of the chest cavity are considered inoperable.

With people whose cancer has spread beyond one lung, the goal is to prevent the further spread of the disease. The nature of the treatment again depends on the stage and cell type of the disease. Radiation is helpful to a significant minority of ill people for a period of time. Frequently some form of chemotherapy is used. The best results thus far are in the treatment of small or oat cell carcinomas with chemotherapy and radiation.

The side effects of treatment for lung cancer are varied. Shortness of breath during exercise or pain at the site of the incision may result from surgery to remove a lung or part of a lung. After radiation, besides the usual side effects,* the ill person may also have difficulty swallowing or may develop pneumonia. In addition to the effects usually found with use of chemotherapy, there may also be constipation, numbness and tingling in the fingers, and possibly heart failure.

The five-year survival for lung cancer is only about 8 percent for men and 12 percent for women. This poor rate is thought to be a result of the inability to detect lung cancer in its early stages. If people did not smoke cigarettes, more than 80 percent of lung cancer would be preventable. Smoking is also linked to cancers of the mouth, esophagus, larynx, pharynx, kidney, bladder, and pancreas.

COLON-RECTUM CANCER

Colon-rectum cancer is the second most frequent type when statistics for men and women are combined. It commonly occurs only after age

*The usual side effects of various kinds of treatment are discussed in the general treatment section, pages 49–50.

forty, and the incidence increases with advancing age. The cause of colon-rectum cancer is unknown. It is suspected that a high-fat, low-fiber diet puts one at greater risk than a low-fat, high-fiber diet. Predisposing factors include a family history of polyps; colon, stomach, or uterine cancer; or a ten-year history of ulcerative colitis.

A one-to-three-year period passes from the time the disease process begins until people become aware of symptoms. Symptoms include persistent diarrhea or constipation, blood in the stool, thin stools of small diameter, cramping pains, excessive gas, weight loss, and abdominal fullness. If a person's intestine is blocked, he may also experience nausea and vomiting.

Accurate and simple diagnostic tests help make colon-rectum cancer a highly curable disease. With a gloved finger, a physician can detect 15 percent of these lesions. The rectum and sigmoid colon can be examined with the use of a proctoscope, a small lighted tube that is passed through the anus into the bowel, and the entire large intestine can be examined with a flexible colonoscope. The colon and rectum can also be examined by x-ray. To enable the colon and rectum to be visualized by x-ray, it is necessary to have the area lined with barium sulfate, a heavy, insoluable powder suspended in a liquid. The barium solution is inserted by enema and acts as a contrast medium. Certain blood tests are useful for aiding diagnostic information, but they are not perfectly accurate. Finally, suspicious tissue is sometimes biopsied. Carcinoma embryonic antigen (CEA) may be measured in the blood and may indicate the presence of a cancer in this area or its level of clinical activity.

Treatment consists of surgery with the addition of radiation and chemotherapy in some instances. Surgery removes the tumor and area lymph nodes to prevent the possible spread of the disease. Most people who undergo surgery do not need a permanent colostomy (an opening in the abdominal wall for the elimination of waste material). After a period of healing, normal patterns of elimination are reestablished. When the rectum must be removed, a permanent colostomy is constructed. Many people with colostomies can learn to regulate their bowel movements by avoiding foods that disagree with them and irrigating their colostomies with enemas every day or so.

Once people with colostomies have adjusted physically and psychologically to this new means of excretion, they can participate normally in all activities. The United Ostomy Association is a self-help organization whose network of local chapters and volunteers helps people to adjust to life with colostomies.

BREAST CANCER

The cause of breast cancer is not known. Predisposing factors include a family history of breast cancer, no pregnancy or pregnancy after thirty and no lactation (secretion of milk from breasts), early onset of menses, or late menopause. There is also a possible increase of risk with the use of estrogen as a treatment for other symptoms. Breast cancer occurs most often in women who are middle-aged or older. It also generally appears in women of higher socioeconomic background.

The latent period for breast cancer is probably ten to fifteen years. There are no symptoms in the early stage. Later symptoms include a lump or thickening of the breast, a change in the contour of the breast, or a lump in the armpit. Although 80 percent of breast lumps are not malignant, it is impossible for a woman to make this assessment herself. Generally lumps that change in size with the menstrual cycle are more likely to be benign. Other symptoms include nipple discharge or retraction, a puckering or dimpling of the skin of the breast, and enlargment of the breast. In later stages symptoms can include pain and swollen glands in the armpit.

Diagnosis is made through examination, x-ray, and biopsy. Women over thirty-five should do a monthly breast self-examination (BSE). In the physician's examination, the breast lump is palpated—lightly touched. The physician may also take some fluid from a cyst and check for evidence of the symptoms described above. Unfortunately, mammography, the x-ray technique used to detect breast cancer, has a substantial percentage of false negative, false positive, and indeterminate results. Recently ultrasonography, which uses sound waves to clarify a pattern in the breast, has been found useful as an adjunct to mammography, especially for women with cystic disease. Finally, if a malignancy is suspected, a biopsy is carried out for microscopic examination of the tissue.

Treatment for breast cancer depends on what stage the disease is in when it is detected. In an early stage treatment can consist of a lumpectomy with a check of nearby lymph nodes for the presence of disease. This treatment can be followed by primary radiation therapy or another type of surgery. If the lymph nodes are involved, total mastectomy or simple mastectomy followed by chemotherapy may be indicated. Since certain breast cancers are dependent on hormones for growth, if a woman is menstruating her ovaries may be removed; if she is past menopause various forms of hormonal therapy may be used. The determination of the advisability of various endocrinologic manipulations may depend on the presence or absence of estrogen receptors and progesterone receptors on the tumor cells when they are examined after surgery. In addition, sometimes chemotherapy and radiation therapy are used in conjunction with surgery.

Side effects of treatment are varied. A feeling of tightness, numbness, and discomfort in the arm and chest may result from surgery. The person's arm may swell as a result of accumulated fluid in the tissue. The actual scar left by the mastectomy is a thin scar that runs from the midpoint of the torso to the armpit. It is said that at that point the woman's chest resembles that of a young boy. After the area has healed, the woman can be fitted with a prosthetic breast, which is indistinguishable from a normal breast beneath clothing. About a year after the surgery, some women choose to have the lost breast rebuilt through implants and grafting by a plastic surgeon.

Besides the usual side effects of radiation some women experience a tightening and thickening of their breast skin. Sometimes, radiation changes the size and shape of the treated breast. In addition to the usual effects of chemotherapy some women experience bladder irritation, fatigue, and cold sores in their mouths. The administration of hormones sometimes is accompanied by side effects. Male hormones which are used much less frequently now, sometimes cause increased sexual desire, acne, and other masculine features, such as increased facial and body hair, enlargement of the clitoris, and a deepening of the voice.

PROSTATE CANCER

The prostate is a small conical gland at the base of the male bladder, surrounding the first part of the urethra. The cause of prostate cancer is unknown. Most cases occur in elderly men who die of other causes. It occurs more among married than single men and is more frequently found in blacks than whites. There are also no known predisposing factors for prostate cancer. It is thought that people with a history of venereal disease or prostate infections are at higher risk. The latent period is presumed to be many years. Prostate cancer in its early stages is difficult to detect except through rectal examination. As the illness progresses, symptoms include continuing urinary difficulties, weak or interrupted flow of urine, the need to urinate frequently, especially at night, an inability to urinate or to begin to urinate, painful or buring urination, and blood in the urine. These symptoms are frequently caused by benign (noncancerous) enlargement of the prostate, which occurs in more than 50 percent of men over fifty years old, or from infection, cysts, or inflammation. In advanced stages of the disease, people often experience pain in the lower back or pelvis.

Initial diagnosis may be made on digital examination, laboratory tests, and tissue biopsy. First, the physician palpates the prostate gland in a rectal examination. Next, he orders urine and blood analyses as well as an x-ray of the area. Finally, through a needle biopsy, he obtains tissue for microscopic examination. Choice of treatment depends on the stage of the disease, the rate of tumor growth, and the health and age of the individual. Treatment ranges from internal or external radiation therapy, through surgical removal of the prostate gland, to the administration of the female hormone estrogen or orchidectomy (surgical removal of the testicles). Most early cases can be controlled through radiation therapy.

Side effects from treatment include the usual side effects of radiotherapy. Fewer than 5 percent of all people treated for prostate cancer experience damage to the intestines. Sometimes people have difficulty urinating because of damage to their urethra. Surgical removal of the prostate may cause urinary difficulties or impotence. The administration of estrogen produces fluid retention, breast swelling, and impotence.

CANCER OF THE UTERUS

The uterus is the womb, the hollow muscular organ that receives the fertilized egg and houses the fetus until birth. Two parts of the uterus that develop high rates of cancer are the cervix (the lowest portion of the uterus and its opening to the vagina) and the endometrium (the mucous membrane lining of the uterine cavity). Causes of both types of cancer are not known. Herpes simplex type II is a suspected cause of cancer of the cervix, and it is thought that cancer of the endometrium might be hormone-related.

Cancer *in situ* of the cervix can be detected early and is 95 percent curable, hence is usually not included in cancer statistics. Thanks to early diagnosis through the Pap (Papanicolaou) smear and improved treatment, deaths from cancer of the cervix have decreased by more than 70 percent in the past forty years.

Factors correlated with cervical cancer include sexual intercourse before the age of eighteen, multiple sexual partners, marriage at an early age, poor male sex hygiene, chronic irritation, more than five completed pregnancies, venereal disease, and vaginal infections. Since this is a slow-growing neoplasm, the latent period lasts for many years. Cancer of the uterus appears most often in women between the ages of forty and seventy. Symptoms include vaginal discharge and vaginal bleeding after sexual intercourse and after periods.

Cervical cancer is diagnosed through pelvic examination and tests of tissue and mucus. In the Pap test a smear is taken from the mucus around the cervix to detect cancer of this tissue. A cervical biopsy allows for microscopic examination of the tissue of the cervix. Treatment for cancer *in situ* of the cervix is local excision. For stage 1 cervical cancer, treatment consists of radiation therapy and/or surgery. Surgery is preferred for younger women, and radiotherapy for older women.

Cancer of the endometrium, the body of the uterus, is highly curable. Predisposing factors include a family history of endometrial cancer, completion of menopause, no pregnancy, diabetes, hypertension, and obesity. Women who have taken prescribed estrogen after menopause are also predisposed toward cancer of the endometrium. Because this is a slow-growing neoplasm, the latent period lasts for many years. Symptoms include an irregular menstrual cycle, vaginal bleeding, and a brownish vaginal discharge.

Diagnosis is made through three techniques: Pap test (only about 40

percent accurate for endometrial cancer), analysis of suctioned uterine secretions, and dilation and curettage (D and C). In dilation and curettage,
the uterus is expanded and tissue is scraped from the walls to be examined
for malignant cells. Cancer of the endometrium is treated with preoper-
ative radiation therapy followed by a hysterectomy, the surgical removal
of the uterus.

Side effects of treatment are varied. In premenopausal women, removal of the uterus obviously causes loss of fertility. In addition to the
usual side effects of radiotherapy, there can also be loss of fertility or a
narrowing of the vagina. Women who have intercourse during the radiotherapy course are less likely to have narrowing of the vagina than those
who abstain. Sometimes the large or small intestines or the bladder is impaired and will have to be surgically corrected. When radiotherapy is used
in conjunction with surgery, the doses of x-ray are smaller and the side
effects are greatly lessened.

Natural History

Cancer is generally described in stages, which relate to the extent of tumor
spread. Stage 0 cancers are *in situ* and are considered by some to be precancerous states. Stage I means that the tumor is localized and that there
has been no spread or metastasis to other areas. Stage II means that the
tumor has invaded the underlying tissue but is still localized. In stage III
the cancer cells have metastasized to regional lymph nodes, and the condition is termed regional involvement. Stage IV means that the cancer has
reached advanced stages and has spread to distant parts of the body. Cancer is most curable in Stage I. As the stages progress, the chances of cure
are lessened.

For each type of cancer staging is described in more specific terms. For
example, in the staging of cancer of the uterine cervix, Stage I is limited
to the epithelial lining of the cervix. It becomes Stage II when the cell
growth extends into the body of the uterus or upper vagina. It is described
as Stage III when it involves the structure of the pelvic wall, and Stage
IV when the tumor has spread to other sites in the body, like the bladder
or the rectum.

The American Cancer Society has established seven warning signals to
alert people to the possibility that they have cancer. The signals are: change
in bowel or bladder habits, a sore that does not heal, unusual bleeding or
discharge, thickening or lump in breast or elsewhere, indigestion or difficulty in swallowing, obvious change in a wart or mole, and nagging
cough or hoarseness.

The symptoms of cancer are associated with the location of the cancer as well as the degree to which it has affected the normal functions of its site in the body. Often, when the disease is in its early stages, symptoms are mild or absent. Sometimes, too, healthy cells will temporarily compensate for abnormal ones, making illness hard to detect.

One of the great difficulties in treating cancer is that often an individual is in Stage III before his symptoms are sufficiently disturbing to cause him to see a physician.

Symptoms are indicative of the damage caused by the disease process. Sometimes tumors obstruct one of the many hollow structures in the body. At other times damage to a particular organ or tissue causes spillage of the contents, which usually remain in the structure. Sometimes, as a result of an excess production of fluid or the blockage of normal drainage pathways, fluid will collect in the chest cavity or abdomen. Excess fluid is sometimes felt by the ill person as increased pressure in his chest or abdomen or seen in abnormal chemical test levels.

Symptoms are also caused when the invasion of an organ by abnormal cells results in changed function or pain. The most common sites are the nervous system, the liver, the lungs, and bone. Invasion of the central nervous system may cause changes in mental status, loss of motor or sensory function, visual changes, or headaches. Cancer of the liver is often asymptomatic until well advanced. At that point symptoms include enlargement, fluid in the pelvic and abdominal cavities, test results of liver function that are abnormal, impaired clotting mechanisms, and jaundice, a condition characterized by a raised bilirubin level in the blood. Bilirubin is the breakdown product of blood. An elevated bilirubin means that the blood is being broken down too rapidly, the liver is not able to process properly, or there is an obstruction from the liver.

Lung involvement may cause chest pain, a diminished respiratory reserve, coughing up of blood, coughing, infections like recurring attacks of pneumonia or bronchitis, and an obstruction in an airway. The invasion of the bone marrow from other primary tumors can decrease the production of blood cells and thus alter blood counts. Malignancies of the blood like leukemia alter the production and function of certain blood cells. This alteration can, in turn, alter the production of all other blood cells in the body. Such alterations often cause increased susceptibility to infection, bleeding, and anemia, a disorder due to a deficiency in the red blood cells or their hemoglobin content. Invasion of the breast can produce lumps or masses, swelling, dimpling, thickening, skin irritation, retraction or scaliness of the nipple, distortion, pain, tenderness, or nipple discharge. Masses can also be symptomatic of some lymphomas. Additional symptoms can include pain, which is the result of pressure on nerve endings or the invasion of cancerous cells in the nerve roots, and electrolyte abnormalities. If any invasive cancer is not treated, it will continue to grow and metastasize and will eventually cause death.

Prevalence and Incidence

It is estimated that there were about 855,000 new cancer cases in 1983. The incidence of nonmelanoma skin cancer was about 400,000. This type of cancer appears on the surface of the skin, is rarely invasive, and is easily excised. The more virulent types of cancer account for the remaining 455,000 new cases. Of those, lung cancer has the highest incidence. It is estimated that there were 135,000 new cases of lung cancer in 1983 and that 117,000 deaths occurred from cancer of the lung in the same period. Figures for colon-rectum cancer were 126,000 new cases and 58,000 deaths; for breast cancer 115,000 new cases and 38,000 deaths; for prostate cancer 75,000 new cases and 24,000 deaths; for cancer of the uterus 55,000 new cases, which would rise to over 99,000 if carcinoma *in situ* were included, and 10,000 deaths; for urinary cancer 57,000 new cases and 19,000 deaths; for oral 27,000 new cases and 9,200 deaths; for pancreas, 25,000 new cases and 23,000 deaths; for leukemia 24,000 new cases and 16,000 deaths; for cancer of the ovary 18,000 cases and 12,000 deaths; and for skin cancer 17,000 new cases and 7,000 deaths. For breast cancer the prevalence is 25 per 1,000. For lung cancer the rate is 1 per 1,000; and for cancer of the cervix, 2.5 per 1,000.

The cancer rate for blacks is higher than that for whites. Blacks have higher increases in lung, colon-rectum, prostate, and esophageal cancer. While cancer mortality figures have increased for both races in the last twenty-five years, rates for whites have increased 9 percent while rates for blacks have increased 34 percent. Twenty-five years ago these rates were almost identical. Some of this increase in rates for blacks may be the result of increased access to medical care, leading to a more accurate reflection of the actual rate of disease.

In 1983 about 440,000 people died of cancer. For many kinds of cancer, like leukemia and Hodgkin's disease, the survival rate has improved dramatically in the last twenty years. For other types, like cancer of the mouth and the esophagus, there has been virtually no change in the survival rate. For lung cancer there has been a small increase in survival time and an increased incidence. Overall, there has been a steady rise in the age-adjusted national cancer death rate.

Populations at Risk

Populations at risk for cancer depend on age, race, ethnicity, sex, and environmental and occupational factors, among others. Several types of cancer are related to particular occupations. For example, benzene workers have a higher rate of acute leukemia than do other occupational groups.

Cancer of the bone occurs more frequently among workers who paint radium dials on watches and clocks. Cancer of the lung is closely asociated with several occupations in which people work with asbestos, chemicals used in the manufacture of textiles, arsenic (used for smelting and the manufacture of insecticides), and chemicals used in the refining of various kinds of ore and petroleum. Skin cancer occurs most often in those who work out of doors, like construction workers, farmers, and sailors. This type of cancer is also related to occupations that use chemicals, such as those involved in the breakdown of coal products.

Other kinds of cancer occur more frequently in one sex than another. For example, four out of every five bladder cancers occur in men, which may be related also to the occupations they represent. Breast cancer obviously occurs over 99 percent in women, but those at greatest risk are wealthy, unmarried, and childless; have rich diets; and have mothers, aunts, or sisters who have also had breast cancer. Cancer of the cervix is also obviously a women's disease; women at greatest risk are those who begin sexual intercourse early in life, have many pregnancies or sexual partners, and have uncircumcised partners. The rate of kidney cancer is much higher for men than for women, and the rate is rising for men. Lung cancer is found predominantly in urban men, but the rate is rising for women. The rate for lymphoma (cancer of the lymphatic system) is higher in men than women, as is cancer of the pancreas and the stomach and vocal cords.

Some kinds of cancer are age-related. Generally risk increases with age. Breast cancer occurs most often between ages forty and sixty-five; colon-rectum between forty and seventy-nine; lung cancer between forty and seventy; prostate cancer in middle-aged or older men, but also relatively frequently in men over sixty; and cancer of the uterus in women between forty and seventy. Elderly people can often survive cancer, so aggressive treatment is rarely ruled out because of age. Some cancers are more predominant in people sharing a group of common factors. For example, cancer of the esophagus is found most often in men between sixty and seventy who drink and smoke heavily.

Etiology

There is no single cause for cancer. It is not directly inherited except in two instances: familial polyposis of the colon, which is a precusor of cancer, and retinoblastoma, an eye tumor that occurs in some families. Cancer is also not a contagious disease, although viruslike particles have been linked to certain tumors.

It is thought now that there are certain predisposing factors that increase the likelihood of one's developing cancer. One such factor is chronic irritation. Examples are melanoma arising in a mole located under a bras-siere strap or a belt, cancer of the lip in pipe smokers, and cancer of the cervix in women with chronic inflammation of the cervix. Another factor is precancerous lesions, benign changes in the body tissue that later be-come malignant. Examples are polyps or elongated growths of the colon and rectum, and pigmented moles. A third factor is exposure to known carcinogens or cancer-producing substances. For example, thyroid cancer is now seen in people who received x-ray therapy years ago for acne, sin-usitis, or tinea capitis, a fungus infection of the scalp. Also, smoking is strongly associated with lung cancer. People who were exposed to high doses of toxic agents in their work have developed forms of cancer asso-ciated with those agents.

The recent discovery of the "oncogene," the first and perhaps most critical step in the transformation of a healthy cell to a malignant one, has led scientists to think they have discovered the essential element in the cancer process. Oncogenes exist in all cells. When certain of these genes are somehow activated, they begin abnormal production of protein. In that way they cause the cell to become cancerous. Although this does not bring science close to finding a cure for cancer, it does present the possi-bility of using the oncogene as an early warning of cancer. Once the com-position of the oncogene proteins has been described, scientists think they will be able to provide chemical probes to detect the presence of the ac-tivated proteins long before a tumor has developed enough to be detected through x-ray or surgery. Earlier detection and treatment mean a much greater survival rate.

Diagnosis

In cancer diagnostic procedures have two purposes: to identity the type of cancer and the stage of the disease process. The identification of the type of cancer, the histological diagnosis, is made through the microscopic examination of a small specimen of the malignant tissue by a pathologist. The specimen is collected through a biopsy, a small sample of tissue that is generally surgically removed from the suspected malignancy.

Determining the stage of the disease process, commonly called staging, is accomplished through a variety of tests and procedures depending on the histological type and the expected pattern of disease spread. Clinical evaluation, blood tests, surgical lymph node or tissue evaluation, micro-scopic study of cells, and various radiographic techniques like radioisotope scans, computerized tomography, and nuclear magnetic resonance, which yields cross-sectional pictures of any part of the body, may be used. These tests determine the spread of the disease and the extent of its involvement in new sites.

Certain tests are used regularly to diagnose or to rule out specific types of cancer. For example, the Pap (Papanicolaou) smear is used to detect preinvasive, microscopic, early cancer of the cervix. It is easy to do, a regular part of most gynecological examinations, and relatively inexpensive. Many colon-rectum cancers are diagnosed through an examination for stool occult blood (blood hidden in the stool) and the use of a proctosigmoidoscopy, in which instruments are used to visualize the rectum and the sigmoid section of the colon. In the detection of breast cancer, mammograms are the specialized x-rays used. Ultrasound may be used to locate tumors deep in the body. Ultrasound also helps radiation therapists to pinpoint a tumor more precisely in order to regulate the placing and dosage of radiation.

A research goal is better means for early diagnosis for all types of cancer. Because lung cancer is relatively asymptomatic until its later stages, it is often incurable by the time it is diagnosed. Researchers are now trying to develop a test for lung cancer that would be equivalent to the Pap smear for cervical cancer in which sputum would be examined for the presence of early lung cancer. Experiments are also being conducted with inexpensive, simple blood tests in which unique antigens, enzymes, proteins, and other substances are identified to determine the presence and location of cancer. Known by such names as CEA, B-protein, and GI-11, these tests have some positive preliminary results in the detection of certain specific cancers like breast and pancreas. Researchers are trying to "profile" individuals according to their cancer risk factors and thereby help them to know what to be screened for, when, and how often. For example, workers involved with the many chemicals that have been found to be carcinogenic should be screened regularly for the cancers associated with those chemicals. Also, women whose close relatives have had breast cancer should be screened regularly for the presence of a malignancy. There is a general need for lifelong detection for recurrences.

Treatment

The purpose of treatment for cancer is to rid the body of tumorous material or at least to stop the growth and spread of tumors. One of the main determinants of responsiveness to treatment is tumor growth rate. Generally, rapidly growing tumors are more responsive to treatment than those that grow more slowly. Still, in advanced stages rapidly growing tumors respond as poorly to treatment as slowly growing ones.

As tumors become larger, they usually grow more slowly. The faster the tumor grows, the shorter the time it requires to double in size. In fact, tumor doubling time varies inversely with tumor size. Before it is large enough to be detected clinically, a single tumor cell experiences thirty to thirty-six doublings. If tumor cells are left behind in rapidly growing tumors, because doubling time is so short, they are likely to reappear within three years after treatment has ceased. Someone who has remained free of tumors for three years after treatment of a rapidly growing tumor is likely to remain free of the disease, because it is probable that all tumors were eliminated. On the other hand, reappearance of slowly growing tumors may occur as long as twelve years after treatment has ceased.

Although it may appear that all evidence of tumors has disappeared, treatment must continue until the last few cells are eliminated. Late recurrence of tumors—1–3 years for rapidly growing tumors, 4–7 years for intermediate, and 8–12 years for slowly growing ones—means that the treatment was stopped too soon for every cancerous cell to be eliminated. Treatment therefore must be directed toward the eradication of cancerous material from body and must continue long enough to ensure that all tumor cells are eliminated.

Cancer is treated with surgery, radiation, chemotherapy, and immune therapy.

SURGERY

Surgery is the oldest form of treatment for cancer. Surgical techniques are used today for the diagnosis of cancer, for establishing the extent of the spread of the disease (staging), for controlling symptoms, for cure, and for reconstructing parts of the body altered by the disease or the treatment. If a tumor is found in the first stage of the disease process and can be successfully removed before the cancer has begun to spread, the surgery has cured the cancer. Except for nonmelanoma skin cancers, this can be a complicated set of procedures. Often massive volumes of tissue are removed. Because cancer spreads so easily to close lymph nodes, those too are often removed to prevent further spread. Because lymph drainage is altered and much dead space is created in operations of this kind, ill people are more susceptible to infection and to poor healing. Radiation to the area, immunosuppressive therapy (which slows the growth of the cancer), and perhaps poor nutritional status often further complicate the healing process.

One of the main questions in surgery is how much tissue to remove to maximize the possibility of controlling the cancer. This has been an issue in breast cancer. For a long time many surgeons thought that only a radical mastectomy could maximize control. A radical mastectomy consists of removal of the breast, the skin, underlying chest muscle, and all the lymph nodes in the armpit. Now that staging, chemotherapy, and radiation have become more exact for breast cancer, physicians can choose with greater assurance among four types of mastectomy: radical; modified radical, in which the breast and lymph nodes are removed but the chest muscles are left intact; total or simple, where the breast is removed but the lymph nodes are sampled; and segmental or partial, in which only the affected portion and a surrounding area of breast tissue are removed. Radical mastectomy is rarely done now. In some kinds of bone cancer, where surgeons previously amputated a person's leg or arm, in some specific conditions they are beginning to replace sections of bone rather than amputating a limb.

Factors besides the impact that the surgery can have on the control of the cancer are also considered. An assessment of the visibility of the change wrought by the surgery, the alteration of bodily functions, and the ill person's emotional investment in the function or the part of the body that will be altered become an important part of the decision. Although cancer patients rarely die as a result of surgery, they often suffer disfigurement. Mastectomy is one operation that is disfiguring but can be disguised through the use of a prosthetic breast and careful choice of clothing. However, surgery of the mouth or throat can deform a person's face in ways that cannot be hidden. Even though reconstructive surgery presents increased risks through anesthesia, the slow healing process, and the opportunity for infection, benefits may be sufficiently important to the ill person to warrent the reconstruction.

Disfigurement is not always a matter of what can be seen or hidden. By shortening or removing the vagina, surgery for cancer of the cervix can alter a woman's sex life. Surgical removal of the stomach or part of the colon can make it difficult for a person to digest food. Thus a decision involving surgery must be based on a consideration of its impact on the cancer itself and on the person who must live with the results.

RADIATION THERAPY

Radiation therapy transmits energy at sufficiently high levels to change the physical and chemical characteristics within cells. It tries to kill cancer cells without destroying the surrounding normal tissue. Rapidly dividing cells are usually most sensitive to radiation, and slowly dividing cells are more resistent. Radiation is most commonly used to treat localized tumors.

Radiation is commonly administered using three basic techniques: external beam, implantation of a sealed radioactive source, and systematic administration of a radioisotope. With external radiation, a beam of x-rays or gamma rays produced by a radioactive source like cobalt 60 or by electrical machines is targeted to the exposed area of the body. An example of the use of external radiation would be to the spine or the brain for a tumor. Generally a series of radiation treatments is needed. Often the radiotherapist will mark the treatment portal with indelible ink or gentian violet, which the ill person is not to wash off. The person feels no sensation during the treatment, which lasts only a minute and a half, with a linear accelerator. After the treatment, the person is not radioactive.

The second technique, implantation of a sealed source, requires that a radioactive source be placed into a body cavity or tissue, left in place usually for a few days, then removed leaving no residual radiation. An example would be radium implants for uterine cancer.

The third technique, systematic administration of a radioisotope, involves hospitalizing the ill person until all radioactive material has been dissipated. An example is the use of iodine 131 for treatment of thyroid cancer.

Reactions to radiation can be acute or chronic. Acute reactions ordinarily appear quickly and subside in a few weeks or months. Irradiated skin is sensitive and must be protected from the sun, heat, tight clothing, or other irritants. Adequate intake of food and liquids can prevent nausea and vomiting and help buttress the immune system. When the throat is irradiated, it may feel sore and there may be difficulty swallowing. When the bladder or rectum is irradiated, the ill person may have cramps, diarrhea, or frequent urination. Nausea may accompany stomach radiation.

Other reactions can be more severe and long-lasting. Head and neck radiation can cause hair loss. Other site-specific reactions are a lowered sperm count or even sterility through radiation of male reproductive organs and the abolition or reduction of ovarian hormone production in women, which can lead to temporary or permanent menopause.

Chronic reactions can also be mild or severe. An example of a mild chronic reaction might be the darkening of the skin in the radiated area. A severe reaction could be an impaired healing capacity, intestinal fistulas, or abnormal passages in the intestines. Among the most serious effects are new cancers caused by the radiation that cured the first. These side effects can develop many years later. However, serious side effects develop in fewer than one out of twenty people treated with radiation.

CHEMOTHERAPY

Chemotherapy is the use of one or more chemical agents to eradicate the disease or to stop its progress. Although ideally they should not effect normal tissue, the chemicals used at this time affect both normal and abnormal cells. These agents are ingested orally or administered intramuscularly or intravenously. Most drugs are not taken orally because they can damage the stomach or may be neutralized by digestive enzymes. Distributed through the bloodstream, they can travel to attack detected and undetected tumors throughout the body, hence can be used to treat cancers like leukemia that are too widespread to be treated with radiation or surgery. There are about thirty FDA-approved anticancer drugs currently used, as well as hundreds of experimental drugs not yet approved for general use.

The drugs can be categorized into four groups: alkylating agents, antimetabolates, antibiotics, and steroids. Alkylating agents prevent successful cell division by interfering with the orderly pairing process. Examples of alkylating agents are Cytoxan, Myleran, and L-PAM. Antimetabolates disrupt the cell's metabolic mechanisms by being absorbed like the vitamins or other nutrients, which they resemble, then acting differently after absorption. Examples of antimetabolates are methotrexate, 5-FU, and 6-MP. Antibiotics disrupt the synthesis of RNA, which the cell requires in order to make proteins. Not all antibiotics work in these ways, but examples used in the treatment of cancer are Adriamycin and Bleomycin. Steroids constitute a lesser category than the first three, with regard to cancer treatment. They are thought to prevent the production of certain enzymes that the cells need. Prednisone is often used in combination with other chemotherapy for treatment of lymphoma, and estrogen is used in treating prostate cancer. By the same token the ovaries are often removed as part of the treatment plan for breast cancer, thus preventing the natural production of estrogen.

Because as yet no drugs that destroy cancer cells and leave normal cells unharmed exist, side effects are a great problem. Some, like hair loss, nausea, vomiting, diarrhea, and loss of appetite, are usually temporary, but they can be sufficiently distressing to make completion of the prescribed regimen difficult. More serious than those side effects is the tendency for many drugs to destroy platelets and white blood cells. Platelets are needed to prevent bleeding, and white blood cells help the body to fight infection. Specific drugs can also damage heart muscle or nerve tissue. Damage can also occur to bone morrow, so the body cannot properly control infection, bruising, or fatigue. Many side effects can be controlled by discontinuing or changing a drug. Other means for controlling side effects are prescribing medication to counter the effects, confining someone who can't fight infection to an isolation room, and giving blood transfusions.

Many new trends in chemotherapy are enhancing the chances for success in either the treatment of the disease process or in relieving the symptoms of the disease. For example, it has been found that intense drug therapy before surgery is successful in the treatment of bone tumors in children. Also retinoids, synthetic relatives of vitamin A, have prevented both bladder and breast cancer in mice and rats. It may be that they will be successful in preventing those kinds of tumors in humans and possibly also in combating cancers of the pancreas, esophagus, and lung. Ways have been found to administer powerful doses of methotrexate safely; in the recent past such doses were considered lethal. Some of the many drugs now considered experimental also hold great promise.

NEW FORMS OF TREATMENT

Immunotherapy, the newest cancer treatment, tries to augment the body's natural immune system's ability to recognize the foreign cancer cells and destroy them. In laboratory animals, substances such as BCG can stimulate immune mechanisms. BCG has been used locally to treat human bladder tumors. Thymosin fraction 5, a partially purified thymosin preparation, has shown promise when used in conjunction with chemotherapy following radiation therapy in treatment of oat cell carcinoma of the lung, as well as head and neck tumors. Thymosin is a biological response modifier produced by the thymus gland, the master gland of the body's immune system. Thymosin fraction 5 has been synthesized with the help of recombinant DNA.

Many treatments now are being developed in conjunction with others. For example, hyperthermia, the superheating of body tissues, has been found to increase the effectiveness of radiotherapy and chemotherapy. The selective transfusion of blood components is becoming increasingly available. Platelets are used to prevent hemorrhaging, white cells are being used to treat infection, and red cells are used to replace lost red cells.

Other treatments are being developed through attempts to understand the development of cancer. The oncogene was mentioned earlier.* Researchers have also theorized that many cancers are caused by a two-stage process through exposure to two kinds of substances known as initiators and promoters. They are exploring ways of interrupting the process and thus preventing the development of cancer. In addition, researchers are trying to fuse cancer cells genetically to produce monoclonal antibodies that would fight the disease by seeking out specific targets on cancer cells. Antibodies that work in this way have already proved effective against hepatitis B virus, various strains of flu, and malarial parasites.

PALLIATIVE CARE

While part of treatment is directed toward curing cancer or causing it to go into remission, another part, called palliative care, is directed toward the relief of symptoms. An important component of palliation is the control of pain. Most prominent in pain control is the use of Brompton's mixture or hospice mix, which combines a narcotic, usually morphine, with other ingredients, like tranquilizers and antidepressants, to free the ill person from pain while allowing him to remain alert. These almost invariably result in cognitive impairment. For certain patients with debilitating pain, a series of chemical injections near the spine can act as a

*Researchers have already learned how to suppress oncogenes in some animals and are determining whether the same approach may be used with people.

nerve block. Sometimes symptomatic relief requires drastic measures. For example, a person's leg might have to be amputated even though it is known that his cancer has metastasized to several other parts of his body, because without the amputation gangrene could cause a deadly systemic infection. Generally relief can be provided by much less drastic measures.

Until cancer has been deemed terminal, care is both curative and palliative. Indications of when to stop curative care and provide only palliative care come when radiation is no longer controlling the spread of the disease, when drugs are no longer effective and there are no new drugs to try, and when surgery cannot be used to excise the cancer cells.

PROGRAMS UNDER FEDERAL AUSPICES

Through the National Cancer Act of 1971 and Amendment of 1974 the federal government has provided for the establishment or continuation of cancer centers in certain areas of the country. The centers are located primarily in the Northeast with another pocket in Southern California, but they generate new knowledge of cancer and accelerate the transfer of knowledge of improved cancer presentation, diagnosis, treatment, rehabilitation, and continuing care to health professionals and the general public nationwide. Laboratory Cancer Research Centers engage only in laboratory research. Comprehensive Cancer Centers and Clinical Cancer Centers provide services more or less comprehensively. The Community Clinical Oncology Program is a major research initiative that tries to involve community physicians in clinical trials through participation in NCI-approved research protocols. Since 80 percent of cancer patients are treated in the community, this tremendously expands the possibility of involving large numbers of patients in clinical research. The cancer centers and the research program are only two of the many National Cancer Institute programs. Essentially, any cancer patient or any physician treating cancer patients can be involved in some part of the research, educational, or other activities of NCI.

Prognosis

Prognosis for those with cancer has improved dramatically in this century. At the turn of the century few people with cancer had hope for long survival. In the 1930s the cure rate was less than one out of five. In the 1960s the rate had improved to one in three. Today, it is expected that three out of every eight people who contract cancer will be alive five years after diagnosis. If factors like accidents, death from heart disease, and diseases of old age are taken into account, the survival rate is almost half (46 percent).

Today, there are more than 5 million Americans alive who have a cancer history. Of this group, 3 million have survived for five years beyond diagnosis. Most of this population is now free from evidence of the disease.

Prognosis for cancer depends on three factors: the stage of the disease at the time of diagnosis and treatment, the type of tumor, and the anatomical site of the cancer. The most significant factor is the stage of the disease. Generally cancers in stages 1 and 2 (mildly invasive or moderately invasive) may be curable; those in stage 3 (regional) are controllable; and those in stage 4 (advanced) are often uncontrollable. The problem is that many kinds of cancer do not come to the attention of a physician until they are quite advanced.

Specific kinds of tumors have different prognoses. For example, a Ewing's tumor of the bone, whose cells are anaplastic (without the distinctive characteristics of a cell), has a poorer prognosis than a chondrosarcoma of the bone, whose cells are well differentiated. Finally, prognosis varies according to the anatomical site of the cancer. Nonmelanoma skin cancer carries a very good prognosis, for example, while lung cancer carries a rather poor one.

Anticipated Course of the Treated Disease

Except for cancers excised *in situ*, the course for the long term is generally characterized by remissions and recurrences. Within five years of diagnosis, two out of every three people develop recurrent disease, which must again be treated.

Just as in any other chronic illness, it is imperative to watch for new signs of the illnesses, even in cases of long remission. The reason for follow-up is to detect any exacerbation of the disease as early as possible so that treatment can proceed. People who have had one cancer have a greater chance of developing a second primary cancer than people who have never had a cancer, and it is also always possible to have missed some undetected vestige of the earlier cancer.

It is suggested that people should be examined every one to three months for the first year after treatment has abated. During the next four years they should be examined every three months. Over the next five-year period, they should be examined once or twice a year. If ten years have elapsed since the initial treatment of the disease, less frequent follow-up is necessary.

Psychosocial Information

Any discussion of psychosocial issues in cancer has first to take into account the stage of and prognosis for the specific type of cancer. Despite personal nuances, much of the response of the ill person and his family will depend on this information. A diagnosis of Hodgkin's disease and *in situ* cervical cancer, for example, means there is a substantial probability of cure. This kind of diagnosis usually brings a determination to manage the disease and to pursue life with renewed vigor. People talk about being given another chance or being given a new lease on life. A diagnosis of a second group of diseases where there is some chance of cure or the prolongation of a reasonable quality of life brings with it a different set of responses. Physicians and family members talk a lot about long shots and odds of success in using this or that treatment. Sometimes, in these instances, physicians are not sure of the primary tumor. This kind of diagnosis has ill people and their families donning battle dress. Everybody is willing to do anything and use every ounce of effort to beat the cancer. Each new treatment is met with hope and willingness to endure great pain and suffering. People still look for cure or at least for a long remission. An example of this might be an oat cell cancer of the lung or a colon cancer.

A third level of diagnosis brings forth still a different response pattern. Examples are widely metastasized disease or cancers for which there is no known effective treatment. The ill person and his family usually hope for a prolongation of life. This quest sometimes seems to come at great cost. To those outside the immediate caregiving system, it seems wild and flailing. Many ill people and their families seem to be saying, "I will try anything just to live another week or even another day." The system of palliative care that has been developed to meet the needs of this third group helps to move people from desolation to peace. It tries to make the dying process tolerable.

Modifications in Life-Style

Many facets of life-style affect an individual's chances of contracting the disease. Examples are the relationship of smoking and lung cancer, and diet and colon cancer. Life-style interventions are also related closely to one's ability to withstand the effects of the aggressive treatments for cancer. A nutritious diet, adequate rest, and exercise all help a person to tolerate radiation and chemotherapy and hasten the healing of surgical wounds. Changes in climate, restraint or restriction from certain activities, and changes in daily schedule do not affect the risk of contracting the disease, the course of the disease, or the ability to tolerate treatment.

DIET

Diet is related to cancer in three ways. First, epidemiologists have shown that certain kinds of diets make specific groups of people more likely to get certain kinds of cancer. Cancer of the rectum and the colon, for example, is common among people who eat low-fiber diets containing large quantities of beef, carbohydrates, fats, and refined foods, and cancer of the stomach is common among people who eat large quantities of smoked foods. Second, a well-nourished body fights infection, aids healing, and deals with the demands placed on it by very agressive treatment protocols better than a poorly nourished one. Third, certain cancers affect one's appetite, ability to eat, and ability to digest. Even if the cancer does not interfere with eating, the treatment often does. Surgery to remove part of the stomach or any other part of one's digestive system means that smaller, more frequent meals will have to be eaten. Often, people receiving radiation or chemotherapy will experience aberration in taste or smell or nausea and vomiting, so they will have little appetite. People often feel tired, experience intestinal upset, have sore, dry mouths, and have trouble swallowing. People often feel full after having eaten only a little. Food tastes change, so that people lose their liking for greasy or fried foods. Sometimes, too, people experience constipation, bloating, and heartburn. These treatments also use a tremendous amount of energy. Because a high protein, high-calorie diet is imperative and eating difficulties are common, several fine cookbooks with simple, easily digestible, high-nourishment recipes have become available for people with cancer and their families.

EXERCISE

The ravaging effects of many kinds of cancer and their treatments make people feel like doing little more than lying around. This kind of immobility only promotes feelings of inadequacy and lethargy. Exercise is a way for regaining one's maximum mobility. If prostheses or other devices are necessary, exercise helps people adapt to the equipment. The use of prostheses, assistance devices, physical therapy, occupational therapy, and other means of rehabilitation are indicated even for people with poor prognoses.

Structural changes in limbs, muscles, skin, breathing, and many other areas mean that old ways of exercising are no longer comfortable. One informant who began to jog again after a mastectomy said she felt she was running lopsided when she first ran with only one breast. Another who had been a champion golfer before losing a leg to bone cancer said he had fallen on his face the first time he had tried to swing a club with one good leg and his prosthesis. Because he could not bear to be less than a champion golfer, he switched to swimming, which would strengthen him but would not require the excellent sense of balance necessary for golf.

Having cancer is stressful, and so are the treatments for cancer, and some say that a high degree of stress makes one more susceptible to cancer. Both relaxation techniques and fitness programs ease tension and stress. Thus exercise is useful for maintaining mobility, for easing stress, for learning new ways to relax, and for adapting to the physical demands of the illness.

Legal Aspects

Legal issues in relation to cancer are primarily in the areas of informed consent and the right to work. The right to work issue is straightforward. The Federal Rehabilitation Act of 1973 states that it is against the law to refuse someone appropriate work if he has or has had cancer or a number of other conditions. The issue of informed consent deals with the amount of information it is necessary for a physician to give a patient so that the patient can agree to the prescribed treatment. This is an issue in health care today partly because it is the basis on which many claims of malpractice are made. It is especially relevant in three areas of cancer care. First, many of the treatments in cancer are considered experimental, so it is imperative that the patient be informed about what qualities in the treatment make it fall into the experimental category. Second, even with today's advanced diagnostic testing surgeons often cannot determine the extent to which the disease has spread until they have operated. That means the patient is unconscious when the surgeon may have to make new decisions about what to do based on what he has found. An informant who had gone to surgery thinking that she was to have a simple mastectomy awoke to find that she had had a radical. She was angry at the physician for doing that to her, although she had been informed that it was a possibility. The physician explained that when he had begun the operation, he had seen that the disease had spread and that he had to remove lymph nodes and chest muscle to be sure that he had removed as much of the cancer as was possible. Now, if a mastectomy is necessary, it is almost always performed as a second operation. It was found that concern about avoiding a second anesthetic was less important than the trauma of a mastectomy at the time of biopsy. Although the two-step procedure is now the standard of practice, two states, California and Massachusetts, have made it illegal to do both procedures in one step.

A third legal issue is referred to as therapeutic privilege, the physician's right to withold information from the patient when it is believed that the information would be psychologically damaging. Today it is unacceptable for the physician to withhold information without which the patient's ability to give his informed consent to the treatment plan would be impaired. Generally the informed consent consideration would outweigh those of therapeutic privilege. Thus considerate caregivers find ways to present information without devastating the patient. It is critical that the ill person and his family ask questions and insist that the doctors explain and discuss all aspects of the illness. Since it is the ill person and his family who ultimately have to make and live with treatment decisions, they must have all the information available to the physicians.

Insurance

Most health insurance policies cover the acute episodes of the disease. There is often a deductible, and some policies cover only a percentage of the total costs up to an established ceiling. People can buy a comprehensive health insurance policy that includes a rider for "excess major medical coverage," which will pay a large precentage of all medical bills beyond the ceiling established by their basic coverage. Because of their comprehensiveness these are considered the best kinds of policies. The riders basically insure against any catastrophic illness.

Insurance companies have been slow to cover some of the less acute needs of cancer patients like home care, long-term care, prosthetic devices, and restorative surgery. This situation is changing, however, partially because people with many kinds of cancer are living longer or being cured of the disease.

In addition to the usual kinds of health insurance policies, many versions of cancer insurance are on the market. They are an example of what is called a "dread disease" policy, a kind of insurance limited to a specific disease about which people are often fearful, ignorant, and overwhelmed. Similar policies for poliomyelitis were marketed heavily in the 1940s and 1950s. Aside from the fact that it preys on a fearful, vulnerable population, the primary problem with cancer insurance is its specificity. Many policies pay only if people are hospitalized for at least ninety days, an increasingly unlikely prospect. Some policies will not pay for the complications, for example, the implantation of a pin in the bone of someone with bone cancer. Some will pay bills only if someone stays in the hospital for the treatment. Others will not pay for illnesses caused by cancer treatment, such as pneumonia in people with leukemia. Time limits in the policies often fail to reflect the needs of cancer patients. One company makes no payments for two years if the cancer is diagnosed within four months after the purchase of the policy. It also stops payments three years after a cancer is first diagnosed.

Applying for new or additional insurance with a history of cancer is sometimes difficult. People find that they face refusal to cover, extended waiting periods, or high premiums. Insurance companies tend to lag behind improved mortality statistics, but they eventually catch up. Coverage is easier to get through group plans than individual ones. Generally people with cancer histories and the probability of cure or long remission can find coverage. Often the fear of losing coverage will prevent people from changing jobs or doing anything else that might jeopardize their insurance.

If a person no longer requires hospitalization but is too ill to be cared for at home or has no one to take care of him, he may be eligible for insured nursing home care. If the person is over sixty-five and needs skilled nursing care, that is, intravenous feedings, sterile dressing changes, morphine injections, and the like, Medicare would finance his nursing stay for a limited time. Medicare will also pay for a specified number of visits to his home by public health nurses, home health aides, physical therapists, and social workers, and for a specific amount of hospice care. Medicare will not pay for intermediate-level or custodial care, so physical incapacitation, even to the point of not being able to walk or prepare food, does not make one eligible for Medicare-funded nursing home care. When people need custodial care, they must either pay privately or qualify for Medicaid, which means they must be almost indigent before the state will insure their care. Each state, at this moment, has its own version of Medicaid.

Life insurance is also a problem, especially in applying for a new policy. Some companies insist that a person be free of cancer for ten years before insuring his life.

The criteria for Social Security Disability Insurance depend on the particular site, stage, and type of disease. Basically the extent of spread, involvement of specific lymph nodes, and expected course of the disease must be specified. There is careful differentiation between the kinds of diseases for which there is increasingly successful treatment and those for which there is not. Once an individual is clear of the disease for three years, disability insurance is canceled.

Work

Cancer *per se* does not interfere with one's ability to work. Once again, the issue is the stage of the cancer, the nature of the treatment, and the kind of work one does. An informant with cancer of the esophagus said that he was very glad that he had his own accounting office in his house, because no one but he himself told him whether he was able to work or not. On the days when he could work, he did. When he was too ill, he called his clients and said he would be back to them when he felt better. In that way he was able to work until almost the end of his life.

Cancer evokes such dread images that many people assume that those with cancer are unable to function just because they have cancer. Obviously a construction worker who has worked on the girders of high-rise buildings would have to change his line of work if he lost a leg, but it would be the loss of the leg that mattered, not the fact that he lost it as a result of bone cancer. Most people who have not lost a particular physical ability needed for their jobs and who do not find treatment so draining that they are too tired to work can and should continue to work as long as they are able. When people are too ill to work because the disease has progressed too far or because they are reacting to certain forms of treatment, they will know it.

Vocational rehabilitation services offer training, financial support, and counseling to cancer patients. Counselors use a variety of testing procedures to evaluate an individual's intellectual capacities, motor skills, and potential for retraining. They can also help a person to polish or relearn skills he might need to resume the job he held before he became ill. Rehabilitation services can be best used when they are offered early and when they can be integrated into a person's total treatment plan. In this area, too, it is vital to see the individual as reaching his own potential, not as living out a prognosis for a particular kind of cancer. When someone whose particular kind of cancer has a high mortality rate seeks vocational rehabilitation, for example, it does him a terrible injustice to assume that he is part of the 80 percent who die and not the 20 percent who live.

Relationships with Family Members

The diagnosis of cancer can be as devastating to family members as it is to the ill person. Around the time of diagnosis families begin to focus on the disease and what it means to the unit. It is a time of bewilderment and anxiety. Family members may become depressed, may be unable to sleep, and may take refuge outside the family or in alcohol. With some presentation of hope, most families can rally around the ill person in order to manage the disease. The hope has at least three parts: that a cure may be found, that the family can manage to live with the disease and its symptoms, and that short-term goals, like coming home after hospitalization or going back to work, are within reach.

In addition to having to deal with the meaning of the disease to the family and to begin to understand the ramifications of having an ill family member, relatives have to begin to manage what are referred to as functional disruptions. There are likely to be periodic hospitalizations, many trips to the hospital for treatments of various kinds, and many days when the ill person will not feel well as a result of the disease process or the treatment. This means a disruption of work outside the home as well. As a result of all of this, role shifts will have to occur, with the well members taking over some responsibilities for the ill member. There is a fine line between assuming responsibilities that an ill member cannot carry and taking away the ill person's independence. Since cancer is often a disease of remissions and recurrences, a person often can resume much of his former life-style and many responsibilities when his disease is in remission.

Open communication is the most helpful device for ensuring that everyone in the family system manages optimally. Sometimes this kind of communication is already part of a family network. At other times families have to learn to relate in this way. Part of the communication means engaging emotions. Dealing with cancer is a volatile, charged, emotion-laden task. Knowing that the expression of strong emotion does not mean loss of control or hope is helpful. Questions of meaning become important to everyone concerned. Sharing the meaning that such an experience has and mutually finding ways to manage even bring some families closer together than they were before the experience.

Just as the ill person oscillates between hope and despair, his loved ones are subject to the same kind of mood swing, but the moods do not always coincide. One patient's wife said that her husband was resigned to death from cancer as soon as he was diagnosed but was quietly determined to live as long as possible and approached his treatments in that way. However, his wife and grown children met each new treatment suggestion with an unmitigated fervor and received word of the lack of success with a terrible despair. The man, with his usual reticence, continued to be an emotional anchor for his family.

The response of the family depends very much on where the ill person fits in the unit. A child with cancer obviously evokes a different response from an adult, just as cancer in a very old person evokes a different set of responses from cancer in a relatively young one.

WHEN A CHILD HAS CANCER

The outlook for children with cancer has changed tremendously in recent years. Not so long ago a diagnosis of cancer in a child meant deterioration and certain death. Today, if the disease is discovered before it has metastasized, it is thought that the disease can be eradicated in more than half of the children. With hope comes a very different kind of adjustment for families. What once was dealt with swiftly now can be seen as a chronic illness with an uncertain outcome. Life becomes a long series of treatments, remissions, recurrences, and more treatments, with an eventual outcome that can be cure or death. Even in the best of circumstances the threat of recurrence and death remains. Through all of this the child must be able to develop psychologically and physically along with his peers. Whatever the disruptions and extraordinary emotional and financial strains, the family must strive for normality for their child. Many parents report that the most difficult period for them was the time of diagnosis. Others, whose children's illness recurred, said that recurrence was the worst period, because they felt that their hope was destroyed. Some have had to deny the diagnosis. Others have blamed themselves or the physician. Parents feel angry, confused, and extraordinarily helpless. They want to protect their child from this awful event but know they are unable to do so. If the parents are given hope, they are able to rally more quickly to help their child. Generally, as soon as the diagnosis is made, some form of treatment is instituted. Since the parents of a young child have to make these treatment decisions for their child, open communication helps them to agree on how to proceed. Having parents disagree about the best course to take is disruptive not only to the care of their child but to the life of the family as well.

It is generally agreed that the child should be told as much about his illness as he can understand. Isolating him from this information will isolate him from his family and his caregivers and will make him feel powerless, fearful, and rejected. Because he must be involved in a protracted treatment situation, because his peers will see that he is different, and because he will feel ill at times, it is unrealistic not to keep him apprised of his illness and its treatment. To refuse to involve him is to worsen the situation. Questions should be answered. Explanations should be given. If children are too young to verbalize their fears, parents should assume that they know that they are different and tell them what they need to know. Openness brings the trust of parents and treatment team that the child needs.

The ill child's siblings should also be included. They must be told not only what the disease is and what the treatment plan is, but also that the disease is not contagious and that it is no one's fault. Siblings should see the treatment center and receive an explanation of the treatment tools. Above all, the parents have to be reminded that they should not abandon or isolate their well children while they are dealing with their ill child. Their well children will be experiencing the same overwhelming and complicated responses as they are.

In this same way, other relatives and friends will have dramatic responses to the illness. Grandparents especially will have a hard time, because they will be experiencing the suffering of not only their grandchildren but also their children. Relatives and friends often want to talk but become overwhelmed with their own feelings of helplessness. By dealing directly with the issues, taking the lead in discussions, and asking for assistance, the parents will keep relatives and friends close. A mother whose son had metastatic bone cancer forced herself to stand up in her church and say, "I know that you all feel terrible about my son's cancer and don't know what to say to any of us. What we need is for people to look us right in the eye when they see us and for some driving help to take us back and forth to the hospital for treatments." She said she was shaking but determined. The result was that people did look her in the eye and gave her the help she asked for, and more. They just had not known what to do.

This direct approach works best when the child leaves the hospital, resumes neighborhood friendships, and, if he is old enough, goes back to school. Very often his appearance will be changed. He may be thinner or rounder, and he may well have lost his hair. Direct discussion of the problem, the treatment, and the side effects smoothes the situation. If there is a recurrence of the disease, the family's original response to the diagnosis also recurs. People feel angry, distraught and powerless. However, with attentive and appropriate care, they may move out of this negative pattern and become involved in the new treatment plan.

WHEN AN ADOLESCENT HAS CANCER

Cancer in adolescence is complicated by the myriad transitional issues of an adolescent. One minute the ill person is a child wanting to be taken care of and protected, and the next minute is an adult wanting autonomy and independence. Much of the control for which they have been striving is taken from them. The authority figures against whom they would like to rebel are responsible for their lifegiving care. Their body image, which is so important for developing sexuality and for feeling good about themselves, may be wrecked through hair loss, amputation, or just the experiences of radiation and chemotherapy. The effect of treatment on sexual functioning is largely unknown. To some extent it depends on the degree of pubertal development at the time of diagnosis and treatment. Adolescents may feel not only depressed but worthless. They may agree to be treated not to help themselves but because family members what them to do it. Again, if a feeling of hope is imparted and if family and friends are supportive and do not isolate the teenager, he generally will recover from his depression sufficiently to go along with a treatment plan. Again, as in childhood, it is imperative for loved ones to allow their ill teenager to mature throughout this process. To treat him like a child in the name of protecting him is a disservice.

WHEN AN ADULT HAS CANCER

When an adult has cancer, work and family roles must often be reconstructed. Ideally, role relationships should be flexible so that in remission, an adult can resume responsibilities he could not carry when he felt ill. The ill person should be able to keep his autonomy, making decisions when he is able. Authority should be shared, and communication, again, should be open. In a time of crisis, however, the ideal is difficult to adhere to. It is easy for everyone involved to want to baby and protect the ill adult, just as it is easy to baby and protect a sick child. In addition to knowing that the person is sick, there are additional powerful messages if the ill person looks emaciated, drawn, and deteriorated. If he also has a kind of cancer that gives him great pain, makes him very weak, or produces smelly discharges, it is even more difficult to allow the ill adult to keep his authority.

Repeated hospitalizations make family relationships difficult. When the adult is in the hospital, all of his responsibilities must be taken by others. When he returns home, if responsibilities are not redistributed, relationships become even more strained.

One informant said that her husband, "a real powerhouse of a guy," felt so dependent in his patient role that he became an authoritarian monster with her and her children. The children had to insist that he think about what he was doing and why. They all cried together, and things improved. The problem is, of course, that few families are so emotionally mature and sophisticated. The relationship of well spouse and sick spouse is very difficult. Generally, role reversals strain the relationship, but also the well spouse is part of the treatment decision-making. He or she becomes the ill spouse's liaison with the treatment team, with family, with friends, with work. In addition, he or she becomes the person to transport the ill spouse for treatments and the giver of the emotional and physical support to manage the treatment.

While these kinds of intimacies are enhanced, the more traditional means of expressing intimacy, primarily the couple's sexual relationship, may wane. Often it is the well spouse's concern for hurting the ill person that exacerbates this problem. Sometimes, too, the ill person does not have enough energy or interest for sexual activity as a result of the disease or treatment process. Questions about ability and risk should be directed to the physician. When people lose interest in sexual activity, however, they continue to want the warmth and intimacy of fondling. As in other parts of a relationship, open communication about physical intimacy is helpful.

The strains are heightened with either of two opposite medical outcomes: impending death or unexpected cure. Families can adjust to dealing with the strains imposed by the illness. When there is a change in the *status quo*, their sense of mastery and control is again shaken, as it was when the cancer was first diagnosed. News of impending death or cure mean readjustment and discontinuity.

One theme that becomes highly important in cancers that are not cured is families finding ways to keep the memory of a well, strong relative alive. Sometimes called framing memories, this means being able to think of the person before his diagnosis was made. Often family members and the ill person cannot remember what the person with cancer looked like before he became ill. They dream about him and visualize him in a wasted and sickly state. Because the cancer becomes so important in the life of the family and the cancer often has such a devastating effect on the appearance of the person, framing memories becomes very difficult. As the illness recedes, through cure or through death, old, healthy memories come back, supplanting the ill ones.

Relationships with Strangers

In the case of advanced cancer, strangers react in two ways: They refuse to relate or they treat the person as if he were retarded or very young.
A man who had been successfully treated for cancer of the rectum said
that people began to speak louder, to laugh in an embarrassed way, or to
run away when he told them he was being treated for cancer. In this
instance strangers were reacting to their perception of cancer rather than
to the person. Thus, relationships with strangers are affected by how the
ill person looks as well as by people's attitudes about cancer.

Psychological Aspects

SELF-CONCEPT AND BODY IMAGE

One's self-concept is severely shaken in cancer. Cancer is such a stigmatizing illness that the diagnosis itself negatively affects self-image. One
informant said that she was successfully treated for endometrial cancer
more than ten years ago. At the time of diagnosis she told a few close
friends whom she thought she could trust. One person asked her if she
thought she had caused it herself. Others asked her to reassure them that
they did not have it. Each of them was unable to relate to her about anything but the cancer. She also told her dentist, who responded by telling
her that he had been successfully treated for rectal cancer but had never
told anyone for fear that no one hearing that would come to him.

Problems with self-concept may be reinforced by the changes in appearance accompanying many kinds of cancer. In the early treatment
phases people may be afraid of organ loss and amputation. Later they may
be troubled by the changes in body image caused by the wasting of the
disease. Some people develop observable masses on their skin, others bruise
easily and widely. Clothes may become too loose-fitting or may fail to
cover up the changes people can see in their bodies. One informant (who
ironically had probably contracted cancer of the salivary glands when she
had x-ray treatments for acne as a teenager) covered the inoperable tumor
on her neck with increasingly large and colorful scarves.

STAGES OF PSYCHOLOGICAL RESPONSE

At the time of diagnosis of cancer people sometimes experience denial.
They simply will not accept the possibility that they or their loved ones
could have any form of cancer. Along with the denial of the illness comes
a need to delay any action to treat the disease. At times this delay comes
before an official diagnosis, when people have symptoms that they know

might mean cancer but choose to delay seeking medical attention. When treatment of a fast-growing or spreading cancer is delayed, it may cost the patient his life. An informant in her late fifties felt a small lump in her breast and waited almost a year to see a physician. In that year many more lumps appeared, and she had begun to have bad back pain. By the time she sought medical attention, the disease had spread considerably and she could receive only palliative care.

Another part of the initial response may be anger and rage at the diagnosis. People with cancer may blame themselves and those around them for their contracting the disease. They may become afraid that they will pass the disease along to loved ones. One informant said that her father refused to kiss her and did not want her to drink out of his glass. When asked why, he said abruptly that no one really knew what this was or how you got it.

Ill people become concerned that they will no longer be able to be good family members or continue working. They frequently begin to worry more about the treatment than the disease. Concern about the disfigurement resulting from surgery can contribute to delay in treatment.

The mood of the ill person and his family seems generally to follow the course of the disease. There may be great depression around the diagnosis. When a remission occurs, the ill person and his family generally feel great elation. If there is a recurrence, there is usually a subsequent matching depression. Everyone involved—the ill person, his family and friends, and the medical team—is deeply disappointed. People may become angry at the physicians and at each other. Families often wonder if they went to the right doctor or the right hospital. If they had gone elsewhere, perhaps the patient would have recovered. People with cancer are sometimes angry that they submitted to treatment that ultimately failed them and other times proud that they gave it their best shot.

Through all of this there is the knowledge that the ill person and the family are still dependent on the treatment team, so they have to behave reasonably and somewhat docilely despite what they feel. If they are not good, the treatment team might punish them for it. For all the disappointment and anger, the ill person, the family, and the medical team have to find a new treatment to slow the next stage of the disease process. This is also a common time for a renewal of the denial process, which serves as a good buffer. Those most directly involved with the cancer may need time to absorb the fact that the disease has spread. They may not be ready for facts or explanations. On the other hand they might want to know every detail as soon as it is available. That kind of stance depends on the individual coping styles of the family network.

One informant, whose father had advanced cancer of the stomach and whose husband is a physician, wanted to understand exactly what was happening to her father. Although the knowledge confirmed that his illness was terminal, it offered her some mastery of the situation. When she passed the information to her mother and brother, they decided that she was cruel and heartless (as was her husband) and they pushed her away from them and her father for several days. They were simply not ready for that kind of information.

As the disease progresses, ill people often become increasingly compliant and passive. The physician becomes increasingly important, and visits from the physician become the markers of the day. If the disease advances, the ill person feels increasingly isolated and rejected. Although by its nature this is a lonely state, relatives and friends can ease it by helping the ill person to stay as involved with his life as he is physically able. An ill person may appear quite depressed at this time. To some degree he is mourning his poor prognosis. Waiting for a new treatment plan is a very difficult time.

When a new treatment is begun, patient and family pitch in again toward using the treatment in the best possible way. The good fight continues. Succeeding remissions and recurrences are met with less expectation and disappointment. The mood continues to be a mixture of battling and resignation until either a cure or dying is confirmed.

Mood is affected by the treatment. Both chemotherapy and radiation can make people feel irritable and depressed. People may tend to be self-absorbed and turned inward toward their bodies, preoccupied with the changes brought on by the disease. People who would never have mentioned anything to do with their bodies tell about blood tests, bowel movements, and vital signs. "How are you?" is answered by, "My hematocrit dropped ten points this week" or "They took my catheter out today." To fight the enemy, which is what one's body has become, one must concentrate on it.

As the disease becomes more advanced, the ill person often may be willing to go along with the suggestions of his physician and may allow his family to do more and more for him. Without discussing the prognosis directly, ill people and their families will sometimes make plans for a future they will not share. People who are dying from cancer often feel abandoned and at the same time want to shield their family members from the tragedy they are sharing. In many ways the dying person is separating from his loved ones before he dies. Family members often need help in understanding that the ill person is not rejecting them. Depending on the psychological make-up of the individual and the family, this can be a time of great verbal sharing or of quiet, tender acceptance of the ill person's inevitable death.

How to Be Helpful to Someone with Cancer

The most important point is not to run away. Cancer is not contagious. What people with cancer need most is to continue to relate to others and to their world as normally as possible. To continue to relate means also the share the uncertainty of the person's future. Cancer and death are no longer synonymous. Physicians can recite the odds, but no one knows whether he will be in the percentage of those who made it or the percentage of those who did not. One is unable to predict not only whether he will live, but how he will live. If cure is not possible but remission is, it might be a remission in which the person is quite incapacitated or mutilated. He may be thrilled to be alive or terribly depressed about the way he looks or his life-style.

It is important to remember that not just the disease but the treatment is difficult to bear. Radiation may make people feel sick, and the skin changes color. Chemotherapy often causes hair loss and makes people feel awful. Amputations are done to try to stem the spread of the disease.

Finally, hope is critical. Increasingly it is possible to hope for cure. Almost 50 percent of the people who are diagnosed with cancer today will be alive five years from now. Contrasted with the 1930s, when only one out of five people with cancer survived for five years, this is a remarkable achievement. When it is not possible to hope for a cure, it is almost always possible to hope for remission. People are living longer with cancer than ever before.

4

The Dementias

DEMENTIA MEANS deprivation of mind. As a term it has referred to any problem of confused sensorium. Rather than a single illness, it is a cluster of symptoms, which can be caused by a variety of diseases, many of them poorly understood. Dementia can thus be defined as a generalized disturbance of higher cortical functions characterized by impaired cognition, including memory loss.

Medical Information

People who have dementing illnesses lose the use of those parts of their brains that direct intellectual skills and abilities. Contrary to popular belief, neither dementia nor hardening of the arteries is a normal part of the aging process. For a long time it was thought that senile dementia occurred only after age sixty-five and was related to hardening of the arteries. Neurological illness that began before age sixty-five was considered a distinct disease and called presenile dementia or Alzheimer's disease. Microscopic postmortem brain tissue examinations have demonstrated that both dementias are one illness, dementia of the Alzheimer type (DAT), also referred to as senile dementia–Alzheimer type (SDAT) or Alzheimer's disease. Alzheimer's disease is not part of the normal aging process, nor is it related to hardening of the arteries. In the population of the United States that is over sixty-five years old, it is estimated that only 5 percent are severely demented and 10 more are mildly or moderately impaired. Because those who are over sixty-five make up the majority of the population with dementia, however, the primary focus of this chapter is irreversible dementia of the later years.

Classification

Dementia is classified by cause. There are three types: Alzheimer's disease, multi-infarct dementia, and dementia pugilistica. The most prevalent type (over 60 percent) is Alzheimer's disease, in which communication between cells in the brain is disrupted, causing a degeneration that affects a person's ability to think.

Changes occur in the proteins of the nerve cells in the outer layer of the brain, the cerebral cortex. Abnormal fibers resembling a tangle of filaments accumulate there. These tangles were first described in 1907 by a German neurologist named Alzheimer. Recent use of more sophisticated magnifying equipment, the electron microscope, has demonstrated that groups of nerve endings throughout the cortex degenerate and disrupt the electrochemical communication between the cells. These areas of degeneration are called plaques. The concentration of tangles and plaques present in one's brain correlate with his symptoms. As the number of plaques and tangles increases, intellectual abilities decrease.

Multi-infarct dementia is caused by a series of strokes, which leave the person increasingly mentally and physically disabled. Infarct refers to dead tissue, which is evidence of the stroke. "Multi-" means that several events are involved, possibly occurring months or even years apart. In this type of dementia a blood clot clogs a vessel or causes a vessel to burst and bleed into the brain. In the case of a large vessel, the resultant stroke can be extremely damaging and can even result in death. A clot or rupture in a smaller vessel causes a smaller stroke with less resultant damage. Multi-infarct dementia accounts for 10 to 20 percent of people with dementia. An additional 15 to 20 percent have both multi-infarct and Alzheimer's.

It is often possible to distinguish between the two kinds of dementia because of differences in the history, progress, stages, and symptoms of each type. Those with Alzheimer's are less likely to have a history of vascular disease, hypertension, or previous stroke. The progression of a person with Alzheimer's is usually more of a steady decline than the stepwise decline of a person with multi-infarct dementia. Because multi-infarct may affect only one part of a person's brain, his symptoms may be more limited than the pervasive symptoms of the person with Alzheimer's disease.

The third type of dementia, dementia pugilistica or "punch-drunk syndrome," results from trauma, particularly the trauma incurred in boxing, where abuse of the head can cause swelling, bleeding, and eventual damage to the brain.

Other causes of dementia include less common diseases of the nervous system: multiple sclerosis, Parkinson's disease, Huntington's disease, Pick's disease, and Creutzfeldt-Jakob disease. In the first three illnesses, dementia sometimes occurs in the final stages. Pick's disease has symptoms similar to those of Alzheimer's. In Creutzfeldt-Jakob disease a long-dormant virus is activated producing a rapidly progressive dementia, changes in gait, and muscle spasms (myoclonus).

The third edition of the American Psychiatric Association's *Diagnostic and Statistical Manual* (*DSM III*) offers a psychiatric classification system for dementia. Many geriatricians and others working with demented people do not find this typology useful. Within the classification "Organic Mental Disorders—Section 1," *DSM III* lists two groups of disorders of organic etiology that are traditionally classified as mental disorders: (1) dementias due to certain neurological diseases characteristically appearing in the senium and presenium, and (2) substance-induced organic mental disorders. Within dementias arising in the senium and presenium are primary degenerative dementia and multi-infarct dementia. The essential feature of primary degenerative dementia is the presence of dementia of insidious onset and a gradually progressive course for which all other specific causes have been excluded by the history, physical examination, and laboratory tests. Primary degenerative dementia involves a multifaceted loss of intellectual abilities—such as memory, abstract thought, and other higher cortical functions—and changes in personality and behavior. The clinical picture can be complicated by the presence of depressive features or delusions, usually persecutory. Primary degenerative dementia is subtyped as senile onset (after sixty-five) and presenile onset (age sixty-five and younger). Within those subtypes are further categories; with delirium, with delusions, with depression, and uncomplicated.

The essential feature of multi-infarct dementia is a stepwise deterioration in intellectual functioning that early in the course leaves some intellectual functions relatively intact ("patchy" deterioration). Focal neurological signs and symptoms can include an exaggeration of deep tendon reflexes, gait abnormalities, and weakness of extremities. Diagnosis is made through evidence from the history, physical examination, or laboratory tests of significant cerebrovascular disease that is judged to be etiologically related to the disturbance.

Disorders of the second group, substance-induced organic mental disorders, are caused by the direct effects on the nervous system of various substances. Within this broad classification is alcohol organic mental disorders, of which one category is dementia associated with alcoholism—dementia following prolonged, heavy ingestion of alcohol and persisting at least three weeks after cessation of alcohol ingestion with all other causes of dementia excluded by the history, physical examination, and laboratory tests. Dementia associated with alcoholism is further classified as mild (no more than mild impairment in social and occupational functioning), mod-

erate (moderate social impairment with inability to function occupation-
ally), and severe (severe impairment of functioning with marked
deterioration of personality [irritability, social inappropriateness] and inability to function independently).

Many of the syndromes that appear to be dementia are not. Since they
must be eliminated as possible diagnoses in order for the physician to arrive at the diagnosis of dementia, they are an important group to consider.
Psychiatric syndromes that masquerade as organic dementia are referred
to as pseudodementia. Pseudodementia is referred to here in this narrow
sense of masquerade and not as a term applicable to various other potentially reversible causes of dementia. Among the psychiatric illnesses that
can sometimes appear to be dementia are depression and paranoid schizophrenia. People who are depressed may appear passive, slow, forgetful,
and confused, much as people with a dementing illness. Depression in older
people is especially confusing for those close to them. The losses and dis-
appointments experienced by many elderly people may result in their
seeming sad or distracted; they may even speak of a dead person as if he
were still living. This kind of reactive depression often develops very
quickly, whereas the onset of a progressive dementia is slower and more
insidious.

Alcoholism can also impair many mental faculties, especially recent
memory. Aside from the brain damage that can be caused by chronic alcoholism, the inadequate diet of an alcoholic contributes to a deficiency
of thiamine (vitamin B), which can result in Wernicke-Korsakoff's syndrome with symptoms including staggering and eye and nerve problems,
as well as forgetfulness.

Drug reactions may also be confused with dementia. They are difficult
to sort out, because they often result from two or three drugs in combination. To compound the problem, the drugs may have been prescribed
by two or three different physicians, each unaware of what other drugs
the patient is taking. Drug use is a particularly difficult problem for the
elderly because of age-related changes in metabolism. An older person
might require a smaller dose of medication. The kidneys and the liver of
an older person may be less efficient in clearing the body of the drugs he
has taken. This, along with a general slowing of the metabolism, may
allow a drug to persist in the body longer. Finally, people often take many
"over-the-counter" drugs in addition to their prescribed medications. It is
common to find that people take laxatives, cough medicine, aspirin, and
alcohol without thinking of the effects of mixing those drugs with others.

Chemical imbalances also produce symptoms that can be confused with
untreatable dementia. Poor eating or problems in food absorption can affect the brain. Many elderly people eat poorly either because they have
little money or cannot get to the store, or because they think that nutrition
need not concern them any longer. Older people also tend to be less active

and sometimes complain that food does not taste as good as it once did. If the brain is poorly nourished, a variety of symptoms can appear for a person of any age. The first symptoms to appear from malnutrition may be mental rather than physical. For example, pernicious anemia is a blood disorder caused by impaired ability to absorb one of the B vitamins (B_{12}); one of the first symptoms may be depression or irritability. An abnormal concentration in the blood of sodium or potassium can affect mood and personality. In the same way, inadequate thyroid hormone can result in memory loss, apathy, or depression. Hypoglycemia, a deficiency of glucose in the blood, can have accompanying symptoms of anxiety, confusion, or delirium. Chemical imbalances can be determined through tests to determine the concentration of the various substances in the blood.

An oxygen deficiency to the brain can also cause dementia-like symptoms. This condition can occur because the heart is not pumping efficiently or because of disturbances in heart rhythm, malfunctioning heart valves, or some other heart problem. Chronic lung disease also can prevent an adequate supply of oxygen from reaching the brain. Thus, problems with the heart or lungs can produce symptoms similar to those related to dementia.

Each of the metabolic or toxic causes of dementia may be treatable. If a person's brain has not suffered permanent damage by the time the condition is treated, the dementia-like symptoms should abate. There are several reversible dementias caused by other conditions. Brain tumors, meningitis, brain swelling, head injury, and poisoning by lead or mercury can cause symptoms of this kind. The expression "mad as a hatter" is supposedly related to the behavior hat makers displayed after long periods of exposure to mercury in their work. Exposure to certain pesticides, carbon monoxide, and industrial pollutants can also cause dementia-like symptoms. Some infectious diseases, too, can cause dementia-like symptoms. Diseases like tuberculosis and cryptococcal infections (fungus infections that attack the central nervous system) have to be viewed as possible causes of dementia-like symptoms.

Etiology

The cause of Alzheimer's disease is not yet known. Basic researchers are seeking to discover why certain neurons or certain locations in the brain die and what can be done to halt the process. They want to understand also why acetylcholine, a chemical substance used by neurons to communicate with each other electrochemically, is lost in those with Alzheimer's disease, and what can be done to replenish or replace it. Loss of neurons seems directly related to loss of mental ability.

A breakthrough occurred when scientists discovered that the source of acetylcholine was not in the cortex where the damage appears but rather in the nucleus basalis, an area of the brain located below the cortex. The nucleus basalis sends information to the cortex through processes which extend to the cortex and carry acetylcholine. The same research group is now trying to find out what the neurons do and how they are organized.

Some researchers are investigating the relationship of aluminum deposits in the brain to Alzheimer's disease. Some brains of people who have had Alzheimer's contain abnormal amounts of aluminum and traces of aluminum in the cells that also contain tangles. Some theorize that aluminum acts as a toxin to cause Alzheimer's. Others think the metal accumulates as a result of other changes associated with Alzheimer's. Other metals as well, most specifically manganese, are thought to be related to Alzheimer's. Measurements of trace elements are being conducted in several research centers in order to define their normal levels throughout life and to note whether the levels go up as part of the normal aging process.

There is also a genetic component in Alzheimer's disease. The risk increases if a close family member has Alzheimer's. The risk of Alzheimer's affecting someone sixty-five or older is about two or three in 100. If someone has a close relative who has Alzheimer's, the risk is raised to about seven or eight in 100. The closer the relationship, the higher the risk. For example, the risk is greater for an identical twin if his twin has the disease than it would be for fraternal twins. It is thought at present that several genes are involved, and these genes may have to interact with certain factors in the environment in order for the disease to develop. Also, a higher than normal percentage of cells of people with Alzheimer's disease have too few chromosomes, too many chromosomes, or defective chromosomes. A high-risk group for Alzheimer's disease is people with Down's syndrome. Autopsies of people with Down's syndrome who were thirty-five or older have found the tangles and plaques indicative of Alzheimer's disease in their brains. If people with Down's syndrome live a normal life span, they will develop the disease. The two conditions, Alzheimer's disease and Down's syndrome, sometimes appear in two people in the same family.

Infectious agents are another area of research. Investigators have observed that plaques like those found in the brains of Alzheimer's patients also develop in the brains of mice inoculated with a virus that causes brain degeneration in sheep. Pairs of twisted neurofilaments similar to tangles have been observed in human brain tissue cultures after exposure to Alzheimer's disease brain tissue.

Scientists are also investigating the relationship of Alzheimer's to possible immunological defects. Some researchers think that the plaques and tangles of Alzheimer's may be signs of a defect in the body's immune system. Others have noted the similarity between the proteins that make up normal neurofilaments found in nerve cells and the abnormal proteins that make up neurofibrillary tangles. They suspect that perhaps the abnormal filaments reflect the working of a defective gene, since genes manage the manufacture of proteins. Another theory in this area says that certain genes that have repair functions become less efficient with age.

Prevalence and Incidence

In the United States more than 4 million people over sixty-five years old have some degree of dementia. An estimated 600,000 people are severely demented. About 10 percent of those who are severely demented are under age sixty-five. Alzheimer's disease, in particular, is the fourth most common cause of death in the United States after heart disease, cancer, and cardiovascular disease. It accounts for 100,000 to 120,000 deaths a year, and it reduces a person's normally remaining life expectancy by half. It also accounts for $10 billion spent annually for nursing home care alone.

Natural History

Although Alzheimer's disease is a progressive illness, it is characterized by an unbelievable lability of cognitive functioning. A person can seem fine one minute or at one point in the day and quite demented at another time. One informant recalled that a friend with Alzheimer's had forgotten the name of one of her grandchildren just after playing a reasonable hand of bridge. People move in and out of lucidity. This range of functioning and its concomitant lability make management difficult.

Alzheimer's disease begins imperceptibly. Symptoms are of the kind that one notices only in retrospect; they may mimic depression. Someone with the disease may not be able to sleep well or may seem to change schedule, going to sleep later and sleeping later. Sometimes there is a flattening of certain personality traits, or the person loses interest in the things that used to fascinate him. A person may appear to withdraw or become confused when he is in unfamiliar surroundings or when he has to do several things at one time. The person can usually see what is happening to him. He knows that he is managing less well and he either denies what is happening to him or is terrified.

A common early problem is recent memory loss. Old memories remain, but events that occurred yesterday are not in a person's memory. A prominent public figure was interviewed one day about a meeting he attended the day before. He denied having gone. The press had not been told of his illness, and he was accused of lying to the public.

Many of the early symptoms are attributed to other physical illnesses or emotional upsets. As the person becomes more forgetful, it is harder to find reasons for the forgetfulness. A patient may keep losing things, forget to turn the stove off, or begin to repeat himself over and over again. He may take much longer to complete a chore than he used to and may have to go back to see if he remembered to close the door or turn off the light when he has just done so. This is far different from the benign senescent forgetfulness that is a normal part of aging. It means that one literally cannot remember what he did fifteen minutes ago: that he plugged in the iron or started to run the bathwater, or that the coffee is still too hot to drink. However, very early dementia may be difficult to separate from the normal process of aging. Often only time provides the answer.

Difficulty with memory increases as the disease progresses. Changes are likely to occur in behavior, mood, and personality. The affected person may become increasingly irritable, confused, restless, and agitated. Informants have said that to avoid outbursts of anger from their sick relatives over minor disagreements, they agree with everything, knowing that the person will forget the whole thing anyway. Even though a person may deny or be unaware of the full extent of his limitations, he is extraordinarily frustrated and confounded at having difficulty with parts of him that he could always take for granted.

Problems with abstract thinking also mount as the disease progresses. The person is likely to have difficulty managing his time, taking care of finances, and sometimes even reading. Some people retain the ability to recognize emotions in others, but others lose that ability. The disease's rate of progression also varies. Some people experience severe and swift losses of ability, then reach a plateau and seem to stay at the same level of ability for a long time.

An informant told of what she now thinks were the first symptoms of her good friend's disease. Although she was managing much of her life so that no one noticed any changes in her manner or ability, seemingly overnight she lost the ability to do arithmetic. She could write checks and hand clerks denominations of money large enough for them to make change, but she couldn't add. She might have been able to continue to manage with most things, but she worked at a very chic shop where mistakes were not tolerated by the boss, who happened to be an old friend. Her friend and boss complained to her children and to all their mutual friends that this salesperson was impossible and said they should do something. Because they knew that the boss was irascible, however, and the salesperson was a sweet, obedient person, they blamed the boss for the trouble until they noticed, after a year, that their friend was mixing up all kinds of things. Other people decline steadily and very slowly. Although there are times when the disease does not seem to get worse, it does not get better.

People often become excessively upset. Their response to incidents they would have thought unimportant when they were well is now dramatic and extreme. A woman who cared little for her jewelry and who often lost earrings swore one day that she had put her earrings on the night table

and that her companion had stolen them. When she became more demented, she accused her daughter of stealing her false teeth, which were
in a glass on the table next to her bed.

As the disease progresses, some people have difficulty with their speech,
and some with carrying out tasks in proper order. Personality characteristics may become exaggerated: Outgoing people become highly assertive,
shy people become reclusive, and people who were always a bit flighty
seem to be all over the place. Some people begin to stoop and walk very
slowly. Others develop what is called the *marche à petits pas*, a walk of
little steps.

Later, people may become disoriented about what month or year it is,
where they live, or where they are at the moment. After a while someone
with Alzheimer's may begin to wander away from home, not knowing
where he is going and not able to find his way back. He may become
unable to engage in conversation, and his mood may become unpredictable. He may also become increasingly uncooperative.

In still later stages people with Alzheimer's become less self-aware and
therefore less frightened of the disease. It is said that they tune out. Thus,
in a paradoxical way, the disease process protects them from having to
face the disintegration of their abilities.

Late in the disease process a person may also lose some involuntary
functions; incontinence is common. In advanced cases people become totally incapable of caring for themselves. In some rare cases people have
also lost the ability to breath unaided and to swallow. Ultimately, people
become unaware of their surroundings. Even at that point some show an
amazing tenacity to continue to live. The specific problems, the rate of
the disease, and the severity of the decline vary according to the individual.

Although the progression of Alzheimer's disease is unpredictable, the
eventual result is complete memory loss, disorientation, and ultimately
death. This stage may be reached in ten years, in five years, or in ten
months. There is no way to predict which faculties will be lost at which
point and which will be maintained.

Diagnostic Procedures

Differential diagnosis of specific kinds of dementia are extremely difficult.
The process is one of ruling out other possible causes for the symptoms.
Most important is differentiating between causes that are remediable and
those such as Alzheimer's disease that, at this time, are not.

Since a definitive diagnosis of Alzheimer's disease is made through a
microscopic examination of brain tissue, at present the diagnosis of Alzheimer's can be confirmed only after death. Much of what a physician

tries to ascertain, therefore, is whether the symptoms could be caused by other diseases. A full diagnostic examination includes a careful history and physical examination, several laboratory tests, and radiographic procedures.

The physical examination helps the physician to rule out other diseases. The physician looks for abnormal eye signs, staggering, abnormal sensation, abnormalities of reflexes, and signs confined to a specific area of the body that may be symptoms of other illnesses. He orders blood tests and tests for liver, kidney, and thyroid functions and sedimentation rate, and determinations of blood levels of electrolytes, blood urea nitrogen, calcium, phosphorus, sodium, potassium, chloride, carbon dioxide, sugar, vitamin B_{12}, and folate to eliminate as many potentially treatable illnesses as possible. If the dementia develops very rapidly over a few months, the doctor may do a lumbar puncture in order to be sure that the dementia is not caused by an infectious disease such as tuberculosis. Electrocardiograms, electroencephalograms, analysis of urine, a test for syphilis, analysis of stool, chest x-rays, and a CT scan should all be carried out in order to rule out other possibilities. After all other diseases have been ruled out, a diagnosis of Alzheimer's disease can usually be made based on the person's history, the results of his mental status examination, and the course of the illness.

For the history the physician consults with the patient as well as a close family member or friend. He asks what symptoms first concerned the patient and whether there were similar incidents or differences that he noticed in the past. In addition to medical history, he may ask specifically about activity level, that is, what kinds of tasks the person is able or unable to do. Some questions may concern self-care and independent living, the answers to which help establish level of impairment. They may include questions like: Is the person continent of bowel and bladder? Can he move unassisted? Can he take care of his hair, teeth, and usual toilet independently, dress and undress properly with no help, bathe without assistance, shop, cook, and do ordinary housework? Can he travel alone by public transportation? People who are moderately impaired will at least be able to wash, dress, and undress themselves. Those who are mildly to moderately impaired will also be able to cook, shop, and bathe, and those who can travel alone have very mild impairment or are not functionally impaired at all.

Some form of mental status questionnaire—a series of questions that indicate a person's orientation to time and place, his recent and remote memory, and his alertness—is also administered. The questions may include: Where are we now? Where is this place located? What is today's date? When is your birthday? Who is the President of the United States? Who was the President before him? What month is this? What year is this? How old are you? In what year were you born? There are many versions of mental status examinations, each with its own scoring system. Additional information may be gathered through exercises such as asking the person to repeat the physician's name a while after he has given it, asking a person to remember three items and repeat them later in the interview, or having the person make change, count backward from 100 by sevens, or explain cartoons or proverbs.

A measure called the face–hand test may help the physician to determine whether the disorder is due to a functional or an organic cause. The physician faces the patient and asks him to close his eyes and to place his hands on his knees. Then the physician strokes the person's cheek and, at the same time, the back of one hand. Alternating hand and cheek positions, the physician tries many combinations, each time asking the person to report which hand and cheek are being touched. Inability to answer correctly may be an indication of Alzheimer's or another neurological disease. All of the devices described—level of functioning examinations, mental status questionnaires, and the face–hand test—are used only as screening tools to add small pieces of data to the diagnostic work-up. None would ever be used to confirm a diagnosis.

Several abnormal (pathologic) reflexes may be indications of Alzheimer's disease. One is the snout reflex, in which tapping the area around someone's mouth and chin causes him to pucker his lips. Another is the palomental reflex in which scratching someone's palm causes the contraction of a muscle in his chin. A third is the grasp reflex, which is elicited through contact with the person's palm. Finally, in the tonic foot response toes turn downward in response to pressure on the sole. The physical examination and the various tests of reflexes, mental status, and activity level are all generally repeated after six months. If the symptoms have not worsened in that time, it may be that another diagnosis, such as depression, should be considered.

Therapies

There is no known cure for dementia. Treatment is basically environmental, keeping the ill person as healthy and as safe as possible. Whenever the person is to be treated for a condition other than his dementia, questions arise about the impact the treatment will have on his cognitive functioning, and, if the person is severely impaired, so do ethical issues concerning the nature of the intervention.

Therapies are directed in two areas: attempts to slow down or reverse the disease process and symptom relief. Neither direction has yet met with much success. Drugs meant to affect the course of the disease process are all still in the experimental stage. Some of the drugs being developed attempt to improve memory. One of them, vasopressin, is a hormone produced by the pituitary gland. Now being tested on patients at the National Institutes of Health, it is administered as an inhalent, because researchers think that nerve endings sensitive to smell may transport vasopressin directly to the brain.

Other drugs are being developed to mimic acetylcholine. One such drug, called an agonist, would work directly at the junction of nerve cells. To date, the few drugs of this type that have been developed have had bad side effects, or their effects have been too short-lived. One acetylcholine agonist, being investigated is physostigmine, which is meant to prevent the rapid catabolism of acetylcholine after it has been released from the nerve cells, so that the transmitter continues to work more effectively. Side effects from this drug, too, may be severe, but there is some evidence that physostigmine is helpful to some patients with Alzheimer's.

Some researchers are treating Alzheimer's disease patients with chelating agents, which bind aluminum, the first step in eliminating the metal from the body. All the drugs described here are in the experimental stages. None is available for use without federal agency permission. All must be administered as parts of registered drug trials conducted by research groups to monitor the efficacy and the dangers of particular drugs.

An attempt has also been made to enhance the amount of acetylcholine by taking choline. This diet therapy has not been found to be helpful.

Sometimes tranquilizers are used to lessen a person's unpredictable behavior, anxiety, and agitation. Sometimes antidepressants and sleeping pills are also prescribed. Use of these kinds of medicine has not been notably successful. Medicine should never be self-administered. The ill person may not remember what the medicine is, how much he should take, or when he last took it. Medicine not prescribed by a physician should never be given to people with dementing illnesses. All medication should be monitored by a physician, because side effects can be dangerous. The presence of dementia or another illness, other drugs in the system, or the age of the patient can make him more sensitive to the sedative.

Psychosocial Information

Irreversible and progressive dementia affects every aspect of a person's life. As his memory, learning, and judgment become increasingly impaired, his ability to relate to others and to work will be diminished. He will no longer be responsible for his own affairs. Either a trusted family member will act for him, or the courts will appoint a guardian to look after his interests. After a period of years the individual will become apathetic, unable to recognize loved ones, disoriented, and uninvolved in the life around him. For the ill individual the stress comes in the early part of the illness, not only in dealing with memory loss and occasional agitation and anxiety as well, but in facing the future. On the other hand, the family begins with the loss of companionship, stigma, and worry about the future and moves into exhaustion and prolonged grieving as the disease progresses. Because eventually the ill person can manage only minimal self-care, the family must shift roles, take up the slack, and begin to resume responsibility for an often physically able, mentally disabled adult. Watching a loved one become a physical shell is a horror. In fact, as the illness progresses, caretakers need as much compassion and support as the ill person. People with Alzheimer's disease do not get better. There may be plateaus, but there are no remissions. It is an unrelenting illness.

Changes in Life-Style

DAILY SCHEDULE

Routine is essential for a person with a dementing illness. It increases predictability in a life that feels increasingly unstructured and amorphous. Changes in time and place are very confusing to a person with a dementing illness. That may be why relatives sometimes notice the dementia for the first time on a trip away from home or during a crisis. Unfamiliar surroundings seem to exacerbate the symptoms.

Not only should meals, bath, exercise, and bedtime be scheduled at the same time every day, but the person's environment should be familiar, comfortable, and uncluttered. One informant said that his wife had been having trouble with numbers and with remembering things for several years, but since they led a very quiet life in the same simple house they had lived in for twenty-five years and he took care of the business of their lives, she was doing quite well. There is nothing asked of her that she cannot do.

DIET

Regular calm, nutritious meals with another person present are the best way to prevent problems of malnourishment or dehydration. Sometimes people with dementing illnesses become dehydrated because they forget that they need more fluids during the summer, or because they are vomiting or have diarrhea. The symptoms of dehydration include thirst or refusal to drink; dizziness; dry, inelastic skin; dry, pale lining of the mouth; fever; rapid pulse; flushing; and confusion or hallucinations.

Ill people sometimes do not eat what caretakers have prepared. It is not uncommon for them to throw away or hide food or to eat it after it has spoiled. Food difficulties must be discussed calmly, because hounding the ill person about eating is a sure way to make mealtimes catastrophic. Instead, mealtimes should be routine, comfortable, and without conflict.

RECREATION

People with dementing illnesses who exercise regularly are calmer, sleep better, and find pleasure in the activity. It is useful for a caretaker to exercise along with the ill person, and activities should be enjoyable for both people. An informant told of a man who left a high-powered job when he realized he was beginning to lose his intellectual abilities. He and his wife decided to retire to a house on a lake in New England, because they thought fishing, which both loved, was something that could be done until almost the end. Each day, for several years, they went out in their rowboat to fish, with the wife gradually assuming their mutual responsibilities and even much of the responsibility for the fishing. They continued this activity for several years, because the man grew more docile as he became more incapacitated, his wife was content to be without other adult company, and they were financially secure.

In exercise, too, routine is very important. A regular exercise time becomes a dependable and soothing part of the day. The activity should be quiet and orderly, or else it may only add to the ill person's agitation. Walking and dancing are activities that people may continue to enjoy. Calisthenics are also a good form of exercise, as long as they have been cleared with the person's physician. It is best if the same sequence of exercises is followed each time. The person should be encouraged to remember them if he is able. If he can't remember or if he is having trouble understanding or completing the exercises, they should be put aside to be tried again another day.

Activity can make a person feel weak and tired. Besides, many older people may have osteoarthritis in addition to their dementing illness, which causes them to have stiff joints. Gentle, regular exercise, taught by physical therapists or other rehabilitation experts, can help prevent stiffness and maintain a person's mobility.

Although regular exercise is important in that it enables the patient to function better, it will in no way alter the course of the disease. It is sometimes said that a person became demented after retirement and that the dementia was caused by inactivity, whereas in fact the dementia was probably present earlier, but the signs were hidden behind everyday work routines. It is more likely that the person retired or slowed down because of his dementia.

Until the last stages of the illness a person with dementia retains his ability to take pleasure in simple activities. Usually people continue to enjoy simplified versions of the same activities they appreciated in the past. Music remains pleasurable. Often people continue to love to sing songs they learned long ago. They enjoy automobile rides and the companionship of a pet. Repetitive tasks like setting the table, working in the garden, stacking magazines, and dusting can also be enjoyable for someone if they are meaningful to him. As the illness progresses, it is important for the ill person's family to find simpler joys. Music, holding something that feels nice and is comforting, and being hugged and touched continue to be important, even in the final stages of the illness.

SLEEP OR REST PATTERNS

People with dementing illnesses often have the greatest difficulty in the evening or at night. Many explanations have been offered for this phenomenon. Some think the twilight itself is responsible for increased confusion. Others note that periods of restlessness and sleeplessness are an unavoidable part of a dementing illness. Also, caretakers may be less accepting in the evening because they are tired.

Whenever possible, less should be required of the ill person in the evening. It should be a quiet, calm time. Complicated activities, like bathing, are best accomplished earlier in the day. Some simple activity that will keep him occupied and close to the person who is caring for him is ideal.

Problems increase with the darkness. People are not able to see as well. Objects and people look blurry. After everyone has gone to bed, there is less stimulation for the person with the dementing illness. He loses the order of the day. Sometimes he will waken during the night, wander around, occasionally leave the house, and often disturb the others with whom he lives. At times he becomes frightened, does not remember where he is, or thinks it's time to get up.

Several very simple techniques can alleviate these situations. Night lights in critical places like bathrooms and reflectors on the bathroom door help orientation. Preparation for sleep is important. Daily exercise enhances sleep, while daytime naps make sleep more difficult. Using the toilet just before going to bed will make it less likely that the person will have to get up at night. A quilt is simpler to manage and becomes less tangled than sheets and blankets. Bedrails are helpful to some people but are confusing to others, who try to climb out over them or who forget why they are there. If the person is taking tranquilizers, it is sometimes helpful if his dosage can be increased at night and decreased during the day.

The caretakers should realize the dangers of a dark house if the ill person wanders at night. They must make sure that doors are locked, knobs on the stove are removed, windows that can present danger are locked, and open stairways are protected with gates. They must also be sure that the tap water is not so hot that the person can burn himself if he drinks from the wrong faucet or decides to take a bath or shower.

If the person does waken at night, calm, quiet support is reassuring. This is an especially difficult time for those who live with someone with a dementing illness, because it is irritating and disconcerting to be awakened. Warm milk and quiet music are suggested as helpful in getting a person back to sleep. If the person insists on getting dressed and sleeping in a chair rather than remaining in his nightclothes and his bed, that should be accepted.

DRIVING

No matter how much of his self-care the ill person retains, as impairment progresses it will not be possible for him to continue to drive. Although driving seems automatic after one has driven for a long time, and there are times when one hardly remembers the trip home from work or the drive to the grocery store, the coordination among eye, mind, and muscle and the ability to respond to new information must be constant in order to drive well. Driving is a complex intellectual endeavor that can be confusing and frightening to the ill person, as well as dangerous to both himself and others.

Sometimes people realize that they are not driving as well as they used to and stop driving of their own accord. Other times, while it becomes clear that the person can no longer drive well, he is unaware of his poor driving. Although his ability to drive is impaired, he may still be well enough to participate in decisions about his life. At that point it is important to talk to the person calmly and point out that he sometimes ignores stop lights or that his reaction times are somewhat slower than they used to be. If the person still insists on continuing to drive, his family must find alternative solutions to the problem. The first is to involve an authority figure like his physician, minister, or counselor whose opinion he respects. At times the word of this kind of outside authority is enough to have the person stop driving. If that approach does not work, the family can take the car keys away or modify the car so that the impaired person will be unable to drive it. For example, a gas station attendant can show a family member how to remove the wire to the distributor or the distributor cap itself so that the impaired person will not be able to start the car. The cap or wire can be easily replaced when a family member wants to drive. The state Department of Motor Vehicles can be brought into the case. Each state has different driving rules, but no state supports unsafe driving. If a physician submits a written opinion saying that the person's driving is impaired because of illness, the Department of Motor Vehicles can investigate and suspend a person's license.

RESTRICTION FROM CERTAIN ACTIVITIES

There are several areas of activity that should be restricted. Decision-making in this regard should be ongoing and should involve the ill person, if possible, as well as his caretakers and experts in each area of activity. As a rule, if something endangers the life of the ill person or anybody else, it should be restricted. If an activity adds to the confusion and disorientation of an ill person, it should be adjusted or omitted. Decisions are sometimes complicated by the fact that the person may not realize he is no longer competent in certain areas and the fact that some of the activities are taken for granted among adults in our society. To lose the right to drive, manage finances, cook, light a fire, or even run a bath is to lose status, respect, and autonomy. Yet to allow people who are moderately demented to continue these activities is dangerous.

One way in which to evaluate someone's ability for self-care is through the assessment of his Activities of Daily Living (ADL). Carried out in a controlled environment by an occupational therapist, the ADL tests a person's ability to manage money, fix a simple meal, dress himself, and perform other routine tasks. All these activities have to be assessed approximately twice a year to be sure that the person's abilities have not deteriorated to the point where activities should be restricted. One informant said that her mother stayed at home alone during the day. The informant had recently become worried about her mother's setting fire to the house, which was heated with gas fires in each room. Because her mother refused to waste a match lighting each fire, she would carry a burning piece of newspaper from room to room. It took the dramatic sight of the open flame to cause the informant to rethink the situation. Even though stories of this kind are alarming, it is also essential not to deprive anyone of responsibilities he is able to manage. Keeping as many adult responsibilities as possible helps the person to use the abilities he has and to maintain contact with the adult world for as long as he can.

Impact of the Disease on Social Life

LEGAL ASPECTS

When the person's thinking has become quite impaired, he cannot retain legal or financial responsibility for himself. He will not be able to manage his checkbook, bankbook, or property, nor will he be able to decide how to spend his money, or to give or withhold permission for medical care. To maintain maximal control over one's future, it is best to make arrangements for the management of one's affairs before becoming too ill to decide. This requires that individuals and families acknowledge the course of the illness and plan for the future.

The law provides several ways to deal with this situation. First, an individual can make a will while he is still legally competent. Called testamentary capacity, this means that the person is making a will under his own direction in which he states the names of and his relationship to the people who will receive his property and what that property is.

While he is still able, a person can also assign power of attorney allowing a specified adult the authority to manage his property. Power of attorney can be limited or broad. A limited power of attorney gives a specific individual the authority to carry out specific transactions, like writing checks, selling a house, or reviewing tax records, but no other authority. On the other hand, a broad power of attorney is intended to allow a specific individual to manage all of the affairs of an ill person. The extent of the power must be clearly stated in writing. This is obviously a serious decision; if he is able, the ill person must think carefully about the right person to act in his best interest.

If a person is already at the stage where he can no longer manage his affairs, his family will have to consult a lawyer and eventually the courts. A conservatorship, also known as a guardianship of property procedure, may be needed. In this procedure a petition is filed with the court asking a judge to decide whether the individual is legally competent to manage his affairs. If the judge finds that the person is not competent, he may appoint a legal guardian to act for the person in financial matters and periodically file financial reports with the court. If the ill individual is incompetent and provision has not been made beforehand, this procedure is necessary even for a spouse to sell any jointly owned property.

A request for legal guardianship is sometimes necessary when a disabled person requires nursing home or medical care and is unwilling or unable to consent to it. This is legally more complicated than guardianship of property. Often the facility caring for the person accepts the permission of the person's next of kin rather than petitioning the court for this difficult decision. If the court is petitioned, a judge may decide to appoint a guardian for the person and order the necessary care.

Most state health departments now publish bills of rights for patients in both hospitals and nursing homes. They serve as promises that the states will protect the rights of patients while they are in a dependent situation. Copies of the bills can be obtained from state departments of health or state health departments' licensed nursing homes. If the patient's rights are not protected, a state health department can review and revoke the institution's license.

INSURANCE AND OTHER FINANCIAL ASSISTANCE

When a person is first diagnosed with a dementing illness, it is important for his family to assess the situation in terms of the expenses that will be incurred as well as the resources that will be available to them as the illness progresses. Assets include savings, property, and Social Security, as well as insurance plans.

Most insurance plans are not helpful to people with a dementing illness. Insurance generally covers acute care and hospitalization. When people insure themselves, they are usually thinking of a sudden medical catastrophe. Dementing illnesses, on the other hand, are long-term and incurable, and often require what the government and insurance companies call custodial care.

Medicare's requirements for coverage almost rule out care of people with dementing illnesses. Only after a three-day hospitalization will Medicare pay for nursing home or at-home care if that care is for the illness that resulted in the hospitalization. Medicare will pay only for skilled care (where medical and nursing care are required), will pay fully only for the first twenty days of such care, and only on a shared-cost basis for a total of one hundred days before another hospitalization is necessary. *The Medicare Handbook* says that when care is primarily for the purpose of meeting personal needs that could be provided by persons without professional skills or training, it is considered custodial. Bathing a person and helping him dress, eat, get in and out of bed, and walk are all custodial tasks.

Policies that are sold as supplements to Medicare also do not pay for custodial care. Health insurance policies often exclude payment for dementing illnesses. Life insurance presents problems also. Some life insurance policies waive premiums when a person becomes disabled, but some companies, not recognizing Alzheimer's as a disabling disease, refuse to waive payments. Family members have to check coverage carefully in order to assess entitlements.

Disability payments are also difficult to obtain. When those who make decisions about one's qualifications for disability payments confront a person with a dementing illness, they simply suggest that the person be retrained to do a simpler job. The fact that the person cannot learn new things and that learning will become increasingly impossible does not change their minds. If disability is denied, it is important for the family to find out exactly what has to be documented in order for the ill person to be eligible for payments and for the family to notify the physician about these requirements. The case can be appealed and reappealed.

One additional source of help is the Veteran's Administration hospitals, which admit patients if their medical problem relates to their having been in the armed forces or if the person is indigent. Admission decisions are made by each individual facility. If people with Alzheimer's do gain admission—and they often do not—their families are told that they will be discharged if the bed is needed for someone with a treatable illness. A representative of the Veterans Administration hospitals has said that if the VA admitted all of the Alzheimer's patients whose families applied, their resources would be depleted.

PAYMENT FOR NURSING HOME CARE

In many states Medicaid will pay a limited fee for Alzheimer's patients in nursing homes. In order to be eligible for Medicaid, however, the ill person must be almost indigent. If nursing home placement is necessary because the person can no longer be managed at home, and there is no insurance coverage for a nursing home, the cost to the person or his family is about $20,000 a year and rising. Thus, if a person lives in a nursing home for a prolonged period, the illness is likely to render the family destitute even before the person dies.

Grown children are often concerned that they will have to pay for the care of an ill parent. Questions regarding a child's responsibility are complicated. If a child cannot pay for his parent's nursing home care, he should not sign a contract saying that he will. That contract is like any other. Signing the contract means that the person acknowledges the responsibility. In some states children are not responsible for their parents' support. In others an ill person cannot be denied access to care because his child refused to pay, but the state can take the child to court to gain reimbursement.

A spouse carries financial responsibility. In all states both the joint assets of a couple and the well spouse's income are considered. In many states, however, after an ill spouse has been in a nursing home for six months, he can be eligible for assistance without draining the assets of his well spouse. If the ill spouse is the man of the house, payment for nursing home care will often cause his wife's income to fall below a certain level. At that time she is eligible for Supplemental Security Income and for other services like Food Stamps. In the same way, the house in which a well spouse lives cannot be sold until after his death if the state makes a claim against the estate for reimbursement of nursing home costs. Questions about transferring assets from the ill person to the well person should be addressed to a lawyer. Likewise, eligibility requirements and nursing home rules and restrictions should be discussed with a social worker.

If, as the disease progresses, the family keeps the ill person at home, there are several services available in the community that support home care. First, health insurance and major medical insurance sometimes pay for certain aspects of home care and for necessary appliances. In addition, many research programs, especially in large metropolitan areas, offer low-cost or free medical care in exchange for the person's serving as a research subject. Most programs have specific requirements for eligibility and have passed standards that assure that the research will not harm the participants. The standards are subject to review by the funding source and the institutional sponsor (usually a hospital). Consent forms explain the nature of the research as well as the risks and benefits that can be expected. Patients and families are given the option to withdraw from the research at

any time with the possible understanding that withdrawal from the research means withdrawal from any other free medical care provided by
the research group.

TAX RELIEF

"Tax Benefits for Older Americans," a pamphlet available from the
Internal Revenue Service, describes some forms of tax relief available to
people with dementing illnesses and their families. A caretaker who hires
someone to care for an ill person while he works may be entitled to a tax
credit for part of the cost of the care. The caretaker may also be allowed
to define the ill person as a dependent and thus gain a tax credit or a tax
deduction for part of nursing home costs and medical expenses. Some state
and federal legislators are now urging tax relief for families who care for
a disabled elderly person. Specific bills are being suggested that would give
specific tax relief to those who maintain an elderly disabled person at home.
At this time, however, financial and insurance relief for those with a dementing illness is limited. The poor prognosis and longevity of those with
the illness make care prohibitively expensive for insurance companies and
for the government. The financial burden falls, to a great extent, on the
family of the ill person.

ABILITY TO WORK

If the effects of Alzheimer's on a person are not obvious in the beginning stages of the illness, they become increasingly apparent as the illness
progresses. Often it is at work that the person with a dementing illness
begins to have difficulty. Either his work involves numbers and he is no
longer able to add or divide, or it involves managing many tasks at once
and he can no longer set priorities or remember complicated directions.
One fourth-grade teacher is managing her life well even though she can
no longer work with numbers. Her pupils, her principal, and her fellow
teachers have not noticed her problem. It is apparent only in her mental
status examination.

Because work is so important to people's identities and retirement often
means decreased stimulation, it is best if the ill individual has an understanding boss who will try to find tasks that he can still manage. Sometimes the people involved are unaware that poor performance is due to
disease, and the person is fired. It is then up to the family to protest and
to help the person to apply for Social Security Disability.

Most people with dementing illnesses are over sixty-five, so many have
already retired. Retired people often assume more responsibility at home.
These responsibilities are work also. In time, a person with a dementing

illness will not be able to do housework either, unless the tasks are simple and present no danger to the person or the family.

RELATIONSHIPS WITH STRANGERS

Relationships with strangers can be difficult, because the person with a dementing illness doesn't necessarily appear ill. His odd behavior is not taken in the context of illness. Again, each brain-impaired person is affected differently. People who are confused will sometimes pick up things in a store and want to take them home without paying for them. At other times they will accuse a salesperson of stealing their money. Sometimes, while making polite conversation, they will say something very insulting. They lose the ability to be tactful, saying whatever comes to mind without being able to consider the impact the statement will have on others. Often they will complain endlessly. When ill people are confused or overwhelmed, the way they dramatically overreact may seem deliberate but is actually out of their control.

Strangers have no way to understand such behavior. It is best for the caretaker to disengage the ill person from the situation quietly. Distracting the ill person from the immediate situation is helpful. Responding to the feeling that one thinks is motivating the ill person to react so strongly is also helpful. A woman and her impaired father were in an ice cream shop. When it was their turn to order, the father became very angry, shouting at the shopkeeper and stamping his foot. His daughter quietly took him by the arm, said to him, "it's hard to pick your favorite, isn't it?" and ordered for the both of them. She responded to his confusion by making the decision. If he hadn't quieted immediately, she would have left the shop with him.

If caretakers choose to explain the problem to strangers, they might simply say that the person has an illness which affects his thinking, that what he is doing is not deliberate, and that he is neither crazy nor dangerous. A caretaker's handling of this kind of situation depends very much on his own comfort with the issues and with the explanation.

RELATIONSHIPS WITH FAMILY MEMBERS

Dementing illnesses place as much stress on caretakers as they do on the ill person. The downward course of the illness, the long time span, and the eventual inability of the sick person to honor the efforts of the caretaker are extraordinarily poignant. At the end loved ones can become unresponsive, unpredictable, incontinent, and unrecognizing.

One woman who is taking care of her very demented father tries to express her anguish by likening the experience to her vision of hell where things look the same but have turned horrible. Her father looks like a healthy elderly man, but where he had once been a quiet, fastidious person, he is now demanding and sloppy. She has found someone to be with her father during the day while she works, but she hates to come home at night. She says that if her father did not look the same as ever, taking care of him would be more bearable, but she is constantly reminded of what he once was. If he weren't her father, however, she says she could never make the sacrifices that she has in order for him to remain at home.

Contrary to popular belief, almost all families in the United States do care for their members as long as possible. Even though grown children and their parents generally do not live together, children remain involved in the lives of their parents. When there is a member with a dementing illness, families carry a heavy financial, social, and psychological burden.

Care of the dementing person deeply stresses the family system. At times families become closer, discovering strength in and through each other. In other cases, old disagreements are raised or children and well parent struggle with each other as much as they struggle with the illness. Family members have difficulty accepting the nature and extent of their loved one's impairment. Divisiveness never helps. Those who are most accepting can help those who continue to deny the changes. In the same way, some people will be able to spend more time with the ill person while others may be able to help by taking on more of the responsibilities outside of the home, like shopping or some facets of the family finances. The family should be careful not to put all of the burden on one person, because that person may be unable to stand the stress for the long term. The primary caretaker must have time for himself, has to be able to leave the house, and must have interests besides the ill person in order to survive this very long, very stressful period. It is important for the family members to talk to each other. They can talk informally about responsibilities and feelings, or they can set aside specific times to have family conferences.

RELATIONSHIP WITH SPOUSE

The life of the well spouse changes in many ways. He is neither half of a couple nor a widower. Friends stop seeing him and his spouse as a couple, and many friends stay away. Because he is not a widower, he is not free to make a new life for himself. Because he needs support and friendship during the illness and after his spouse dies, he must somehow maintain a social life. This is extremely difficult, because the spouse with the dementing illness takes so much of the person's energy. Friends who remain play a critical role in helping the well spouse to maintain himself.

Despite the illness, the meaning of the marital relationship continues for most people. The commitment can be kept only if the well spouse adjusts his expectations to the diminished abilities of the ill person. One man related with great pride that, although doctors had told him to send his wife to a nursing home, he had deferred that decision. She kept herself clean, she helped him by dusting and doing other small chores around the house, and she watched television with him in the evening. Before she became ill, his wife had been a real "powerhouse." She was a dynamic organization volunteer, a wonderful mother, and a terrific cook. Because he loved her very much and because her personality pattern allowed him to maintain a quiet, orderly, and warm life, the husband was offended that anyone could think him capable of putting his life's companion in a home.

Other well spouses find the strain too much to bear. A nurse at a county home said that the majority of her patients have Alzheimer's disease. Some have visitors, but they either have no idea who the visitors are or mistake them for someone else.

Sometimes, too, the marital relationship was unhappy before the person became ill. This places an added strain on a very difficult situation. Whatever the previous situation, it is tremendously complicated by the pressures of a dementing illness.

SPECIFIC FAMILY RELATIONSHIPS

The relationship of young children to a person with a dementing illness also changes radically. Children often are afraid that the condition is contagious or that they have somehow caused the illness. Children are astute observers. To try to hide the facts makes them more confused and frightened. They must be taught that much of the ill person's behavior is not willful. This is difficult to understand for young children; while they are being taught to control their own behavior, they learn that an ill relative cannot control his. They are to be nice to Grandpa no matter what he says to them. They are to be respectful to Grandma even when she forgets why she is there with them. Children are often in competition with the demented person for the caregiver's attention. The problem is heightened in the evening, when everybody's energies are low; the impaired person is often at his most confused, and the whole family is together.

Children do best when they can be involved. Very small children, who expect little except to be loved and are no threat, often get along very well with those who are impaired. The more the caregiver understands and accepts the illness, the better he is at explaining it so that children can accept it. Children also need help in explaining the impaired person to their friends. If they do not learn to find the person acceptable, they will not be able to teach their friends the same thing or have friends come to the house.

Teenagers also do best when their help is enlisted. Adolescence is an unpredictable time. Teens are working out their own issues about independence. They may see adults as weird and lacking in understanding.

Dementia is an embarrassment. One very perceptive teenager talked of driving to a nursing home to see her very demented grandmother every evening after dinner. Her grandmother did not know her or her father. The old woman would giggle and speak Polish, the language of her girlhood, which neither the teenager nor her father understood. The granddaughter resented those visits terribly. It was embarrassing to see this once powerful woman reduced to her present state. But after some time, without discussing the matter with her father, the young woman came to realize that her presence was vitally important to her father. After that, the visits were easier.

Ultimately the caretakers of people with dementing illness must face their feelings about the illness: what it is doing to a person they love, and what it is doing to them. Feelings of guilt, loss, and anger can so overwhelm the caretaker that he is unable to care for his ill relative or himself. Understanding the illness can help people to manage their guilt. Loss is real. The caretaker and the family are losing a companion, someone who fulfilled important roles in their lives, someone who is cherished. If the ill person is a married man, his spouse may lose much of her status in the community. Children who depended on a parent who is now a caretaker may lose her attention because she has turned away to help her own parent or her spouse. If the ill person had been working, people lose income and the status of the job. Usually people lose friendships, too, because many people avoid illness in others.

Anger remains a problem. It is terribly difficult not to be angry with someone who is making your entire life hard. An informant said that he has learned to watch for certain words he uses when he is beginning to get furious with his mother. He's not cursing or carrying on; rather, he's choosing words that imply that his mother is in control of her behavior and that much of what she does is directed solely at making his life miserable. When that happens, he knows he must go off to another room and discuss the matter with himself. If he doesn't, he will begin to shout at his mother. Shouting upsets her terribly; she gets more confused, and the whole situation becomes a nightmare.

The grieving process with its recurrent feelings of guilt, loss, and anger, remains a theme for caregivers. It is woven throughout all stages of the illness. In the early and moderate stages, while the ill person retains insight into his plight, the person and the family grieve together. As the illness progresses, the family is left to grieve alone.

As the illness progresses and the ill person becomes increasingly dependent, isolation and confinement can easily become the plight of both the caretaker and the ill person. The ill person will feel more comfortable at home in familiar surroundings, and the caretaker will feel more comfortable not having to worry about the ill person's getting lost or behaving badly. Everybody tends to become confined and isolated.

Caretakers have to watch for signs of their own isolation. Examples of warning signs are drinking too much; using tranquilizers and sleeping pills regularly; screaming or crying too much; feeling out of control; feeling very stressed, panicky, nervous, or frightened; thinking about suicide; overeating; increased smoking, or drinking too much coffee. These warnings are signals that caretakers are not caring for themselves. If they cannot improve the situation, they should seek outside help.

One retired man, who had hired someone to spend working days with his ill wife, used to leave his apartment every morning to spend the day at his club. When he arrived at the club, he went right to the bar, where he got blind drunk. None of his friends tried to help him. They all thought that his plight was so awful that he was doing the best thing by drinking himself into oblivion. Finally a neighbor convinced him that he was drinking to block the situation from his mind and that he needed help in accepting his wife's illness.

Psychological Aspects

Since dementia means loss of mind, the psychological aspects of dementia are the essence of the illness. Dementia severely affects the psychology of an individual—self-concept, mood, affect, ability to express oneself, ability to relate, the very persona. In our society what you are is the way you think, how you use that thinking to relate, to work, to spend your day. Without thinking you are a shell, a body without a mind.

STAGES OF PSYCHOLOGICAL RESPONSE

The loss of recent memory and the ability to do simple arithmetic and changes in mood and personality are early symptoms, which often begin before the diagnosis is made. Since they are unexplained, friends, relatives, and co-workers get angry at what is thought to be volitional carelessness or moodiness.

In the early stages of the illness many people are able to conceal their declining abilities and forgetfulness. They keep lists, try to maintain a rigid schedule, and deny any problem by brushing off or joking about memory loss or mistakes with money. People's social skills and personality often stay intact while their memory and ability to learn deteriorate. With skill and luck, they can conceal the extent of their disability for a long time. When their family members finally become aware of the illness, they are usually dismayed by the extent of the problem.

Other symptoms include the inability to concentrate, anxiety, withdrawal, petulance, and irritability. Soon judgment becomes impaired. People also lose the ability to understand complex messages like jokes, double entendres, or meanings behind words. Later in the process of the disease people require simpler and simpler messages in order to understand how to respond. Some people experience radical personality changes, but many do not. Generally people's dominant personality characteristics become exaggerated: A talkative, friendly person will become more outgoing.

Depression is a part of the illness until the very last stages. At first people are depressed at the symptoms they are experiencing. Memory loss and the inability to calculate are extremely frightening and saddening. People become even more depressed when confronted with the diagnosis of and prognosis for the disease. The disease process itself seems to cause an endogenous depression in certain people. A man whose wife is quite impaired at this time reports that she has started each day for the last few years by crying. At first she cried at her frightening symptoms. Then she cried about the diagnosis. Now she cries and does not know why.

Confusion, disorientation, and restlessness are all signs of dementing illness. People pace around the house a great deal. Sometimes, too, they will wander around the neighborhood. Wandering seems to exacerbate demented people's confusion. When they wander at night, which they often do, disorientation is further heightened.

As the disease progresses, ill people's memories become increasingly impaired. They often lose things and think that they have been stolen, or they hide things from themselves, forget where they have hidden them, and again accuse the people around them of theft. Also, because they forget what has just taken place, people tend to repeat themselves over and over again. Either they tell the same story repeatedly, or they ask the same question over and over. Someone might ask his caretaker what time it is ten times in five minutes. Each time he has forgotten not only the answer, but the fact that he has already asked the question. In the same way people who are quite ill sometimes repeat the same action over and over. They can become frightened or fretful when a caretaker leaves the room because they have forgotten why or where the person is going. When one considers how frightening life would be without memory, it is easier to understand the dependence on and fear about losing one's caretaker.

The timing and sequence of ability loss vary from individual to individual. In the final stages of the illness people have similar symptoms of apathy, lack of involvement with others, and disorientation. They sometimes become incontinent. They sit alone, unresponsive except for smiles or sounds. Some begin to shuffle when they walk. They deteriorate until death.

PANIC REACTIONS

At times a demented person will experience rapid changes in mood or will become excessively upset. This happens primarily when he is confused, disoriented, or overwhelmed. Either he cannot manage what he thinks he ought to, he finds himself in strange surroundings, or he has been made anxious by something in a situation. When this happens, an ill person overreacts by shouting, accusing people around him, refusing to move, or even striking out at those who are trying to help him. An informant recounted taking his ill father to a concert. They were both thoroughly enjoying the music when the fire alarm sounded and people began to leave the auditorium. First his father refused to leave his seat, saying that someone would take it if he got up. Then, when his son insisted that they leave, the father began to shout and scream that he was not going. The father had to be carried out forcibly by his son and several members of the audience. While his father soon forgot about it, it took hours for the son to calm down.

There are instances when such panic reactions are the first signs to a family that something is wrong. Because a dementing illness is so frightening to an individual, it is probably impossible to avoid these kinds of reactions altogether, but much can be done to limit or minimize them. First, when the individual is mildly impaired and a panic reaction occurs, it is best to reassure the person and to move on from the experience. Routine helps, as does predictability. Remembering to simplify tasks is important. If a person has forgotten how to button but can still don a slip-on shirt himself, his family should supply him with slip-ons. If crowds are overwhelming, they can be avoided. Allowing the person more time to complete tasks than he previously needed sometimes helps to avoid a catastrophic reaction. Speaking calmly and firmly and refraining from asking questions of the ill individual also minimize the possibility of panic reaction.

Often distraction will calm someone. At other times, quietly removing the person from the upsetting situation will help him to feel better. Touching is also sometimes very soothing. Some people respond positively to being rocked or held. Others feel restrained with this kind of touching and will become even more upset. If the caretaker becomes upset and shouts angrily, the ill person will often become more upset. It is impossible for a caretaker always to respond calmly and firmly to what can be intolerable circumstances. If the caretaker's responses can be generally firm and comforting, however, she can avoid escalating the reaction. It is helpful, once again, to remember that an ill person generally resorts to this behavior when he is confused, overwhelmed, and panicked. It is not volitional.

SELF-CONCEPT

Nowhere is a dementia more apparent than in relation to self-concept. In the course of the illness one loses one's sense of self. In losing memory, a person loses his ability to be competent as well as his ability to relate to anyone or anything. Independence, skill, and a sense of the future are all lost. There is no answer to the question, "Who am I?" Feelings remain, but they are increasingly difficult to interpret. Throughout, the caretaker must remember the basic need to be assured, to be comfortable, and to feel safe. The perpetual questions, "Am I losing my mind?" and "Am I going crazy?" must be met with warmth, caring, and understanding.

APPEARANCE

Such is the nature of dementia that, while people are losing their memories and their ability to reason, they look normal. In the early stages of the disease people are quite capable of caring for themselves. As the illness progresses, people often begin to neglect themselves. Grooming, bathing, and dressing have to be encouraged. Later in the disease process, people will need help in all of these areas. Caretakers should have their ill relative care for himself as much as he can. Praise and encouragement become a part of the routine.

SEXUAL BEHAVIOR

If the ill person lives with his well spouse, their sex life will eventually be changed radically by the illness. Some people experience a diminished sex drive, whereas some become more interested in sex. Someone's sexual behavior may also change in ways that are difficult for his partner to accept. The person may still be able to make love but may not remember foreplay or the ways that the couple cuddled or talked after they made love. The ability of the well partner to make love may therefore be diminished. Sometimes, too, a formerly gentle and sensitive lover may become sexually demanding, just as he becomes more demanding about so many other things in relationship to his spouse.

What is deemed inappropriate sexual behavior can assume several guises. Sometimes a demented person will wander naked into a living area of the house or outside. He may take his clothes off because he thinks that it is time to go to bed or because his garments are uncomfortable. Simple, comfortable garments that button at the back will solve this problem. Sometimes, too, very confused people expose themselves or fondle their genitals in places where such behavior is socially unacceptable. It is most important to remember that these behaviors are rarely done in order to attract the attention of other people. The meaning of the action is comfort, not sexual arousal. Distracting the person is an effective means of changing his activity.

SUPPORT SERVICES FOR FAMILY MEMBERS

Because the illness is devastating and long-lasting, it is critical that family members help each other and enlist whatever outside social and emotional supports they can. Of all such help, the ones that seem effective are the support groups organized through ADRDA, the Alzheimer's Disease and Related Disorders Association. Addresses of local groups may be obtained through the national or local office. The groups are used for both information and informal sharing; people support each other, give each other tips for managing their impaired person, suggest additional resources, and allow each member a kind of "gallows humor" outlet for talking about the crazy things that go on in their houses. Members stay involved with the groups as long as they like and come whenever they can. People have said that without their group, they would have felt that they were going insane.

Various in-home services for the aged are also helpful. State, county, and federal offices for the aging can provide information about the services available in particular areas and the conditions for elibility. In addition, local community mental health centers provide counseling and, in some cases, day hospitals or activities for the intellectually impaired. Rehabilitation centers assess an individual's ability to live independently. Meals on Wheels, in some areas, can provide for meals. Other services may be available through local religious groups or social service agencies.

One resource with great potential for dealing with Alzheimer's is day care. Although there are not many day care programs available yet, it is thought that more will be developed in the next few years. In one such program, the Alzheimer's Disease Day Treatment Program at the Wisconsin Regional Geriatric Center, twelve patients spend two and one-half days a week at the center. The focus of the program is therapeutic recreation. The atmosphere is calm, structured, and predictable. Patients help with lunch, exercise, sing, dance, paint, and are involved in a program to maintain good physical health. The staff has found that use of physical touch—hand-holding, stroking, and hugging—is extremely important to people with dementing illnesses. The program also educates and supports family members, primarily through a weekly support group meeting led by a social worker, a nurse, and a psychiatrist. One strategy, described in another program, is to help change the way family members interpret behavior. Family members are asked to describe a behavior that is painful, sad, or infuriating to them, then are helped to reinterpret the behavior. For example, a physician said his mother insisted on taking off many of her outer clothes in hot weather. He had found that almost unbearable to watch until a helper pointed out that his mother was perfectly comfortable and was much more comfortable than when she had been fully clothed. The lack of some clothing became a signal that she was making herself more comfortable.

If the family can afford it, it is helpful to have someone come in for several hours a day to be with the ill person so that the caretaker can leave the house. For this solution to work, the sitter should be educated sufficiently about the nature of the illness and how to manage the crises that will surely arise. Often the ill person will be insulting or suspicious of the sitter. He will tell her that she is not needed any more or will wonder out loud why there is a stranger in his house. If the sitter is calm, understanding, and patient, the confused person will most probably adjust to her. In that way the sitter can become part of the week's routine. This "time out" should be arranged for whichever times would best support the family—day, evening, or night. Other care arrangements are night care in which someone comes in to stay the night with the ill person, and board-and-care arrangements in which the ill person moves out of the home temporarily to offer respite to the family. As the problem of dementia grows, more services will be developed to serve the population. For now, creative facilitation of support for the family is critical.

NURSING HOMES

The decision to place a relative in a nursing home is very difficult. Even the words used to describe the action are different from the terms usually used for making living arrangements. "Place," "put," and "send" are words of disposal in which the ill person has very little to do with the decision. Some professionals think families should consider institutionalization before they have reached the point of emotional and physical exhaustion. Many informants say that the decision is made when the caretakers just cannot take it any more. Either the caretaker himself realizes that he is exhausted and out of control, or not strong enough to manage, or else someone who is close to him does. Since the ill person's physical needs often escalate, it becomes exceedingly difficult to care for him.

The decision is complicated by the fact that each nursing home has its own strengths and weaknesses. The only way to learn about nursing homes is to visit them and talk to relatives of similarly ill people who live in the homes. The caretaker must educate himself about the levels of care for which nursing homes are licensed, as well as the level of care to which his ill family member will be assigned. Unless they are otherwise ill, most people with a dementing illness will be assigned to the intermediate level of care. Those choosing a nursing home also have to investigate application procedures, costs and methods of payment, and affiliation of the homes. Costs are high, and most insurance plans do not pay for intermediate-level care. Some nursing homes have additional funding sources.

Each nursing home also has its own style. Some relate better to people with dementia than others. Some might be cleaner or neater than others. Some welcome the involvement of relatives, and others discourage it. Although style is somewhat a matter of taste, calm and routine are tremendously important to a person with a dementing illness.

How to Be Helpful

Helping Someone Who Is Demented

Primarily the goal is to help the person to be more secure, less confused, and less dangerous to himself and others than he would be without your help. Be sure that the person is wearing an identification necklace or bracelet that includes his name, the fact that his memory is impaired, and the telephone number of someone close to him. Learn to listen to more than the person's words. Even if he is acting as if someone who had died forty years ago was right in the room with him, perhaps he is also saying that he is lonely or sad. Think about what you say before you say it so that you are communicating as simply and as clearly as possible. Simplify questions and requests. Don't ask someone to do something until you have broken it down into the smallest unit of activity.

To help a person orient himself, keep clocks and calendars with the day and the date in full view. Remember also that people become more disoriented in the dark; use night lights in all habitable rooms. If a person with dementia visits you, think about what aspects of your environment could be dangerous to the person. Swimming pools, open fireplaces, a pot of water boiling on the stove, and very hot water in the faucets are all potentially dangerous to someone whose memory and judgment are impaired. Smoking is also very dangerous, because the person may forget that he is smoking or where he left a burning cigarette. Driving is hazardous as the disease progresses. A person is likely to lose his way, forget how to operate the car, or become confused about signs and signals. A regular schedule helps a person with a dementing illness. It is also best if he has to conform to the same schedule as others in his home. If he stays awake all day and is involved in some activity, he is more likely to sleep through the night.

Helping the Family of a Demented Person

When, in the course of any chronic disease, someone reaches the point of severe disability, his family needs a great deal of help. However, the need is different for the family of the demented person. First, when the person is severely demented, he needs little from anyone but his primary caretakers. His body remains, but his personality is not there to befriend. Second, since dementia attacks personality, the response is most devastating to loved ones. To care for someone who has lost his personhood, his ability to reason, to remember, to know you is shattering. Finally, people can live for a long time with severe dementia. As years go by, they can become increasingly regressed and confused. The sheer length of caring for a progressively diminished person is frustrating, enervating, and exhausting.

Thus, to be of greatest help to someone with a dementing illness, it is critical to support his family. The illness takes such a tremendous toll on loved ones, especially those who try to care for the ill person at home, that any relief or encouragement you can give the family is a direct help to the ill person. Above all, family members need some time to themselves. In addition they need the outside stimulation of work, hobbies, or time with friends in order to manage each day. Thus, helping to do or find respite care and keeping caretakers involved and active is paramount.

Throughout these long and devastating illnesses, two themes remain constant. First, the ill person's actions and thoughts are often not volitional. In the early stages of his illness he will be frightened and depressed. To manage these terrifying feelings, he may deny problems, become cantankerous, or find some other psychological means for comfort. As the illness progresses, the person will gradually regress in his intellectual and social abilities. he will not be able to learn new things, will lose his recent memory, and will eventually even forget the identities of those closest to him.

The second theme is the extraordinary amount of stress borne by the caretakers of the ill person. Because the person is often depressed in the beginning of his illness and later loses his social skills, it is easy to abandon him and his family. Ultimately care becomes the responsibility of loved ones, who generally manage at home as long as they can and finally place the ill person in a nursing home, when the individual becomes very demented and no longer recognizes friends or loved ones. At that point caretakers need support, understanding, and comfort more than ever. They are mourning the loss of a loved one years before his death.

5

Diabetes

DIABETES IS a condition that does not allow the body to convert food into energy properly. When food is digested, a form of sugar called glucose is released into the blood and normally moves into the body's cells for energy use or to the liver, where it is stored for future use. The regulation of the flow of glucose depends on the hormone insulin, which is produced by the pancreas. When insulin production is not sufficient or when the body is not able to use the insulin produced, there is a high buildup of sugar in the blood, because the glucose continues to circulate without being used. Eventually the glucose is filtered from the blood by the kidneys and eliminated via the urine. The disease is diagnosed by determining the level of glucose or sugar in the blood. An abnormally high glucose level indicates an insulin insufficiency. Diabetes is treated through a combination of diet, exercise, stress management, and, if needed, insulin or oral medication.

To some extent diabetes affects all aspects of a person's life. The fact that an insulin-dependent diabetic is governed by the clock and remains subject to insulin shock must affect her relationships with others, the kind of work she does, and the ways in which she chooses to spend her leisure time. She is reminded that she is diabetic each time she eats, exercises, makes love, or injects herself with insulin.

The single most important facet of treatment for diabetes is self-management. That notion distinguishes diabetes from any other chronic illness. Except for regular medical consultation, a person with diabetes cares for herself. Family also becomes involved in the management of the illness if a child has diabetes or when a diabetic goes into shock. Social support is necessary for understanding, forestalling complications, and sometimes even physical survival. With effective self-management and good medical and social supports, most people with diabetes can lead rich and active lives.

Medical Information

Etiology and Classification

The cause of diabetes is not known, but factors contributing to its development include heredity, obesity, aging, physical and emotional stress, pregnancy, and perhaps viral infections.

There are basically two kinds of diabetes. Type 1, also called insulin-dependent or ketosis-prone, was previously called "juvenile-onset," because it generally begins in childhood or adolescence. In insulin-dependent diabetes, the pancreas produces little or no insulin, and the diabetic must therefore, inject the insulin in order for the sugar her body requires for energy to be utilized properly. Insulin must be injected because it would be destroyed by the digestive juices if taken by mouth. In type 1 the untreated disease can progress rapidly to a gravely imbalanced metabolic state, ketoacidosis, which can result in coma and death unless controlled by the administration of insulin and fluids.

In type 2—also known as non-insulin-dependent, "maturity-onset," or non-ketosis-prone diabetes—the pancreas produces some insulin, but the amount is insufficient. Onset is usually later in life, generally after forty years of age, and it can often be managed through weight reduction and limitation of carbohydrate intake. Sometimes a drug is taken to stimulate the production of insulin by the pancreas.

Prevalence and Incidence

In 1983, according to the American Diabetes Association, there were approximately 11 million adults plus children with diabetes in the United States, including 600,000 people newly diagnosed. Two million people under thirty have type 1 diabetes. The National Center for Health Statistics reports a 1981 prevalence of 5,499,737. The discrepancy in the statistics is accounted for by the American Diabetes Association's assumption that there are more than 5 million Americans with undiagnosed type 2 diabetes.

Natural History

The course of the illness must be looked at separately for the two types. Before the discovery of insulin, most type 1 diabetics lived less than five years after onset and died of ketoacidosis or infection. Those with type 1 diabetes today who do not take insulin follow the same course. For people with type 2 diabetes, the course of the unmanaged, very poorly managed, or unmanageable disease entails progressive neuropathies with possible resultant gangrene and leg amputation, visual loss and blindness, and eventual death from kidney failure or infection.

At present about 75 percent of people with diabetes die of cardiovascular-renal complications like heart attack, kidney failure, or heart failure, but death comes on an average thirty years after onset, and the average life span is increasing. An increasing number of juvenile-onset, insulin-dependent diabetics live for more than forty years after diagnosis, but with greater blood vessel disease, for example five times as many leg amputations, than experienced by nondiabetics. People with diabetes are also hospitalized two and one-half times more frequently and have longer average hospital stays.

Thus, heightened morbidity leads to a shorter life span, and there is greater likelihood of permanent physical disability and loss of independence. The life expectancy for someone with type 1 diabetes is one-third less than that for the rest of the population. With treatment and good self-management, most people with type 1 diabetes can live well into middle age; those with type 2 can have a normal life span. Diabetes cannot be cured at present, but in most cases the complications of the illness can be lessened.

Symptoms at Onset

Common symptoms of the onset of less severe type 2 diabetes are weakness and fatigue, aching, numbness and tingling of the fingers and toes, blurry vision, or skin infections. Symptoms of severe or type 1 diabetes are very frequent urination, intense thirst, rapid weight loss, extreme hunger, weakness and fatigue, itchy or dry skin, blurry eyesight, and skin infections. Those groups of symptoms are what cause people to seek medical attention. Many diagnoses of type 2 diabetes are made through a routine physical examination when the patient is presymptomatic.

Crises

The two kinds of crises that can occur with type 1 diabetes are ketoacidosis or diabetic coma and insulin reaction or hypoglycemia. In ketoacidosis, an inadequate supply of insulin prevents the body from using blood glucose for energy. In order to get the energy it needs, the body begins to burn fat, which results in a buildup of substances called ketones.

Some of the symptoms of ketoacidosis are like the ones described for type 1 diabetes, which first bring the diabetic to see a physician; excessive urination and thirst, fatigue, and weight loss. Additional symptoms are abdominal pain, nausea and vomiting, blurred vision, rapid and deep breathing, fruity odor of the breath, drowsiness, and unconsciousness. Ketoacidosis is treated with insulin and fluids.

Insulin reaction occurs when there is too little sugar and too much insulin in the blood. The symptoms of insulin reaction—irritability, dullness, headache, crying, change in mood or behavior, shaking, sweating and lightheadedness, hunger, numbness of tongue and lips, pale or moist skin, and weakness—develop very quickly. If the symptoms are not treated immediately, they may progress to dizziness, slurred speech, loss of coordination, confusion, and unconsciousness. An insulin reaction that occurs at night may lead to excessive sweating, dreaming, morning headache, or confusion upon awakening.

Treatment depends on quick intake of sugar in any form, which should be repeated in fifteen minutes if no improvement is seen. If the diabetic person is unable to swallow, a drug called glucagon can be injected under the skin; it releases glucose into the blood. If that is unavailable, intravenous glucose can be administered. After the reaction is over, eating some slow-digested food like bread, crackers and milk, or a regularly scheduled meal or snack will prevent a second drop.

For insulin-dependent diabetics, the problems of managing diet, insulin, exercise, and stress are much like a balancing act. People hate to get "shocky," but because some of the factors that contribute to shock, especially stress, cannot be fully predicted, insulin-dependent diabetic and those close to them have to learn the signs of shock. Irritability is high on the list, with the patient becoming quite intransigent in her actions as shock progresses. For example, a family member might see a diabetic becoming shocky and insist that she drink a glass of orange juice, which should bring her out of it in ten minutes. The diabetic person might become quite negativistic and refuse, saying she's just fine when she and the family member know she's not fine at all. Many diabetics tell stories of being dragged to the emergency room or forced to drink orange juice by frantic family members.

Complications

Diabetes can affect the eyes, the kidneys, the circulatory system, and the nervous system. The most common eye complication is diabetic retinopathy, a deterioration of the small blood vessels that nourish the retina, the light-sensitive internal coat of the eyeball. It usually does not occur until the patient has had the illness for at least ten years, and it does not occur at all in many people with diabetes. Of the 85 percent with a retinopathy, 80 percent have background retinopathy where vision is not impaired. Another 15 percent have some visual changes, and only 1 to 3 percent have advanced proliferative retinopathy, causing profound visual loss. Some of these problems can be treated with laser surgery by ophthalmologists who have special retina training. Blindness is found in people with diabetes at twenty-five times its rate in the nondiabetic population. In fact, diabetes is the greatest cause of acquired blindness in the United States. Every year approximately 5,000 people with diabetes become blind.

The complication that affects the kidneys is called diabetic nephro-pathy, in which the person may develop protein loss (proteinuria) and fluid retention (edema). Over several years the person may develop renal failure. Once renal failure is complete, the person must be on kidney dialysis, receive a successful kidney transplant, or die. Each year, about thirty diabetics per 2 million population require renal dialysis or transplantation as a result of kidney failure. Diabetics account for 25 percent of the renal dialysis slots in the United States. Kidney failure is the cause of death for 6 percent of the adult diabetic population and about 50 percent of the juvenile diabetic population.

A third complication is peripheral vascular disease, disease of the blood vessels of the limbs. For people with diabetes, gangrene—death of parts of the tissues of the body as a result of inadequate blood supply—is about twenty times more prevalent than in the nondiabetic population. In order to try to save the limb, arterial bypass surgery is performed, in which an attempt is made to bypass arteries that are not functioning and essentially replace them with artificial or transplanted parts. Many people have small vessel disease and are not candidates for bypass. If bypass is successful, an individual may lose a limb in steps in order to save at least part of the leg and increase the opportunitites for rehabilitation. In this process the studies used to direct the surgery present their own set of dangers. To enable the physician to visualize the arteries, contrast material is injected into the arterial system. The introduction of the contrast material increases the risk of kidney failure or stroke. Chiefly because of blood vessel complications, diabetes is a leading cause of death in the United States. Another common complication, diabetic neuropathy, involves the peripheral nervous system and has several manifestations. The first is the possibility of injury or ulceration because of sensory loss. For example, the person cannot feel the pain of a blister on the foot or a cut and so may continue to walk until the unprotected injury has become extensive. The combination of peripheral vascular disease and neuropathy account for the majority of amputations in the United States. A second manifestation of neuropathy, the inability to know where one's legs are, leads to difficulties in walking. A third is foot drop, which can impair walking, increase the chances of injury, and cause a floppy or slapping gait. A fourth is severe pain due to incorrect impulse transmission by the damaged peripheral nerves. A fifth is the inability of the male to have an erection. This last manifestation also has a strong psychological side effect as anticipation of possible impotence may become a self-fulfilling prophecy. Bladder and gastrointestinal mobility problems may also occur as part of the neuropathy, as well as loss of control of blood pressure with change in posture.

Another group of complications relates to heart and blood pressure. After thirty years of diabetes, hypertension is found in 50 percent of diabetes patients. It is estimated that between one-quarter and one-half of the adult diabetic population has coronary heart disease. Diabetic women are at higher risk for coronary heart disease than nondiabetic women.

Another group of complications is related to pregnancy, which affects the body's ability to handle sugar even in nondiabetics. Many women with diabetes can have healthy pregnancies; however, fetal mortality for people with type 1 diabetes is ten times higher than in the nondiabetic population. (Almost all type 2 diabetes is diagnosed after the childbearing years). Several factors are important in regard to pregnancy and diabetes. One is that although the exact pattern of inheritance cannot yet be drawn, heredity is a factor in diabetes. One researcher reports if both parents are diabetic, there is approximately a 50 percent chance that the child will develop diabetes. If only one parent has diabetes, the chance is very small (about 1 percent) that she will develop diabetes before the age of twenty and approximately 10 percent that she will develop the disease in her lifetime. A second factor is that birth defects in infants of diabetic mothers are seven to eight times more frequent than in nondiabetic pregnancies. Costs of pregnancy for a diabetic woman are higher because she must see her physician frequently for adjustments of her insulin and will probably spend more time in the hospital. Another area of difficulty is in managing diet. During the first three months of pregnancy, nausea and vomiting often make it harder to eat properly. Lower caloric intake could lead to insulin reaction, so it may be necessary to lower the insulin intake. Also, since greater amounts of glucose will be present in the blood and urine during pregnancy, more frequent testing is necessary. It is important for the diabetic woman to consume enough calories to keep herself and the fetus healthy without gaining more than about twenty pounds in total. Thus, healthy pregnancy is certainly possible in most situations, but it requires increased effort and scrutiny.

Most patients do not develop complications with either type until fifteen or twenty years after onset. Generally with careful diet, a good exercise program, good care of the extremities, and, if necessary, well-managed insulin or oral medication, chances of complications are greatly lessened. As the patient lives longer with the illness, particularly with in-sulin-dependent diabetes, complications increase.

Diagnosis

For the physician to diagnose a patient as diabetic, blood sugar tests must demonstrate levels above the range considered normal for nondiabetics of the same age. The test results are age-related. For everyone, blood sugar levels rise about 6 to 10 milligrams per decade of life. Patients who have such symptoms as extreme thirst or excessive urination will usually display blood sugars that are significantly elevated following either a meal or fast-ing. Milder diabetics will display normal blood sugars after fasting but elevations after a meal.

Nondiabetics have blood glucose levels of 100 milligrams of sugar per 100 milliliters of blood, or less when tested after fasting overnight. After a meal the blood sugar rises for everyone, but in the nondiabetic person the blood sugar will drop to normal levels in two hours, and in the diabetic person it will stay elevated. A postmeal blood sugar of 120 will make a physician suspect diabetes, and a 200-milligram level will mean a clear diagnosis.

If the physician needs further documentation, a glucose tolerance test is administered: A subject drinks a 75-gram or 100-gram glucose solution. This test is carried out first to establish the diagnosis of diabetes in patients whose fasting blood sugars are borderline; second to test those with normal fasting blood sugars who have disorders of the kidneys, nerves, or eyes that are associated with diabetes; third, to evaluate those who are at risk for the disease, such as relatives of diabetics, obese people, those taking cer-tain drugs, and pregnant women who previously delivered large babies; and fourth, to further evaluate those with unexplained sugar in their ur-ine. In the glucose tolerance test, blood specimens are collected to measure the sugar level in the blood before the person drinks the solution and at half-hour intervals for three to six hours after to test for hypoglycemia (low blood sugar), which is sometimes seen in early diabetics.

Certain procedures must be followed to ensure accurate results from a glucose tolerance test. First, a high-carbohydrate diet must be followed for three days prior to the test. Second, during the test the person must rest and abstain from smoking. Third, the person cannot have been ill for several weeks previous to the test. Fourth, drugs such as Dilantin, steroids, and birth control pills may have to be discontinued previous to the test.

Other diagnostic tests have been developed for diabetes, but they have not been shown to diagnose diabetes more accurately than the standard glucose tolerance test. Three of those tests, primarily research tools, are the intravenous glucose tolerance test, the tolbutamide tolerance test, and the cortisone glucose tolerance test.

Measurement of glycosylated hemoglobin gives a good indication of the presence of the clinically high blood sugar over a long period of time. Glycosylated hemoglobin is the respiratory pigment in the red blood cells to which glucose has attached. The pitfall of using urinary glucose is the variable renal threshold for glucose in different patients; that is, some patients develop glycosuria (glucose in the urine) at a blood sugar of 150 mg%, while others not until 300 mg% or more. For this reason and because blood sugar determinations are easy to do at home, urinary glucose measurements are gradually becoming obsolete.

Therapies

Treatment prescribed for diabetes attempts not to cure the disease but to make up constantly for the deficiencies caused by the disease and to slow the rate of complication. The possibility for cure is in two areas, one still a dream and the other in the experimental stage. If the pancreas could be made to begin to produce and keep producing its own insulin again, that would be the dream cure. If experiments in the transplantation of a healthy or artificial pancreas bear fruit, that could become a cure.

At this time, however, the goal of treatment is to control blood glucose. Control is maintained or restored by balancing food, exercise, stress, and sometimes insulin or oral medication. Surgery is sometimes indicated in the case of severe complications. Life-style interventions regarding food, exercise, and stress will be discussed later, although they are certainly an integral part of the medical regimen. This section will describe insulins, drugs, and surgical interventions.

INSULIN

All type 1 diabetics must take insulin every day. Insulins are categorized according to how long it takes them to begin to act and how long they will continue to act. The three types are short-acting, which have a rapid onset of action and are effective for a short period; intermediate, which have a delayed onset and are effective for about twenty-four hours, and long-acting, which have a slow onset and are effective for about thirty-six hours.

Physicians mix the kinds of insulin they prescribe according to the needs of the particular patient. Although long-acting insulin seems more palatable because it requires fewer injections per day, a short-acting or intermediate insulin may be used by itself or paired with long-acting to ensure better control of the blood sugar.

Injecting itself can produce side effects such as lipoatrophy (wasting of tissue at the injection site) or hypertrophy (thickening of tissue at the site). Both effects can be minimized by varying the site of the injection, using many sites. A third side effect is a possible allergic reaction to certain kinds of insulin. Insulin is generally made from the pancreas of cattle and/or hogs. Some people are allergic to the insulin made from one or the other of those animals, and in those cases it is important not to use the mixed insulins or those made from the animal to which the person is allergic. Human insulin is also now available.

HOME BLOOD TESTING

One of the most revolutionary breakthroughs in diabetic management is the capacity for the diabetic to test the glucose level in her blood as needed. Home monitoring helps the diabetic to adjust blood sugar levels, diet, exercise, and insulin. In the past only home urine testing was available. Because there may be a considerable delay between the time blood sugar rises and the time the rise appears in the urine, if it shows up at all, urine testing is a far less accurate reflection of the current level of control. Diabetics and nondiabetics have varying thresholds for glucose in the urine, so that similar blood levels may correspond to very different urinary levels of glucose.

To measure blood sugar levels, the diabetic needs an implement with which to prick her finger and a strip of chemically treated material on which to place a drop of blood. There are devices available (Autolet and Autoclix) that she can place on her finger and press. They automatically pierce the finger with a lancet and release only the necessary drop of blood. This drop is placed on treated material (Chemstrip or Dextrostix). By matching the color that the treated material has turned from the drop of blood with an accompanying chart, the diabetic can measure her blood sugar level within 10 or 15 points.

If the diabetic has trouble interpreting in this way, or if she must know her exact blood sugar, she can purchase an Ames glucometer, which will give a readout of blood sugar when the Dextrostix is placed in the meter. Only Dextrostix can be used with the meter, and Chemstrips or Accucheck can be used without water. Other machines are available for the same purpose.

ORAL MEDICATION

Some type 2 diabetics take oral hypoglycemic agents, which help stimulate the pancreas to increase its production of insulin. These patients, too, must balance the amount of insulin taken with regular meals and exercise in order to avoid low blood sugar. If they do not, because their pancreas has been stimulated to produce more insulin than they can use, they can have a reaction similar to an insulin reaction. Most type 2 diabetics can manage their illness through careful diet, regular exercise, and monitoring of their blood sugar level to be sure that it remains within the normal range.

THE INSULIN PUMP

The insulin infusion pump has been hailed by some as creating a revolutionary means of supplying insulin. It is basically a battery-driven syringe for continuous injection of insulin, which can achieve normal or near-normal glucose levels in selected patients. To be used successfully, it demands careful monitoring of blood glucose levels and consequent adjustment of the dosage pumped. Its value is that it allows the diabetic more freedom and assurance of proper management. An important concern has been the question of advancing retina disease. As of May 24, 1982, the Disease Control Center in Atlanta reported 4,000 to 5,000 pumps sold in this country and twenty-four deaths in insulin pump treated diabetics. None of the deaths resulted from mechanical failure. Several were due to hypoglycemia. Success of the pump seems to require careful patient selection, individualization of glycemia goals, and intensive patient education.

SURGERY

Surgery is indicated in two instances. First, in cases of impotence an inflatable penile prosthesis can be implanted. Second, in cases of severe vascular disease by-pass surgery is attempted; if by-pass surgery fails, amputation of some part of the leg is performed in order to prevent gangrene.

Looking to the future, there is great hope for the possibility of pancreatic transplant, which theoretically should cure the illness. A healthy pancreas would regulate the production and distribution of insulin. It would also entail the problems of harvesting and dealing with immune systems that the transplantation of other organs has brought.

Psychosocial Information

Modifications in Life-Style

Diabetes, especially insulin-dependent diabetes, can affect every aspect of one's life. It is always there. Because the metabolism depends on so many factors, the person with diabetes is constantly in a balancing act. Once she has taken insulin, she is governed by it. She must eat enough of what she is supposed to eat, when she is supposed to eat it. She must exercise enough, but if she exercises more than the necessary amount, she will have to eat more, but not too much more. In addition, she must allow for the stresses of the day, but there are always stresses that can not be antici- pated—on the job, in family life, driving, or many other areas.

For example, what if a person with diabetes decides to save some of her fruit and fat exchanges from lunch for an ice cream snack in the after- noon? Her boss then calls an emergency meeting before she can have this snack, in order to call the diabetic and her section on the carpet. After the meeting the person, now very anxious, eats too much, trying to prevent shock. As a result she needs a bolus of insulin, and so the day see-saws. One diabetic informant used the analogy of the bumpy road. If a non- diabetic is driving along and notices a funny change in her driving, she says, "Is this the car, or is it the road?" In the same situation, a person with diabetes says, "Is it the car, is it the road, or is it me?" There is always the factor of diabetes to consider. Since no insulin-dependent diabetic can live forever shock and complication free, the person with diabetes ulti- mately organizes her own risks and satisfactions.

DIET

Because the effective conversion of food into energy is the focus of the treatment of diabetes, diet is the pivot on which the rest of the treatment plan turns. If one is a type 2, non-insulin-dependent diabetic, the point of careful diet is to keep the intake of carbohydrates low in order for the moderately functioning pancreas to put out enough insulin to match the output of glucose. If one is a type 1, insulin-dependent diabetic, the point of careful diet is to take in enough carbohydrate for the insulin injected to be used and, on the other hand, to see that no more carbohydrate has been ingested than could be matched by the amount of insulin ingested. More carbohydrate than can be processed by the amount of insulin present can produce hyperglycemia and ultimately diabetic coma. More insulin than is needed to process the amount of carbohydrate present can result in insulin shock. Type 2 diabetics generally experience only hyperglycemia or diabetic coma, although those on oral medication can experience some shock. Type 1 diabetics can experience insulin shock as well as hypergly- cemia or coma.

The importance of diet was recognized early in the treatment of dia- betes. However, in an effort to keep the intake of carbohydrates low, pa- tients in earlier times were keeping their total food intake exceedingly low and literally starving themselves to death. Today two points about diet are generally agreed upon by diabetologists. First, regular, well-balanced meals help control the amount of sugar in the blood. Second, maintaining ideal body weight is very important. In fact, in overweight non-insulin-dependent diabetics, risk for type 1 diabetes doubles for every 20 percent of excess weight.

The aspect of diet about which diabetologists do not appear to agree is the strictness with which it is necessary to follow a prescribed diet. Some say that avoidance of foods high in sugar content and in saturated fats and cholesterol, and a regimen of regular meals, are critical. Others say that the tightest control of food intake with no cheating is the only way to control the disease and avoid complications.

The diet indicated for type 1 and type 2 diabetics is basically the same. However, type 1 diabetics are governed by the insulin they have injected. Once they have given themselves the shot, they must feed the insulin or will develop some of the symptoms described earlier.

The "Exchange Diet," which is distributed widely, is a technique for grouping foods of similar values so that the diabetic can plan and vary meals while still maintaining the prescribed diet. The exchange diet divides all permitted foods into six groups depending on the amount of carbohydrate, protein, and fat they contain. The six groups are milk, vegetable, fruit (sugar), breads (starch), meat (protein), and fat. Listed under fats are butter, dressings, and other foods high in fat content like avocado, nuts, and bacon. Listed under bread are cakes, breads, cereals, and such vegetables such as corn, baked beans, and potatoes. Correct portions are indicated, as are miscellaneous foods that cross groups and so count as two types of exchange. For example, one-half cup of vanilla ice cream is equal to one bread and two fat exchanges, and two tablespoons of peanut butter are equal to one meat and two fat exchanges. Certain additional foods are allowed in reasonable amounts. This category includes seasonings like vinegar, garlic, and pepper as well as coffee, tea, bouillon, and unflavored gelatin.

The accompanying table shows a day's meals for a 1,500-calorie diet. By following the exchange diet, modified for her life-style, the diabetic is receiving the correct amount of fat, protein, carbohydrates, and calories, eliminating concentrated sweets and maintaining a regular meal schedule.

FOOD	AMOUNT	EXCHANGE	LIST
Breakfast			
Orange juice	one cup	2 fruit	3
Cereal, dry	3/4 cup	2 bread	4
Toast	1 slice		
Egg	1	1 meat	5
Margarine	1 tsp	1 fat	6
Skim milk	1 cup	1 milk	1

Continued on next page

Continued from previous page

FOOD	AMOUNT	EXCHANGE	LIST
Lunch			
Cold cuts	1-1/2 oz sl.	2 meat	5
Cheese	1 oz.		
Bread	2 slices	2 bread	4
Carrot and celery sticks	1/2 cup	1 vegetable	2
Apples	2 small	2 fruit	3
Mayonnaise-type dressing	4 tsp	2 fat	6
Dinner			
Chicken, baked	3 oz.	3 meat	5
Peas	1/2 cup	2 bread	4
Potatoes, mashed	1/2 cup		
Tomatoes	1 cup	2 vegetables	2
Lettuce, etc.	as desired		
Fruit cocktail	1/2 cup	1 fruit	3
Margarine	1 tsp	1 fat	6
Skim milk	1/2 cup	1/2 milk	1
French dressing, low-calorie	1 tbsp.		
Bedtime snack			
Graham crackers	2 squares	1 bread	4
Skim milk	1/2 cup	1/2 milk	1

EXERCISE

Exercise is also critical in the life of the diabetic. Sufficient exercise burns calories, so that less insulin is required to process food into energy. Increased exercise requires an increase in food intake in order to avoid insulin shock. It is thought that exercise improves circulation and therefore inhibits peripheral vascular disease.

Diabetics face the same dangers from exercise as anyone else but must take extra precautions. For example, skiing, expecially cross-country skiing, is fine, but because there is always the possibility of shock, the diabetic should not ski alone, should have sufficient food available for regular meals and emergencies, and should take extra care that his feet are warm, without blisters or abrasions. In fact, it could be said that exercise is even necessary, but the diabetic must be most careful.

FOOT CARE

The foot is an area where small problems that are inconsequential for the nondiabetic can wreak havoc in the person with diabetes. Because peripheral nerves may not function normally and sense injury, the diabetic may not notice a blister that would cause pain to a nondiabetic. In a short time that blister can become an open sore. Because the healing process requires a good flow of blood and the diabetic may not have a good flow, healing may be slow. Increased sugar in the blood also allows infection to breed, as does the warm, dark moist air found in a shoe. Thus, a cut or sore on the foot is more likely to become infected, and the diabetic is less able to fight infection. Daily inspection of the feet is required; shoes and socks should be properly fitted; nails should be trimmed straight across, and other precautions should be taken, including regular visits to a podiatrist.

DENTAL CARE

Because diabetes lowers the resistance to infection and retards healing, extra care must be taken concerning the teeth and gums. Without care, periodontal disease can be severe enough to destroy gums and even supporting bone. Once teeth lose supporting bone, they can become loose and eventually fall out.

In addition, those with diabetes can also have tooth decay, dry mouth, degeneration of the nerves of the tooth, and ulcerations of the oral mucous membranes. Finally, in periodontal treatment, extensive dental care, or surgery diabetes must be well managed, and the person must receive preventive antibiotic premedication.

RESTRICTION OF CERTAIN ACTIVITIES

Restriction relates entirely to physical changes. It would be dangerous for a diabetic to be without the necessary food groups for a long period or without insulin if she is insulin-dependent. Likewise, it would be dangerous to engage in activities with inflexible timing. If the diabetic's proprioceptive responses are affected or if her peripheral nerves are damaged, she should not engage in activities that depend on those facilities. For example, boxing, hot dog skiing, motorcycle riding, and long-distance trucking would be dangerous choices for at least insulin-dependent diabetics, although some, through extraordinary discipline and precautionary measure, could master them all.

SLEEP OR REST PATTERNS

Because sleep is related to the ways in which the body metabolizes food and to stress and relaxation, it is important for the person with diabetes to have sufficient rest and sleep. In some cases of type 1 diabetes sugar will drop during the night, and the person will wake up hypoglycemic or shocky. If that is a pattern, the insulin should be checked by a physician. Regular patterns of shock should not occur.

STRESS AND RELAXATION TECHNIQUES

Along with insulin maintenance, diet, and exercise, stress is a critical factor in the management of diabetes. It is also the most difficult factor to anticipate. Stress occurs when a change in a person's environment causes a particular response in her body in which the nervous system is activated and certain hormones are released. When a person with diabetes feels stressed, it is also harder to recognize the beginning signs of shock, such as sweating or experiencing a change in emotion, because they resemble normal reactions to stressful situations.

Thus, stress can interrupt the control of diabetes leading to metabolic decompensation (the rise of glucose and ketones) and ketoacidosis (diabetic coma). At times severe stress can upset control to the point where a diabetic who does not require insulin may need it until the stress is over, or a very stressful period may signal the beginning of insulin dependence.

It is important, then, for those with diabetes to learn to control the impact of stress. A variety of different relaxation techniques have been espoused. In biofeedback, feedback from a monitor allows the person to see how her thoughts and feelings can control her inner responses; yoga involves techniques of deep breathing, stretching, and concentrating on one's heartbeat; in self-hypnosis, the person repeats and concentrates on a short sentence until her body responds to suggestion and relaxes. Another technique involves progressive relaxation, in which the individual is taught to relax one set of muscles at a time, working through the body. In meditation, the person focuses on a single word, phrase, or image in order to relax; and in guided imagery, someone helps the individual to imagine herself in pleasant situations. It is recommended that people think through the ways in which they handle stress as well as the situations in which they feel the most stressed, so that they can lower their own responses.

DAILY SCHEDULE

Regularity is critical to self-management. One diabetic informant says that diabetes imposes a grid over one's life. Particularly with type 1 diabetes, an individual must live by the clock. If she complies with the treatment plan, the clock becomes like another person organizing her life. "It can be like a sentence. Now you have to . . ." The diabetic must schedule insulin or oral medication, meals, exercise, and sleep in ways that might be good for everyone but to which no one else must adhere. The difference, of course, is in the consequences, in weighing the risks. If the diabetic does not conform to a daily schedule in which the amount of insulin or oral medication, food, exercise, and stress are the same as that of the day before and the day after, she runs the risk of getting sick. Thus, there are parameters with which the diabetic must comply in order to maximize her chances of getting through a day without feeling sick.

Social Aspects

LEGAL ISSUES

Diabetics are not restricted by law from operating a motor vehicle or from marriage. Their rights to training and to work are protected through federal regulations making it illegal for most large employers to reject diabetics unless diabetes would make the work hazardous (see "Ability to Work"). In many states the person with diabetes is considered handicapped and is thus eligible for a wide range of services. The many Developmental Disabilities Acts also have increased available services for diabetics. One thinks of developmental disabilities often in terms of retardation, but in fact the term refers to conditions that originate during the developmental years.

INSURANCE

Once an individual has been diagnosed as having diabetes, particularly type 1, insurance is difficult to obtain except in group plans. Medical, life, automobile, and mortgage insurance all present problems in acquisition. In each case companies differ in their attitudes toward diabetes, and it is always important to approach several in order to find the most favorable plan. The Diabetes Group Insurance Trust has established a range of insurance programs for diabetics underwritten by the Sentry Life Insurance Company.

Diabetics are eligible for a range of federal insurance plans, among them Medicare, the End Stage Renal Disease program, Medicaid, Crippled Childrens Services, and Vocational Rehabilitation Services for Blind and Visually Handicapped. Finally, Social Security and Disability Insurance is available for the severely disabled.

FINANCIAL ASPECTS

The financial burdens of diabetes are significant. They are greater, once again, for type 1 diabetics than for type 2. Type 1 diabetics must pay for insulin and syringes, which average from 60 cents to $1.05 a day. Assuming that they have some sort of insurance coverage for their major medical expenses, they still have significant preventive medical expenses. Regular medical examinations by internist, endocrinologist or diabetologist, ophthalmologist, dentist, and podiatrist may be supplemented with visits to a dermatologist, and to a urologist for male patients, and very frequent visits to a gynecologist–obstetrician for a pregnant or prepregnant female. Dietary instruction is necessary at several points in the life of a diabetic, because nutritional needs change as one ages, and the diabetic diet often requires that the individual spend more for food.

In this era of home blood glucose monitoring, the diabetic also must pay for the costs of testing, including a monitor for readings.

But the costs of complications are by far the greatest. Loss of vision, cardiovascular impairment, and loss of all or part of a limb or limbs cause the person to add tremendous costs to even her daily living expenses. Financial burdens are even greater for the elderly. All told, money spent for preventive care may save or forestall expenses incurred by later complications.

RELATIONSHIPS WITH OTHERS

Family Members.   Because diabetes affects activities of daily living and often "runs in families," it becomes a family issue. Adaptation is related to many factors, particularly age of onset and type of diabetes. Type 2, non-insulin-dependent diabetes, makes far less demands on the lives of the diabetic and her family than does type 1. With type 1 the presence of the insulin and the knowledge that one has to "feed" it properly or feel unwell changes the place of diabetes in the life of the family.

In terms of age of onset, a very sick child who is dependent on family members for care changes the life of the family. Obviously, the younger and more dependent the child, the more difficult it is for the family to make a healthy adjustment. Some families deal with this situation very well, and others become "diabetic families," whose identity is the illness. Much of the individual adjustment depends on strengths and weaknesses present before the diabetes was detected.

The prime social issue, responsibility, has two sides. The first relates to feelings of guilt that family members may have because someone, especially a child, contracts the disease. Parents will note that there is diabetes on one side of the family or the other, or mothers will say they have not properly cared for the child or she would not have become diabetic. That problem also exists for spouses who sometimes think that if something had been different in their lives together, their wives or husbands would not have become ill. The second responsibility issue concerns who takes charge of monitoring and maintenance. When the diabetic is in shock, knowledgeable people around her—adults or children—must assume some responsibility. However, in most situations when a person is healthy in other respects, she can administer insulin and check blood glucose levels by the time she is ten years old. Ironically, parents will often allow the child to take responsibility for those facets of her treatment but will not expect her to monitor her own diet, exercise program, and stress management. All these factors are equally important in what must clearly be a self-managed disease. The sooner a child is able to take responsibility for the management of her illness, with consultation and monitoring by physician and parents, the better are her chances of developing as a person with diabetes rather than a person whose sense of self has been totally shaped by diabetes.

Onset of diabetes during puberty is common. During this period, hormonal, social, and psychological adjustments are difficult even for teens with no physical difficulties. Moreover, diabetes affects those activities in which teens are most usually engaged. For example, going out with friends at nine o'clock at night for a pizza and a coke is considered harmless by teens and parents. As a matter of fact, parents today would breathe a sigh of relief knowing that that was how their teenagers were entertaining themselves. However, the type 1 diabetic would have to be thinking about food exchanges and to have eaten less dinner in order to take part in a pizza party.

The teen years are times when many are experimenting with alcohol, yet all but an occasional glass of wine is forbidden to the diabetic. Teens begin to smoke, too, and smoking for people who are more prone to cardiovascular disease is really courting danger. Some teens may more or less casually experiment with drugs, but diabetics cannot experiment without risking the delicate balance of food, insulin, exercise, and stress with which they are living. Drugs may not only have an effect on blood sugar but also impair the ability to react to an emergency, such as insulin shock. If the adolescent's diabetes is not controlled, she cannot drive. The risk of shock is too great. Thus she must postpone obtaining her driver's license, her badge of young adulthood, until her diabetes is controlled.

The teenage years, then, are especially difficult for diabetics. At a time when most are allowed to be a bit wild, free, and experimental, teens with diabetes are told to be careful, controlled, and disciplined. Of course many, probably most, are not as careful as physician and family would like. It is the period in which noncompliance rates are highest. Denial of the illness and living for the present help the adolescent to pretend that she is no different at a time when it seems critical to be like everyone else.

Sexual Activity.   Diabetes does not affect a person's sexual desire or fertility. Because sexual intercourse is a physical activity, it is best to eat extra carbohydrates to avoid an insulin reaction, just as one would before engaging in sports or other increased exercise. One of the recognized complications of diabetes for males is impotence, which can occur fifteen or twenty years after onset. As mentioned previously, anticipated impotence also can create psychological problems. Sexual response in women is not affected generally, but psychological problems can occur, especially when onset is coupled with adolescence.

Strangers. The relationship of the diabetic to strangers seems to depend on the type of diabetes. With type 2 diabetes, if one can maintain diet, there is no reason to discuss the illness. With type 1 the insulin and the illness enter much more into the life of the person. If there is a possibility of insulin shock, and no friend or family member is around, a stranger should be informed about possibilities. Since diabetes does not "show," however, it is up to the person with diabetes whether to discuss it or not.

Dependence/Isolation. To some extent, because of the possibility of insulin shock, there is increased dependence. However, except in rare cases of highly labile diabetes or severe complications, there should not be increased confinement or social isolation. If the diabetic is physically able, confinement and isolation would reflect a poor self-image, which should be improved with counseling.

ABILITY TO WORK

As was mentioned before, the only situations in which a type 1 diabetic is restricted are those in which insulin shock would endanger her or her co-workers. The federal government does not allow insulin-dependent diabetics to pilot airplanes, join the military, or drive buses or trucks interstate. Some jobs, like policeman or fireman, are hazardous because of long, erratic hours and the possibility of emergency situations and high stress. Others, like working on high scaffolds or around high-speed machinery, do not allow necessary flexibility. Otherwise the ability to work is the same as it is for the rest of the population.

DIET AND SOCIAL LIFE

To see the relationship of social life and diet, one has only to think of the place of food in any social occasion from Baptism to marriage to burial. Still, the current fashion of slim bodies and nutritious meal planning has come close to the ideal diabetic diet. One middle-aged informant who is a type 2 diabetic reports that it is easy to dine out at friends' houses and keep to her diet, because everybody is dieting, and broiled chicken and vegetables seem to be the dinner of choice. Of course, the real issue is that others can cheat and not pay so dearly. Diabetics can cheat a little, but if they cheat too much they pay with the symptoms of high sugar. If they cover the high sugar with too much insulin, they pay with the symptoms of insulin shock.

RECREATIONAL ACTIVITY

The issue with recreation is whether the activity can endanger the diabetic or anyone around her. If there is no danger, the activity is fine. If the danger is only to the diabetic but, through social supports and precautionary measures, she can protect herself, the activity may be relatively safe.

Unless the person with diabetes gets sufficient exercise from her work, it is essential for her to engage in a regular recreational exercise program every day. Suggestions about the form this exercise should take have run the gamut from jogging to tennis to weightlifting to strenuous walking. Regular strenuous exercise helps convert food into energy, may reduce the insulin requirement, and at best reduces or defers the possibility of cardiovascular complication.

DAILY SCHEDULE

Diabetes makes the clock a member of the family. In order to make the metabolism of food as predictable as possible and to take every precaution against either insulin shock or an elevated blood sugar, a regular daily schedule of meals, exercise, and, if necessary, insulin or oral medication is necessary. Just as foods can be exchanged for those of similar value, so can exercise. Type 1 diabetics also say that occasionally they have to compensate for eating something extra, increased stress, or a change in exercise pattern with a compensating or covering dose of insulin. If such an adjustment becomes part of the daily pattern, the physician should be consulted about adjustment of dosage or type of insulin.

Psychological Aspects

SELF-CONCEPT

Because type 1 diabetes becomes a central part of one's life, it must dramatically affect self-concept. Age of onset is important. A child with diabetes grows up with the illness as part of her. By the same token, if a teenager becomes diabetic, she adds diabetes to her adolescent development.

An adult who has a lifetime of experiences and a developed idea of herself makes diabetes part of an already established identity. Again, previous experiences, social supports, and the psychological state of the person before diabetes is detected all contribute to the effect that the illness will have on the person.

There are some type 1 diabetics who have diabetes as their identity. When asked what they are, they will probably say diabetic first and describe other roles like daughter, student, or friend after. For others, the illness is something that must be managed but is a small part of the sense of self.

Still, one informant who is a successful professional with a rich personal life says that when he uses the expression, "I don't know where I am" he means, "I don't know at what level my blood sugar is." Thus, even in well-adjusted people with type 1 diabetes, the illness, and particularly the continuous measurement and management of it, becomes a significant part of identity.

STAGES OF PSYCHOLOGICAL RESPONSE

Often the diagnosis of type 1 diabetes occurs in the hospital. The patient is overwhelmed with the diagnosis and especially with all medical personnel telling her that she can live a normal life because a TV star, Mary Tyler Moore, and a hockey player, Bobby Clark, both have diabetes. The patient's response is first to be very passive and accepting in order to try to handle the news. It has been suggested by diabetic informants that to tell a type 1 diabetic that she will be able to live a normal life is a lie. To stay well, she will have to live by the clock, eat by the book, inject herself every day, and exercise vigorously every day, and she will still have bouts of insulin reaction. Such a life-style, though it would be healthy for everyone, is not normal.

The diabetic's next response is either to get angry that this has happened to her, to deny that she is ill, or both. If social supports are understanding and if there is someone with whom the diabetic can talk, she can move through this stage to the time when dealing with diabetes becomes a part of her life. One informant said, "You get tired of constantly attending to yourself." People resent having diabetes, but they can learn to live with it.

CHANGE IN MOOD OR AFFECT

Some mood swing, especially an irritable time late in the afternoon, is common. Of course, that is a low time for many people, but it is a time when many type 1 diabetics get a little shocky. Irritability is also an early sign of insulin reaction. Informants say that they become negative and will refuse to let people help them because that is part of their reaction.

How to Be Helpful to Someone with Diabetes

A person with insulin-dependent diabetes is governed by the clock. She must eat a restricted diet and is to some extent subject to insulin shock. Helping the person to manage this part of her life and not trying to promote breaches of the restrictions are important. The theme of self-management extends to exercise and handling stress as well. All aspects of a person's life that affect the production of insulin have to be

juggled and balanced to achieve the best control. Note the signs of beginning shock. If the person does get shocky, offer her a piece of hard candy
or, even better, some orange juice. Primarily, to be most helpful one should
respect the illness and the place it must have in the person's life, then
assume that, except in the case of shock, the person will manage her illness
as she manages the rest of her life.

6

The Epilepsies

EPILEPSY IS a collective term for a group of disorders caused by abnormal brain cell electrical activity. Each disorder of the group involves some sort of seizure associated with either loss or disturbance of consciousness, an abnormal psychic experience or behavior, or abnormal motor or sensory phenomena. Usually, but not always, epilepsy involves convulsive movements of the body. Sometimes it involves uncontrolled hyperactivity or only momentary inattention. In fact, epilepsy is not a disease but a set of symptoms.

The term epilepsy is derived from the Greek meaning "to be seized" or "to be laid hold of." Twenty-five centuries ago Hippocrates denied the "divine" or "sacred" nature of epilepsy, but even today myths and fears about epilepsy persist. In these times particularly, when 90 percent of people with epilepsy can have their seizures controlled through medication, the greatest problem is ignorance about the manifestations and ramifications of the illness.

A compounding common problem is the confusion of epilepsy with other impairments of the brain such as mental retardation and cerebral palsy. People with certain forms of mental retardation or cerebral palsy are more likely to have a seizure disorder than the rest of the population, but people with other forms of these disorders do not have a higher incidence of epilepsy. For example, spastic diplegia, a form of cerebral palsy involving weakness with spasticity in the legs, and choreoathetosis, a spontaneous movement disorder resulting from the involvement of deep gray matter structures in the brain, are not generally associated with seizures.

In the same way, having epilepsy does not increase one's likelihood of having cerebral palsy or of being mentally retarded.

Medical Information

In epilepsy the specific nature and frequency of seizures is more important to understanding the impact of the disease than the diagnosis itself. For example, frequent psychomotor seizures will affect someone's life differently from absence seizures or even very infrequent grand mal seizures. As a rule, epilepsy is neither fatal nor progressive. Although its course, in most forms, is predictable, its crises are not. In fact, the inability to predict the onset of a seizure is an important factor in the lives of people with epilepsy and those around them. Many people with epilepsy say no matter what else they are doing, the question remains, "Will I have a seizure today?"

Classification

Seizures are classified as either generalized or partial. It is common for people with epilepsy to have had both kinds of seizures at some time in their lives. Generalized seizures involve both sides of the brain and a disturbance of consciousness. If the abnormal activity is confined to only part of the brain, the seizure is described as partial and the area of the brain involved is called the epileptic focus.

Tonic-clonic (grand mal), absence (petit mal), infantile spasms, and some others are considered generalized seizures. Tonic-clonic seizures involve loss of consciousness, motor convulsions, and some amnesia. They may or may not begin with an aura, a warning or premonition comprising noises in the ears, flashes of light, olfactory hallucinations, vertigo, or myriad other neurologic signs. The first movements in the seizure are tonic, that is, stiffening and contracting. The next are clonic—shaking movements in which the muscles contract and relax. At times people bite their tongues, lips, or cheeks; lose sphincter control; or, very occasionally, even fracture their vertebrae. A tonic-clonic seizure can last from a few seconds to fifteen or twenty minutes, but the average length is about five minutes. People rarely survive a seizure of fifteen or twenty minutes' duration. Bystanders should move things out of the way that could hurt the seizing person but should not move the person until the seizure is over. The period following a seizure, called the postictal phase, can be characterized by any neurological deficit, depending on the part of the brain where the seizure originated. The most common symptoms are extraordinary fatigue and confusion. This period usually lasts fifteen to thirty minutes, but it can last up to twenty-four hours.

Absence seizures are characterized by very brief losses of consciousness, often associated with fluttering of the eyelids and mild twitching of the mouth. Infantile spasms usually occur in the first year of life and are characterized by clonic seizures of short duration.

Partial seizures occur with less frequency than generalized seizures. They are classified as simple partial seizures, complex partial seizures, and secondarily generalized seizures. Simple partial seizures may involve disturbances in motor or sensory function. They may begin with an unusual sensation or movement of some part of the body or with visual or auditory sensations. Complex partial seizures are characterized by subjective symptoms like feelings of strangeness or inappropriate familiarity, illusions or visions, or involuntary and apparently purposeful activities, followed by amnesia for these events. The now-outdated terms for these seizures were psychomotor seizures or temporal lobe seizures. Secondarily generalized seizures begin as partial and become generalized.

Etiology

Different types of seizures occur for a variety of reasons. Generalized major motor seizures, for example, may be caused by toxic-metabolic disturbances, structural lesions of the brain like tumor or stroke, or high fevers in young children, or the cause may be unknown. Absence seizures tend to have no identifiable cause. Often focal or partial seizures are caused by specific structural lesions.

The age at which the person begins having seizures is often very helpful in determining the cause of the seizures. For example, generalized seizures that occur in the newborn are often of metabolic origin, specifically due to hypoglycemia (decreased blood sugar) or hypocalcemia (decreased calcium in the blood). Seizures that occur in the newborn may also be due to an infection like meningitis or generalized sepsis. They may be the result of very high fevers in young children or of congenital lesions occurring prenatally or caused by a birth injury. Seizures that occur for the first time in childhood or adolescence are usually of idiopathic (unknown) origin.

Seizures that begin in the third or fourth decade of life are particularly ominous. Trauma is one of the most common causes of epilepsy in young adults. About 5 percent of people with severe closed head injuries have epilepsy within two years of the trauma. If the injury penetrates the skull and the dura matter, the outer fibrous membrane surrounding the brain, the incidence rises to 30 to 50 percent. Seizures are most likely to occur within the first year following the injury; 90 percent of the risk of post-traumatic epilepsy is over by the end of the second year.

Sometimes generalized tonic-clonic seizures develop during chronic alcohol or barbiturate intoxication, almost always in periods of reduction or withdrawal from the substance. Over several hours the person experiences one or more seizures or short bursts of two to six seizures. After barbiturate withdrawal convulsions can recur for several days. Alcohol or its withdrawal can also precipitate seizures in anyone with epilepsy after an evening or a weekend of heavy social drinking. It is important to distinguish between alcohol-precipitated epilepsy and withdrawal seizures. The long-term management of withdrawal seizures consists of continued abstinence from the drug. Long-term use of antiepileptic medicine is not helpful and can be dangerous, since drug abusers often stop their treatment abruptly also and can thus accentuate the risk of precipitating a withdrawal seizure.

When there is no history of head trauma, substance abuse, or withdrawal, these seizures are often due to brain tumor, stroke, or other structural lesions of the brain. When a seizure disorder begins after age twenty, the person has a 10 percent chance of having a brain tumor. The risk changes a little with advancing age: 11 percent after age forty, 15 percent after age fifty, including primary tumors as well as those which have spread from other sites. In 50 percent of people with brain tumors, epilepsy can be halted by removal of the tumor.

Arteriosclerotic cerebrovascular disease is the most common cause of seizures in people over fifty. Approximately 4 percent of people who have brain infarction and about 10 percent of those with bleeding within the brain have seizures accompanying the stroke. Another 3 percent of people with stroke have recurrent seizures in later life, possibly generated by the cerebral scar. Hypertension—high blood pressure—predisposes one to cerebrovascular disease (disease of the blood vessels of the brain), especially bleeding within the brain. Seizures occur in about 20 percent of people with hypertensive encephalopathy, a disease of the brain that results from accelerated hypertension. Other vascular causes of seizures at almost any age include collagen vascular disease. In 15 percent of people with systemic lupus erythematosus, the first manifestation of the illness is a seizure. In heart disease, emboli to the brain can produce a stroke, which may cause seizures. Transient cardiac arrest or cessation of breathing with subsequent deficiency in oxygen to the brain may result in seizures. Aneurysms represent a much less common but potential cause of seizures.

Infections of the central nervous system, such as certain forms of meningitis occurring in newborns and in the six-month to five-year age group, may cause seizures. Status epilepticus, in which one seizure follows another almost continuously, is a common complication of meningitis and has a high mortality in this age group. Seizures are a frequent manifestation of brain abscess.

Although no single factor has been identified as the primary cause of epilepsy, several factors have been identified that may precipitate seizures in susceptible individuals. Such factors include hyperventilation (rapid, deep breathing), sleep (usually within the first thirty minutes or just before waking), sleep deprivation, certain sensory stimuli (such as flashing lights), reading, speaking, watching television, coughing, laughing, touch, pain, and specific sounds such as music or bells. Hormonal changes such as puberty, menses, or those caused by adrenal steroids may also be predisposing factors. Fever, emotional stress, and drugs such as phenothiazines, analeptics, tricyclic mood elevators, alcohol, antihistamines, and overdoses of anticonvulsants may also lead to seizures.

Prevalence

The fact that epilepsy is a set of symptoms rather than a single disease accounts, to some degree, for the great difficulty in obtaining statistics relating the prevalence and incidence. The National Institute for Health Statistics reports a prevalence of 966,082 for 1981. Using that figure, approximately 5 out of every 1,000 people in the United States have epilepsy. On the other hand, the National Institute of Neurological and Communicative Disorders and Stroke reports a prevalence of 2,135,000. Epilepsy is the second most prevalent neurological disorder after stroke.

Peak incidences for the onset of epilepsy in childhood are the first two years of life, ages five through seven, and, especially in girls, early puberty. Incidence is said to be highest in the first year of life, then diminishes with each age group until age sixty, at which point it begins to increase again. Both incidence and type of epilepsy are related to age of onset, because the developing brain has more limited reactions to injury and because the inherited predisposition is most often expressed in childhood. As the brain grows and matures, the developmental patterns of epilepsy change both electrically and clinically. Thus the same stimulus, such as hypocalcemia (decreased calcium in the blood), can cause a partial seizure in the newborn and a generalized seizure in the adolescent or adult.

Most studies show that mortality rates for people with epilepsy are age-related, with the highest mortality rate being for those under age five and the next highest for those over sixty-five. The third highest mortality rates are for those between twenty-five and forty-five. Generally the earlier the age of onset, the higher the mortality rate. Onset after age thirty generally means normal life expectancy. Those with severe and uncontrolled epilepsy have a higher death rate than other groups. As a rule, the average life expectancy for people with epilepsy seems to be slightly lower than that of the general population.

Populations at Risk

Epilepsy knows no cultural, national, or racial boundaries. The particular populations at risk for seizures include only ones with specific predisposing medical bases. For example, people with histories of birth injuries, trauma, substance abuse and withdrawal, or structural brain lesions are all more likely to have seizures. One does not inherit epilepsy *per se* but rather a predisposition. The risk of idiopathic epilepsy through age twenty among children and siblings of people with epilepsy was three times the rate of the general population. Having two parents with epilepsy increases the chances of the child's having the disorder. Generally genetic factors are most important when epilepsy begins in childhood and decrease in importance with age. In a study entitled *Genetics of Epilepsy: A Review*, Newmark and Penry say that 30 to 40 percent of unselected patients with seizures, including people who have had only one seizure, will have had someone else in their family also have seizures. Up to 10 percent of the offspring of such patients may have epilepsy, with the highest rate present in the offspring of affected mothers. Males have a higher rate than females, supposedly because men have been subjected to more head trauma. Finally, more than 75 percent of those with epilepsy have their first attack before age eighteen. Conditions associated with high risk of late epilepsy include a depressed skull fracture, an acute blood-filled swelling in the brain, partial or complete loss of memory lasting more than twenty-four hours after a trauma, and tears in the fibrous outer covering of the brain (the dura), or specific neurologic signs.

Natural History

If left untreated, repetitive seizures may result in a lowered level of oxygen in the blood and thus in the brain. An insufficiency of oxygen to the brain can result in brain injury, which can result, in turn, in more seizures. Except in the case of status epilepticus, where epileptic attacks follow each other almost continuously without the person's regaining consciousness, seizures are not constant even though the lesion causing the epilepsy is constantly present and the electroencephalogram may be consistently abnormal.

The natural history of epilepsy depends to a great extent on its etiology. Young children who have febrile seizures generally are free of seizures later in life. Seizures of metabolic origin may not recur once the metabolic problem is identified and treated. Seizures due to structural lesions of the brain behave variably, and the issue of greatest concern is the behavior of the underlying disease. Occasionally prolonged seizures may precipitate a heart attack or disturbance in heart rate.

Association with Other Diseases

Epilepsy is associated with several other disorders that involve the brain. As was mentioned earlier, those who are mentally retarded or who have cerebral palsy have a higher rate of seizures than the population as a whole. Also, seizures are often the initial clinical presentation or a subsequent complication of stroke. People who are hyperglycemic (elevated blood sugar) or hypoglycemic (abnormally low blood sugar) as a result of diabetes or its treatment may have seizures as a presenting symptom. Disturbances of sodium and calcium metabolism are also associated with seizures. Seizures of various types may be clinical manifestations of infections that occur in children and adults such as meningitis (an inflammation of the surrounding membranes of the brain and spinal cord) and encephalitis (an inflammation of the brain). Finally, head injuries can result in structural lesions of the brain associated with seizures, either at the time of the injury or as long as years later.

Diagnosis

Diagnosis begins with a medical history, including details about the birth process and the health of other family members. Questions are asked about substance abuse and head trauma, either of which can be a basis for seizures. Developmental milestones, such as when someone began to walk and talk, are reviewed to measure the person's development in relation to a normal time frame. People are asked to describe any warning symptoms they have about the onset of a seizure, how long it lasts, and how the person reacts afterward. This information helps to identify the area of the brain in which the seizure originates. Also recorded is the relationship of seizures to specific precipitating factors such as lack of sleep or flashing lights.

In addition to the general medical examination, a neurological examination is performed. This includes a careful examination of the head and neck for abnormal sounds that occasionally occur with blood vessel malformations in the brain and can cause seizures. An individual's mental status is assessed (for a fuller explanation, see Chapter 4, "The Dementias"), the twelve cranial nerves are examined, including tests of the ability to smell, vision, appearance of the optic nerve (the nerve connecting the brain to the eye), eye movement, facial motor and sensory function, taste, and the muscles of articulation, chewing, and swallowing. The tongue and neck are examined as well. Next, the motor examination assesses balance and the part of the brain that coordinates motor function by having the person walk normally, on her heels, on her toes, and in tandem. Motor function is tested more specifically, often comparing one side of the body with the other. Reflexes are checked, using a rubber hammer. A sensory examination is carried out as well, looking for impaired sensations to hot, cold, pain, and pin prick or disorders of perception, vibratory sense, position sense, and higher interpretive sensory modalities.

Diagnostic Procedures

The most secure confirmation of the diagnosis of epilepsy is through observation of a seizure, together with an electroencephalogram (EEG), a recording of brain electrical activity. Twenty or more electrodes are positioned on the person's scalp in the form of either small disc paste electrodes or small subdermal needles. The test is neither painful nor dangerous. During a part of the EEG, the person is asked to pant rapidly and deeply; at another time a bright light is flashed in front of her eyes at various speeds. While EEG contributes to the diagnosis of epilepsy, it is not meant to be conclusive, for it will show mild, nonspecific "abnormalities" in 15 percent of the normal population and the interictal EEG may be normal in people with epilepsy.

For people whose pattern of seizure is difficult to document, telemetry allows the recording of EEGs using a small radio transmitter placed on the person's body and connected to EEG scalp electrodes through which waves are transmitted to a receiver and recording equipment in the EEG laboratory while the person moves about. Seizure discharges, their duration, and the timing of seizures can all be recorded, allowing for the localization of the origin of the seizures and documention of subtle or unexpected seizures.

Computerized tomography (CT scanning), a highly refined computerized x-ray of the brain, is often used in the diagnosis of epilepsy. The person is usually examined lying down with her head placed through an opening in the machine. X-rays are taken of her brain, and a series of pictures of transverse slices of the brain result. A CT Scan can reveal excess fluid in the brain (hydrocephalus) or a tumor, a cyst, a stroke or hemorrhage, an abscess, or some other structural lesion. This test can be done with or without the intravenous injection of contrast material. The contrast material can result in potentially dangerous allergic reactions, but such reactions are rare and may be related to previous allergies. The contrast injection may help identify a lesion that would not otherwise be defined. People who are claustrophobic or who become anxious when put into confined spaces will find it uncomfortable, because the head is often surrounded by rubberized sandbags, and the person may be unable to see as the test proceeds.

The next test that might be done is a lumbar puncture or spinal tap, the removal of fluid from the spine, which can give evidence of infection, inflammation, or nonspecific changes. Cerebrospinal fluid bathes the brain and spinal cord and serves metabolic as well as mechanical functions. For the spinal tap, a needle is placed between the third and fourth or the fourth and fifth lumbar vertebrae, and a small amount of fluid, usually less than 5 percent of the total available volume, is removed. This amount of fluid is ordinarily replenished in less than one hour.

The only common complication of this test is the appearance of post-lumbar puncture headaches in a small number of people, which is related to the leaking of spinal fluid after the tap; leakage can be minimized by using a small-caliber needle and restricting activity soon after the tap. Ordinarily it is recommended that the person remain in bed for the better part of a day after the spinal tap to minimize the chances of a headache.

Treatment

The purpose of treatment is to achieve the best possible control of seizures with the least side effects. Once a diagnosis of recurrent seizures that are expected to respond to antiepileptic drugs has been reached, treatment consists of at least two to four years of daily medication. There is some debate in the literature about treating a person who has just had her first seizure, because all antiepileptic drugs have some side effects, and many untreated individuals may experience no further seizures. The decision of whether to start antiepileptic therapy depends on the seizure type, other associated illnesses, other medications, and the patient's life situation. If the seizure was tonic-clonic, treatment is usually begun after one seizure, because a second seizure may occur when the person is vulnerable to injury. If the event was absence or a certain type of partial seizure, the physician may suggest waiting. Often, if a person has absence seizures, she may not see a doctor until she has had repeated episodes. Most recent studies indicate that early treatment may be beneficial in preventing progressive development of a seizure process from repeated electrical stimulation of vulnerable portions of the brain.

The main principle of therapy is that initially a single drug be used in moderate dosage. Therapy is generally started with one drug, because that is often sufficient for control, and if a person develops a reaction to the drug, the cause will be clear. If seizures continue, the dose of the drug may be raised until the concentration of the drug in the blood has reached levels that are effective in the majority of patients. If the dosage begins to reach a level that is possibly toxic, it may be discontinued or reduced, and another drug may be introduced. Generally multiple drugs are more difficult to manage and are avoided if possible.

The anticonvulsant medication must be carefully chosen depending on the type of seizure. The most commonly used drugs for seizures that originate in the cerebral cortex (the brain's surface), which include most grand mal and partial seizures, are phenytoin, phenobarbitol, and carbamazepine. The ability to measure the amount of medication in the blood (commonly referred to as blood levels) has improved recently, allowing maximum seizure control and avoidance of toxicity. Thus, the time it takes to reach therapeutic levels can be measured accurately, individual differences in people's ability to metabolize the medicine can be established, and the half-life of the medication can be measured. Half-life is the time it takes for the serum level of an anticonvulsant to drop to half its steady-state level after it has been discontinued. Since phenytoin and phenobarbital have a half-life of more than twenty-four hours, they need not be taken more than once a day. People are more likely to take medicine as prescribed if it does not interfere with their daily schedules (as would a child's embarrassment at having to take medicine in the middle of the school day), hence they will be more likely to hold to a prescribed dosage if it is less frequent.

Side effects vary to some degree. Phenobarbital tends to make people sleepy. Sometimes the sleepiness decreases after a while; in other cases people find the drug interferes with their activity level, slowing them appreciably. Phenobarbital also may cause hyperactivity or behavioral disturbances in children or older adults. Phenytoin (Dilantin) may cause drowsiness and unsteadiness of gait in excessive doses. It frequently causes excessive hair growth in undesirable places as well as hypertrophy (increase in the size of the tissues) of the gums. Although it is highly effective for seizures originating in the cerebral cortex, it can make absense seizures worse. Carbamazepine (Tegretol) is highly effective against generalized and complex partial seizures. It often causes nausea and dizziness in older people. In rare instances it can also cause bone marrow suppression, a cessation of the soft, pulpy substance in the bones that is concerned with blood formation. Because the timing of dosages depends on the half-life of a particular drug, phenytoin and phenobarbital with half-lives of more than twenty-four hours can often be taken once a day. In contrast, carbamazepine has a shorter half-life and must be taken three times a day to maintain therapeutic blood levels. Another drug, used more commonly to treat absense seizures in children, is ethosuximide (Zarotin), which is very effective but may exacerbate generalized seizures and can cause gastrointestinal problems.

Valproic acid (Depakene or Depakote) was developed recently, primarily for the treatment of absense seizures and secondarily for all generalized motor seizures. Unlike the earlier drugs, which were discovered by chance or represent minor variations of earlier drugs that were known to have anticonvulsant qualities, valproic acid was devised as a rational compound that might have anticonvulsive activity because of its chemical composition. It makes people less sleepy and has minimal adverse effects, especially if it can be used alone. When used with other antiepileptics, the interaction is pronounced and at times unpredictable. Because of large interpatient variability (partially because it is often used with other drugs), it is not yet possible to define a characteristic level-dose ratio. Side effects include nausea and vomiting, which can be managed by taking the drug with or after meals or by reducing the daily dosage for one day. Rare instances of potentially fatal liver damage have been reported with valproic acid.

People whose seizures are well controlled for many years are sometimes taken off anticonvulsant drugs because daily medication might not be warranted. This is a calculated risk taken with the understanding of both the patient and physician that seizures might recur, but with an awareness that every anticonvulsant has side effects so if the person can do without the medication, she should. EEGs may be done prior to the discontinuation of medication and sometime subsequent to the medication. If unacceptable side effects occur from any particular drug, an alternative drug is substituted.

PREGNANCY

A woman who has epilepsy and requires medication has at least a 90 percent chance of having a normal child. The decision to become pregnant is one that should be made in consultation with the woman's physician, since epilepsy can affect pregnancy and pregnancy can affect the disease by increasing or decreasing the frequency of seizures. The hormonal changes caused by the pregnancy and birth can affect the way the anticonvulsants are metabolized, so blood levels will have to be monitored closely.

Both epilepsy and the anticonvulsants can affect the baby. Women taking anticonvulsants face a two to three times greater risk that their infants will have congenital malformations, while women with epilepsy who are not taking anticonvulsants have up to two times greater risk. The causes for the increased risk are not completely understood but are thought to relate to genes common for epilepsy and congenital malformation or to a specific effect of the drugs. Most malformations occur during the first three months of pregnancy. Cleft lip or palate, in which there is a congenital failure of fusion between the right and left palatal processes, and congenital heart disease are the most common malformations.

Drugs thought to cause severe congenital problems are trimethadione

(Tridione) and paramethadione (Paradione). A woman should probably avoid pregnancy while taking these drugs. Phenytoin (Dilantin) slightly increases the risk of cleft palate and heart disease as well as "fetal hydantoin syndrome," which includes growth deficiency, small head size, abnormalities of the nails and fingers, and other minor problems. Most of these babies have normal intelligence. Problems associated with phenobarbital are less frequent than those with phenytoin, and this may be the drug of choice for a pregnant woman with epilepsy. Depakene may increase the risk to 1 to 2 per hundred for spina bifida, and pregnant women taking this drug should consider prenatal testing for neural tube defects. Finally, although medications are carried in the breast milk, it is thought that the doses passed are so low that they will not harm the infant. Occasionally women taking more than 90 mg. of phenobarbital may find that their babies are drowsy and should discuss this with their physician.

SURGERY

Most seizure disorders can be controlled through medication. For those few severe disorders for which control through medication is not possible, there are three principal surgical approaches: the removal of actual epileptic brain tissue, commisurotomy, and implantation of electrodes. The removal of epileptic brain tissue is sometimes indicated when there are uncontrolled focal seizures, that is, seizures whose single precise origin in the brain can be identified. Multifocal seizures will probably not be corrected through this approach. In commisurotomy, the corpus callosum and sometimes other tracts that connect the right and left hemispheres of the brain are severed. This operation has been performed on about one hundred high-risk or "last resort" patients in the last fifteen years. It works best in people with infantile hemiplegia in which a sunken, scarred hemisphere that serves no other function than to cause generalized seizures is separated from the normal hemisphere. In the third type of operation, the implantation of electrodes, which was introduced in 1973, electricity stimulates several electrodes for a ten-minute period several times a day for up to eight months. Resultant data are conflicting and difficult to interpret.

TREATMENT FOR OTHER CONDITIONS RESULTING IN SEIZURES

The therapy for any specific metabolic or general medical condition resulting in seizures is to treat the underlying problem. For example, hypoglycemia should be treated with sugar; hypocalcemia should be treated with calcium. People who are withdrawing from barbiturates or alcohol should be withdrawn slowly so that seizures do not occur. Removal of blood clots that have occurred through trauma on the surface of the brain may halt seizures.

Two sorts of precautions should be taken when someone has a seizure: preventing the person from harming herself, and preventing other people from harming the person. The person should be placed in a position where various physical movements will not result in injury to her body. Her airway or breathing passage should be maintained, preferably with a plastic airway if an experienced person is present to insert it. Insertion should not be attempted by anyone who is not experienced. Contrary to popular thinking, the person will not swallow her tongue, so there is no reason to manipulate her mouth. Great harm can be done by putting things in the ill person's mouth during a seizure. After a seizure, the person should be allowed to rest.

ANTICIPATED COURSE OF THE TREATED DISEASE

The prognosis for epilepsy depends on the presence or nature of the underlying disease. An infant may have one isolated benign seizure associated with a fever, or an adult may have seizures as part of the symptomatology of a malignant brain tumor. Obviously, the prognosis for the child is excellent, while that for the adult with the malignant brain tumor is poor. In general, if the person with epilepsy follows the correct medical regimen, the probability of good to excellent control of seizure disorders is better than 90 percent. The remaining 10 percent may have ever more frequent seizures, may suffer significant side effects from their medications, or may require more complicated therapy than the usual oral medications.

The prognosis for the intellectual, performance, and behavior abilities of someone with epilepsy depends very much on the conditions associated with the epilepsy. People with epilepsy of unknown origin whose seizures are under good control with usual doses of anticonvulsant medication usually have normal intellect and behavior. When seizures are difficult to control and multiple medicines are administered in high doses, side effects including lessened functional ability and frequent seizures may contribute to behavior problems and poor performance. When people are brain-damaged and/or have neurologic deficits, prognosis depends on the underlying problems in the brain. Life expectancy is greater in people with epilepsy of unknown origin, generalized tonic-clonic or absense seizures with infrequent seizures, and normal intelligence. Mortality for people with epilepsy is thought to be greater than the general population.

Psychosocial Information

Epilepsy affects the lives of the ill person and his family through its symptoms, through the side effects of treatment, and because of society's often archaic views of the disease. Until the discovery of modern anticonvulsant medication (phenytoin) in the late 1930s, there was little that could be done to control symptoms other than the use of barbiturates with all of their associated side effects. Today symptoms are generally controlled, but there are still powerful memories of people locked away or in voluntary hiding when they thought a seizure was beginning. Because epilepsy is sometimes associated with retardation and psychosis, ignorance leads some people to believe that everyone with epilepsy has many psychosocial problems. One informant even repeated the classic story of being told she didn't look like an epileptic after telling an employer she had epilepsy.

Modification in Life-Style

Generally a moderate life-style with a nutritional diet, regular meals, a reasonable schedule, and sufficient sleep and activity is best for those with epilepsy, as for everyone else. The difference is that for people with epilepsy, excesses that would be unimportant to a completely healthy person could cause seizures. For example, sleep deprivation may precipitate seizures. Sometimes EEGs are recorded during sleep after a night of sleep deprivation to increase the probability of finding paroxysmal activity. Drinking to excess can exacerbate seizures. People with seizure disorders are generally advised not to drink alcoholic beverages or to use alcohol very sparingly, perhaps having no more than one light drink or one glass of wine a day.

Some seizures are evoked by watching television, coughing, or other specific sensory stimuli, hence persons thus affected are urged to avoid these stimuli. Children who have frequent and potentially injurious seizures are often supplied with football helmets to wear to prevent significant injury to their heads when they fall. People who have frequent or unpredictable seizures may have special instructions for avoiding activities that would be dangerous to them. Thus, activity is restricted both to decrease the possibility of having a seizure and to avoid injury.

Legal Aspects

For those with epilepsy legal restrictions fall into four areas: education, driving, eugenic marriage laws and eugenic sterilization, and workmen's compensation and unemployment. With regard to education, a student with epilepsy has the right not to be segregated unless her seizures are part of a brain abnormality that also causes retardation or unless emotional problems do not allow her to learn in the average classroom.

Driving is a more complex issue. In this automobile-oriented society, it is very difficult to carry out adult responsibilities without being able to drive. There is no question that people whose seizures are uncontrolled should not drive. State driving codes differ in regard in epilepsy. Generally, in order to obtain a driver's license a person must remain free of seizures for a specific period of time, which varies from six months to two years. Several states make the physician responsible for informing the state if a patient has a seizure. Approximately three-fourths of the states require periodic medical reports. If the patient does not tell the physician, the physician cannot report it, and even if the patient does tell the physician or the physician treats the patient for a seizure, the physician often leaves the driving decision to the patient. Most people do not inform the state. A social worker in an epilepsy center reports that the staff likes to restrict people as little as possible. Restriction interferes with the ill person's life and her relationships with clinic staff. If a person who needs to drive tells you that she has had a seizure and you respond by reporting the incident, she may decide not to tell you about the next seizure.

If someone is denied a license, the action is subject to administrative review in most states. The review findings are binding, subject to judicial review. If an epileptic driver is involved in an accident, a number of legal questions affect her liability for damages. To avoid liability she must conform to the standard of conduct of a reasonable person who has a similar disability. If she knows she is subject to sudden losses of consciousness, she may be found negligent and held responsible. The primary question is the foreseeability of the lapse of consciousness.

There are no longer any state laws forbidding marriage to or annulling marriages of those with seizure disorders. However, some states still have eugenic sterilization laws on their books for epileptics who are institutionalized. Such laws have rarely, if ever, been enforced. Employment remains difficult. Social stigmas and misunderstandings make employers hesitant to hire those with epilepsy. Primarily employers are afraid that people with epilepsy will have more accidents and that employing them will result in increased workmen's compensation insurance premiums. Neither notion is accurate. When working in jobs that take their impairment into account, epileptic workers have an accident record that compares favorably with that of other workers.

Some states have tried to prevent employers from using compensation premiums as an excuse for not hiring those with epilepsy. Several permit a "partial waiver" of compensation benefits by a worker for injury caused by a pre-existing condition. Almost all states have now adopted the "subsequent injury fund," which spreads the risk of hiring handicapped people among all employers in the state.

The areas of "search and arrest," adoption, and sterilization continue to be significant for people with epilepsy. In two states epilepsy in the adopted child is still the basis for annulment of an adoption. In three states laws authorize involuntary sterilization of people with epilepsy. In forty-three states arresting officers are not required to search people for emergency medical information prior to making an arrest for "drunk and disorderly" conduct. The Epilepsy Foundation of American and other groups continue to lobby for changes in thes archaic laws.

Insurance

Obtaining adequate insurance at reasonable rates is very difficult. The Commission for the Control of Epilepsy and its Consequences found that 52 percent of the respondants to its survey on insurance had difficulty obtaining life insurance, 37 percent had problems getting accident insurance, and 32 percent had trouble getting automobile insurance. It has been suggested that the difficulty in obtaining most kinds of insurance arises from the fact that insurance tables are based on obsolete data. As seizure control continues to improve and as medications are developed with fewer side effects, the improved statistics are expected to demonstrate that people with epilepsy are more insurable.

Since people with epilepsy generally fall into the category of people who represent a higher than average mortality potential, they will probably have to pay a high premium for an individual life insurance policy. The premiums will vary according to the individual's health history; type of seizures, length of time the person has been seizure-free, the person's age, and the age at which the first seizure occurred. For example, life insurance is generally more available for those with absence seizures than it is for those with tonic-clonic seizures. The National Epilepsy League now offer group life insurance policies for those people with epilepsy who are employed and who do not have a life-threatening disease.

Automobile insurance is also very difficult for a person with epilepsy to obtain. Generally she has to pay higher premium rates as an "assigned risk." Assigned risk coverage lasts for a limited period, after which a person must apply for another assigned risk plan if she has not been able to obtain standard coverage. She cannot choose her insurance company; rates are usually 25 to 50 percent higher than standard coverage; and the amount of coverage is customarily the minimum required by the automobile financial responsibility law in the particular state. Many states specifically exclude people with epilepsy from their assigned risk plans. Available data show that while the overall accident rate for people with epilepsy may be greater than for the general driving population, certain groups of drivers with epilepsy have a much lower than average accident rate.

Because the costs of medical care for people with epilepsy are substantial, health insurance is also difficult to obtain. Many insurance companies do not issue major medical insurance to people with epilepsy. Those that do generally provide time-limited, cancelable coverage. Coverage is easier to obtain when seizures are controlled and the patient is employed. Employment is a sign of some stability and adjustment to the illness. Group health coverage is more easily obtained, raises rates for those with epilepsy only slightly above average, and does not exclude people with epilepsy from hospital or medical coverage. Usually it is best to maintain a policy if one was covered before epilepsy was diagnosed, even if it means higher premiums.

Social Security Disability Insurance is available for a former contributing worker with recurrent seizures or for survivors who may be similarly disabled. To be eligible one must be unable to do any kind of gainful work. Severity is determined by type, frequency, duration, and sequelae of seizures. At least one detailed description of a typical seizure is required, including presence or absence of aura, tongue biting, sphincter control, injuries associated with the attack, and postseizure events. Documentation of epilepsy should include at least one EEG. People whose seizures can be controlled are ineligible unless the amount of medication required to control the seizures is toxic. Where documentation shows that alcohol or drug abuse affects the therapy or contributes to the precipitation of seizures, this information is considered part of the overall assessment of the impairment severity. Eligibility for Social Security Disability Insurance and Supplemental Social Security Income also makes one eligible for other programs such as Medicare and Medicaid. Medicaid provisions vary by state, and Medicare covers medication only on the inpatient basis. If people are sufficiently impaired to receive disability payments and their seizures become controlled, they are no longer considered disabled, their disability income is discontinued, and they are no longer considered a priority group for vocational rehabilitation. Closing basic eligibility also means the health coverage that pays for anticonvulsant drugs is lost, and without these drugs seizures may recur, creating a frustrating but currently unavoidable revolving door.

Relationships with Others

The effect of epilepsy on relationships is often related to the kind of seizure as well as to age of onset. For example, a person with infrequent absence seizures may be seen by her family and friends as absent-minded or a daydreamer. On the other hand, someone with tonic-clonic seizures that occur a few times a year may have to explain them to new friends and colleagues so that they will understand and be less alarmed if one occurs. Someone who has a tonic-clonic seizure once every five years may assume that she will seize sometime in some place, but she will not disclose her condition, preferring to take her chances rather than have people think of her as an epileptic. After she has a seizure, she knows she will have to help people around her deal with what they saw.

When epilepsy begins in infancy or childhood, the family's response to the illness is very important. Many parents interviewed about their response to a first tonic-clonic seizure expressed horror, a worry that the episode was an indication of mental disorder or retardation, and concern that the condition was inherited. Mothers of children with febrile seizures at first thought that their children were dead or dying.

Children with epilepsy are aware that they are different, because they have to take pills every day and because parents worry about them and seem to be more protective of them than they are of the other children in the house. They generally feel isolated and confused. Teachers often reinforce the feelings of vulnerability and difference by avoiding the child or keeping her from activities or stresses they think might provoke a seizure. Concern over the dangers of physical exercise like gym and swimming compounds the anxiety. The other children in the class then become fearful and wary, isolating the child with epilepsy even if they have never witnessed a seizure. When children are also educationally subnormal, parents' and teachers' level of expectation falls lower than should, thus making it less likely that a child will learn to live independently. In contrast, those who are less disabled because they have normal or above-normal intelligence generally aspire to a normal social and work life.

If they do not understand the illness, other children can be cruel. They may jeer and call the child with epilepsy crazy. In order to avoid this spiraling isolation, parents, teachers, and the child need realistic limits and expectations as well as knowledge of what to do in case of a seizure. Representatives of the Epilepsy Foundation and hospital epilepsy centers as well as other health professionals with expertise about epilepsy can provide audiovisual materials and explain the illness to school personnel, parents, and children.

People who have had epilepsy from infancy or young adulthood seem most dependent and enmeshed with their families. Parents are often overprotective and frightened, feeling responsible for and guilty about their child's disorder. For example, one informant said that her mother was sure that she had seizures because she was allowed to take acrobatics as a child. A man in his middle thirties who had graduated from high school and held a responsible job lived with his mother, who doled out his pills each morning and reminded him to come right home from work so that she would not have to worry that he had had a seizure and was lying in the street.

Those whose onset was in late adolescence seem more independent despite problems in dealing with adolescent issues like dating, driving, and choosing work. A man in his early twenties said he would rather not think about it. He takes his pills, and if he has a seizure, he has one. All of his friends know he has epilepsy, and he expects them to look out for him. He wears his symptom like a military decoration, with a great deal of bluster and swagger. A young woman about the same age has a very different reaction. She has had very few seizures, but she considers sharing knowledge about her condition a sign of intimacy in a relationship, a test to see if people care enough not to run away from her. When she has a seizure, she feels apologetic. Not knowing what she did during the seizure makes her feel out of control.

Adults with epilepsy have to concern themselves with different kinds of relationships. Married people who have had epilepsy for many years find that spouses generally take the illness in stride. One woman reported preparing her latency-age children for her seizures in much the same way as she would prepare them for another kind of emergency. The children were shown pictures of what someone looked like during a tonic-clonic seizure. She explained many possible effects, such as loss of sphincter control or postseizure aphasia as well as the importance of moving things on which she could hurt herself. She posted telephone numbers of people they were to call, including the local emergency squad, her mother, and a neighbor. In the past few years the children have witnessed two seizures with no perceptible negative effects.

Adult-onset epilepsy is thought to present few problems if the person has a stable home and work life. A woman who was involved in highly visible community work was found to have complex partial seizures at age thirty-three. At first she was quite depressed at the diagnosis, but knowing that she had probably had the seizures for many years, she and her husband decided that this new information would not change their lives significantly. Still, it is an added stress and stigma for some spouses. One woman said that although her friends, colleagues, and children had been able to accept her epilepsy, her husband had not. She had two seizures, neither of which he witnessed, and he told her he could no longer live with her in such an unpredictable situation. A social worker in an epilepsy clinic said a woman was referred to her in regard to finding a different kind of work. When she called, the woman said she could not come in during the day because she was not allowed to cross the street when her husband was not at home. She had had her first tonic-clonic seizure in her husband's presence, and his solution to his terror was to keep her a prisoner in what he deemed to be a safe environment. Before she could help the woman to find work, the social worker had to help the couple to resume their lives.

Ability to Work

Generally work in which a seizure could prove dangerous to a person with epilepsy or her co-workers is inappropriate. The military and the police and fire departments generally will not employ people with epilepsy. Those with seizure disorders are generally discouraged from working at heights or in jobs that call for driving motor vehicles. Often, however, employers make little distinction between those whose seizures are well controlled, nocturnal, or confined to distinct stimuli and those whose seizures are not controlled. Large studies of workers in industry have shown that epilepsy does not play a significant part in accident causation.

When looking for a job, the person with epilepsy must decide whether to tell a prospective employer that she has epilepsy. To tell means that she might not be hired, but not to tell means risking having a seizure on the job and being fired for not disclosing medical information. An informant says that she tells her employers after she has been employed for about six months. That way, if the employer fires her, at least the employer knows that he is firing a good worker. When asked what she would do if she had a seizure on the job before the six-month period was over, she said she would take her chances. Another informant says he is always careful to explain the nature of his seizures to a prospective employer, because he would not feel comfortable working in a place where he could not alert his co-workers to a possible seizure. Both of these people have had seizures once every four or five years, yet their way of dealing with the issue of work is very different. Although those with controlled seizures can do almost any job, many more positions are closed to them than need be because employers are ignorant about epilepsy. Therefore, more people with epilepsy tend to be underemployed or unemployed than necessary.

Relationships with Strangers

Epilepsy is hidden as long as one does not have a seizure. When a seizure occurs, it can easily be mistaken for something else. The person may appear inappropriate, drunk, crazy, or inattentive. Thus, it is easy for strangers to misjudge the symptoms or their significance.

Psychological Aspects

Some important psychological issues for those with epilepsy are dependence, control, anger and aggression, depression, the myth of the epileptic personality, and the relationship of epilepsy to specific psychiatric disturbances. In some ways a person with epilepsy must be dependent on her medication and on people around her when she has a seizure. Dependence is often reinforced when family members are overprotective. For those whose seizures are not well controlled or who have major health problems to which the seizures are secondary, dependence may be necessary for survival.

Control is also an important issue, because a seizure means loss of control, that is, loss of consciousness and of the means of assessment, self-regulation, and communication. Control is so important in this society that we measure maturity by it. Self-discipline, fine manners, and the ability to keep a cool head no matter what is going on around you are admirable traits. With epilepsy, people must know that at some unpredictable time they will be totally out of control. They will not even know what has happened to them unless they ask someone who witnessed the seizure. Even then they can never be sure that the person will tell them what really happened. Sometimes a person who has had a psychomotor seizure is picked up by police officers on charges of being drunk and disorderly. For that reason and others, people with epilepsy should consider wearing bracelets or necklaces identifying them and their illness.

ANGER AND AGGRESSION

Anger is a threefold issue. People say that they are angry at having epilepsy, that they become angry at other people for being ignorant of and insensitive to the symptoms, and that the epsodes themselves feel like "little rages" in which one loses control, then is depleted. Aggression is another trait associated with epilepsy. Some clinical studies have shown excessively aggressive behavior in about 25 to 35 percent of some groups of patients with partial complex seizures, and others have shown no association between violence and psychomotor seizures.

Such dramatic variation can be accounted for to some degree by the way the terms violence and aggression are defined and by the reasons for which people are referred to the institutions or programs that are presenting the statistics. Some studies have reported a relatively high incidence of epilepsy among prison inmates with a documented history of violent assaults against other individuals and psychomotor seizures in violent individuals referred from juvenile court. Many of these studies suggest that violence may sometimes have neurological determinants, not that people with epilepsy are violent. Generally, directed violence during a seizure is rare for most people with epilepsy. It more often happens that during or just following a seizure some people thrash around in a nondirected, aggressive manner if restrained.

DEPRESSION

Depression can be a significant problem for people with epilepsy. It is not known whether it is part of the symptom configuration or part of the impact of the symptoms and limitations. Some people also report that rapid changes in mood, lasting from minutes to hours, are part of the onset of a seizure. There is also a high rate of postseizure depression, but again it is not known whether the depression is part of the symptom configuration or, rather, a psychological reaction to having had another seizure. Suicide occurs more commonly among people with epilepsy than in the general population. The highest increased risk has been associated with temporal lobe epilepsy

EPILEPTIC PERSONALITY

In the past many personality characteristics were attributed to people with epilepsy. They have been described as preoccupied with religion, prone to outbursts of aggression, paranoid, pedantic, egocentric, and obsessive. Very few people with epilepsy have all these traits, and the traits are also present in many other populations. Therefore, the so-called epileptic personality, which has never been documented, is not only useless but counterproductive in understanding people with epilepsy.

PSYCHIATRIC DISTURBANCES

Although the reasons are not understood and there is not one personality pattern associated with epilepsy, people with epilepsy do have a higher incidence of personality disturbances and intellectual difficulties than the general population. Contributing factors are thought to be the presence of an abnormal physiological state in the brain's limbic system, the ring of gray matter and tracts bordering the hemispheres in the medial portions of the brain that play a role in emotions; a disturbed psychological response to ignorant societal attitudes; the effects of repeated, uncontrolled seizures leading to brain damage; and/or the presence of an underlying degenerative disease.

Another area of concern in the psychiatric literature is the cause of a schizophrenia-like psychosis that sometimes occurs in people with epilepsy. Studies have shown people with epileptic psychosis to have a history of prolonged use of anticonvulsant medication and an incompletely controlled seizure disorder that preceded the psychosis and usually involves the limbic system. One theory suggests that chronic anticonvulsant therapy may have a toxic effect on mental functioning. Another hypothesizes that the psychosis is the result of chronic abnormal electrical activity in limbic structures. Basically, the relationship of epilepsy to psychosis remains undefined.

How to Be Helpful to Someone with Epilepsy

Because seizures are controlled for 90 percent of people with epilepsy, you will probably never witness a seizure whether you are a colleague, neighbor, counselor, or friend. If you are with someone who has a seizure, try to move out of the way anything on which the person might hurt herself and then call for help. Most seizures are over in five minutes, with some additional time for post seizure reaction. Then the person will want to know what happened and be assured that you were not so horrified you will not be able to continue your relationship. Often the person will be very tired and may have some other neurologic deficit like an inability to talk or walk for a while.

   Remember that a person with epilepsy should be careful to avoid specific stimuli that may provoke seizures, such as inadequate sleep and immoderate amount of alcohol. If seizures are uncontrolled, she should avoid endangering herself or others by declining certain kinds of activities. Otherwise, she can live normally. Her epilepsy need not be a hindrance to work or social life.

7

Heart Disease

HEART DISEASE IS any abnormal condition of the heart or its function in maintaining blood circulation. It is the most prevalent of all the life-threatening chronic illnesses. Almost 50 percent of deaths in the United States result from some form of heart disease. However, the control or reduction of risk factors like hypertension, smoking, and high-fat, high-salt diet has resulted in a 30 percent decline of deaths from heart disease over the past twenty years.

The several types of heart disease and treatment are confusing. Some terms, such as heart attack (myocardial infarction), sound familiar and ominous. Some treatments, like bypass surgery, sound familiar and magical. Confusion arises from similarities in terminology and from the fact that many of the types are not mutually exclusive. Some are the result of others, some are manifestations of others, and many can be present in the same person at the same time. Although the types will be more thoroughly explained later in the chapter, a brief introduction to classification and treatment may be helpful.

Four of the most common forms of heart disease—heart attack (myocardial infarction), angina (angina pectoris), stroke, and heart failure (congestive heart failure)—are manifestations of atherosclerotic heart disease. Atherosclerotic heart disease can cause a heart attack, in which part of the heart muscle dies; angina, in which there is a certain kind of pain; stroke, in which part of the brain tissue dies; or heart failure, in which fluid accumulates in certain areas of body tissue.

Other important forms of heart disease are arrhythmia (deviation from the normal rhythm of the heart); hypertension (high blood pressure), in which the blood circulates through the arteries at a higher than normal pressure, which can damage the arteries; rheumatic heart disease, in which a specific kind of infection has caused rheumatic fever and the untreated fever has damaged the valves of the heart; congenital heart defect, in which someone was born with a heart defect that to some degree impairs blood ,flow; and peripheral arterial disease, which affects the flow of blood from the heart.

Surgery is used to replace certain valves of the heart as well as to aid its pacemaker function. If disease is present along with the structural problem, surgery cannot control the disease process. Medicine is used to treat many heart conditions, including hypertension. Hypertension presents a special problem, because it is generally without symptoms, so people are not highly motivated to take the medicine necessary to treat it and to prevent damage. Untreated hypertension can cause atherosclerotic heart disease and thus heart attack, stroke, heart failure, and angina. This example underscores the point about a complicated classification system and a confusing nomenclature.

Heart disease often becomes a heavy physical and emotional burden. Heart damage or its possibility is frightening. The symptoms of heart disease, particularly chest pain and shortness of breath, are in themselves anxiety-provoking. In addition, one worries not only about becoming increasingly disabled but about the threat of sudden death.

Medical Information

The heart is the pump that operates the system of vessels transporting vital materials through the circulatory system—the network of arteries, arterioles (small branches of the arteries), capillaries, venules (small veins), and veins. A constant pressure (diastolic) forces the blood forward, and the contraction of the heart adds extra pressure (systolic). The arteries provide oxygenated blood from which the wastes and carbon dioxide have been removed to all of the organs of the body. Red blood cells pick up oxygen in the lungs, then carry the oxygen to individual cells, picking up the carbon dioxide that they release as waste when returning to the lungs. In the same way, substances like hormones are moved from one part of the body to another, metabolic waste products are removed from cells, and nutrients are carried to the cells. Thus the heart is the pump for the transportation system between specialized tissues in the body.

A hollow, muscular organ, the heart has four chambers: two collecting chambers called the atria and two pumping chambers called the ventricles. It is divided into two sides. The right atrium receives the blood that has been depleted of oxygen and is filled with carbon dioxide. When passed to the right ventricle, the blood is pumped into the lungs to eliminate the carbon dioxide and pick up oxygen. This oxygen-rich blood travels to the left atrium and then to the left ventricle, from which it is pumped to the rest of the body. Backward flow of blood is prevented by the presence of valves at the entrance of each of the chambers. The coronary arteries circulate the blood needed for the heart muscle.

The pumping action of the heart is controlled by the sinoatrial (SA) node or natural pacemaker, the small bundle of muscle fibers and nerves that send out electrical impulses at regular intervals and thus cause the heart to contract. The SA node sends an impulse through the atria to the atrioventricular (AV) node, which sends impulses into the ventricular muscle via a bundle of nerves called the bundle of His. When the heart relaxes, valves that allow the flow of blood from atria to ventricles are open, and the fall in pressure causes blood to flow in. Having received the impulse to contract, the atria help to move the blood to the ventricles. As the ventricles receive the message to contract, the pressure closes the valves between the atria and ventricles, and the blood is squeezed from the right ventricle to the lungs and from the left ventricle to the body via the aorta.

In addition to its pumping function, the cardiovascular system uses sensors and monitoring devices in other parts of the body to help it adjust the circulatory system. For example, the primary regulator of blood pressure is the brainstem, in which groups of cells determine the diameter of the blood vessels (vasomotor center) and activate or inhibit the working of the heart. On the one hand, blood pressure is augmented when the cardiac-activating center commands the sympathetic nervous system to increase the heart's activity and the vasomotor center commands the sympathetic nervous system to constrict arterioles and veins. On the other hand, heart activity is slowed and blood pressure is decreased when the cardiac inhibitory center conveys commands to the pacemaker. When the blood pressure rises, sensors from the heart and carotid arteries in the neck send messages to the brain, which inhibit the activating and vasomotor centers and stimulate the inhibitory center. Other sensors monitor the volume of blood and the oxygen content of the blood, sending messages to the brain with information necessary for adjustment. The nervous system's regulatory activity is augmented by hormones secreted by specialized cells in the endocrine glands. The activity of the cardiac-activating and vasomotor centers is sustained and prolonged by increased secretions of specialized cells in the medulla of the adrenal gland. Also, blood volume can be increased by a chemical substance produced in the walls of the kidneys, causing greater reabsorption of salt and water from the kidneys. This same substance also causes the arteriole walls to contract and increase their resistance.

When any part of this system malfunctions, some kind of heart disease may ensue. The focus of the disease process can be the pacemaker, the conduction system, the valves, the blood pressure, the muscle, or some other aspect of the circulatory system. Because this group of diseases can affect the entire circulatory system, they are grouped under the name cardiovascular disease. "Cardio" refers to the heart, and "vascular" to the blood vessels. These diseases can damage not only the heart but also the brain, the kidneys, and other organs and tissues as well.

Natural History

The natural history of heart disease depends on the form of disease and the kind and extent of damage it causes to the circulatory system. Some forms of heart disease, like a very slowly progressive angina pectoris, may hardly interfere with a person's life. Others, like severe angina, can cause sufficient damage that the heart can no longer maintain itself and the person dies.

Symptomatology

The symptoms of heart disease may be invisible. Chest pain is the most common. It can be caused by an insufficient amount of blood flowing through the coronary arteries or by injury to the heart muscle. The pain of a heart attack is more severe, usually lasts longer, and can radiate through the left shoulder and arm, up the neck to the jaw, and to the back. Anginal pains are usually temporary; occur at times of physical exertion, emotional stress, or after a heavy meal; and are sometimes relieved through rest. Chest pain may also be related to other causes, like diseases of or injury to the bones and muscles of the chest or abdomen, or anxiety. The pain associated with anxiety is often related to a specific upsetting situation, is less affected by physical exertion, and lasts longer. The pain of musculoskeletal distress or inflammatory conditions often increases with deep breathing or other chest wall movement.

Shortness of breath (dyspnea), another symptom of cardiovascular disease, can be due to impaired pumping of the heart causing fluid retention in the lungs. Shortness of breath can occur even when a person is resting. Often a person will find that this symptom is relieved when he sleeps sitting up or with his head resting high on several pillows. Sometimes he will find relief by putting his head out the window to catch his breath. Sometimes people awaken suddenly in the middle of the night because of shortness of breath (paroxysmal nocturnal dyspnea). Shortness of breath can also be a symptom of other conditions like lung disease, anemia, or pregnancy.

The retention of fluid (edema) is also a symptom that the pumping action of the heart is failing (congestive heart failure). Excessive retention of fluid is generally evidenced in swelling of the ankles, feet, and abdomen. These symptoms, too, can be indicative of other diseases. Fainting (syncope) can also be due to the failure of the pumping action of the heart, irregularity of the heartbeat, or the narrowing of the arteries that supply the brain. These symptoms can often be relieved by lying down. Blueness of the skin (cyanosis) is another symptom which indicates that the supply of oxygenated blood is being diverted from the surface blood vessels to supply other parts of the body. The lips and skin, and skin under the nails, take on a bluish tinge. It is because of these symptoms that newborns with congenital heart defects are sometimes referred to as "blue babies."

Rapid, forceful beating of the heart (palpitations) may be a symptom of cardiovascular disease, but it can also be indicative of anxiety. Other symptoms include pains in the legs and feet caused by narrowing of the blood vessels in the legs and abdomen, and headaches and dizziness caused by hypertension. Finally, fatigue can be a symptom of heart disease, as it can be indicative of many other illnesses. Other symptoms can include blood spitting (hemoptysis), cough, indigestion, dizziness (vertigo), sexual impotence, depression, insomnia, apathy, and poor memory.

Some symptoms are related to particular forms of heart disease. In addition, each of the symptoms already discussed is part of a total symptomatology for a particular form. These more specific groups of symptoms will be discussed later in the section headed "Classification."

Confusion with Other Diseases

There are many conditions with which heart disease can be confused because of a similarity in symptoms. One such condition is esophageal spasm, an irritability of the esophagus that can produce pain similar to angina. This kind of pain, however, is usually of shorter duration than angina, has its onset when someone is at rest, and is often relieved through walking. Pain in the muscles of the chest can also be mistaken for angina, as can mild rib inflammation, arthritis of the joints between the spine and the ribs, and gall bladder disease.

Chest pain can also come from pleurisy, an inflammation of the linings of the lungs; from shingles when nerves are irritated by a herpes virus infection; or from a rib broken inadvertently through coughing. In addition, bursitis of the left shoulder, aching from arthritis in the area of the neck, and even aching caused by poor posture can mimic the symptoms of coronary heart disease. Emotional distress, particularly depression, sometimes triggers angina-like pain. Finally, there is a condition called cardiac neurosis in which people who experience chest pain, palpitation, or breathlessness become erroneously convinced that they have heart disease. These people often become acutely aware of the beating of their hearts and think that their hearts are beating irregularly, too rapidly, or too loudly. They become alarmed, particularly when they are in a very quiet situation like having gone to bed for the night. As they become increasingly aware of their beating hearts, they become more frightened that if they fall asleep, they might not awaken. Life becomes a cycle of fear, anxiety, and fatigue. If people with cardiac neurosis are not treated successfully psychotherapeutically, they are likely to become invalids.

Predisposing Factors

A large number of predisposing factors place people at greater risk. The factors are cumulative; that is, the degree of risk increases with the number of risk factors present. If the average risk is 100 and a forty-five-year-old man has normal blood pressure and cholesterol levels and does not smoke, his risk is 77. As risk factors are added, the risk rises. The Framingham Heart Study reported that cigarette-smoking raises the risk to 120, the addition of an elevated cholesterol (310) raises the risk to 236, and the addition of hypertension (180 systolic) raises his risk to 384. A family history of premature coronary artery disease or early death from heart attack places one at great risk. White men have a greater incidence of heart disease than women. There is a much closer ratio between non-white men and women. It was thought that before menopause women were protected from heart attacks by the existence of estrogen, a female hormone; however, even after menopause, when the death rate from heart attack increases for women, it never reaches the rate for men. It has recently been reported that estrogen given to postmenopausal women may increase their risk of disease. Coronary artery disease affects ten times as many men as women under age forty-five, but among the very elderly the rate is almost the same.

Certain factors also contribute to a higher risk among certain groups of women. For example, women who use oral contraceptives are at greater risk for heart attack, particularly if they also have a family history of heart disease, smoke, have hypertension, or have high cholesterol levels. The use of oral contraceptives has been related to increased frequency of high blood pressure and blood clots.

The cardiovascular system undergoes greater stress during pregnancy. Pre-eclampsia, a disease of pregnancy whose cause is unknown, can cause hypertension, the accumulation of fluid, and the loss of protein in the urine. If this condition is not treated, it can threaten the health and life of mother and fetus. In addition, pregnancy sometimes causes phlebitis, inflammation and clot formation in the veins. If blood clots break off and enter the circulatory system, they can lodge in the lungs; if they are of any substantial size, they can interfere with blood flow. Finally, if a woman contracts rubella (German measles) in the first three months of pregnancy, her child may be born with congenital heart disease, among other problems. Other infections, and certainly many drugs, may affect the health and viability of the developing fetus. Black women who are poorly nourished are also at greater risk for peripartum cardiomyopathy, in which a gradual softening, thickening, and dilation of the heart muscle causes congestive heart failure at the end of pregnancy or in the first five months after delivery. Women with malfunctioning hearts, such as a congenital heart disease or rheumatic valvular disease, are at increased risk for problems such as heart failure, rhythm disturbances, and an increased incidence of fetal death. Race is also a factor in heart disease and in hypertension, which increases one's risk for heart disease. Black men have three times the rate of hypertension of white men, and black women have twice the rate of hypertension of white women. It is thought that this is due more to environmental than hereditary factors, since research has demonstrated that crowding, continuous social and psychological adjustments, and living in socially subordinate positions can contribute to high blood pressure. Death rates from stroke are much higher in blacks than whites, as is the percentage of known cases of rheumatic fever. Heart attacks and sudden death from coronary events are more common among whites than blacks. Heart attacks occur less frequently among Orientals in the United States, but it is thought that the rate is affected by living in the West, since rates are higher than they are for Orientals living in their homelands.

National origin and early cultural influences are also related to the risk of cardiovascular disease. The frequency of heart attack can vary as much as tenfold from country to country. However, within a few years of migration from countries with a low incidence of heart disease to one with a high incidence, immigrants demonstrate increased frequency. In addition, education, social mobility, marital status, and social status are all thought to be associated with the risk of heart disease, but the relationships have not yet been clearly demonstrated.

Certain psychological factors are also thought to place one at increased risk for heart disease. Competitiveness, intense striving for achievement, urgent sense of time, easily provoked impatience, overcommitment to vocation and profession, excesses of drive and hostility, and abruptness of gesture and speech characterize a coronary-prone behavior pattern known as Type A. This pattern has been found to be associated retrospectively and prospectively with angina pectoris, myocardial infarction, and advanced coronary arteriosclerosis. (The matter is discussed further under "Psychological Issues.") Anxiety, depression, and neurosis have been found to be prospectively associated with the development of angina pectoris, but not with heart attack. When clinical coronary disease is present, all these emotional states appear at a higher than average rate. Chronic conflict and life dissatisfaction have also been found to be related to heart disease, as has chronic interference with sleep. Age is also a risk factor. Three out of four heart attack deaths occur after age sixty-five. The presence of diabetes can also increase one's risk of heart attack.

Cigarette smoking, obesity, lack of regular exercise, and stress all place one at increased risk for heart disease. These risk factors, all of which relate to life-style, will be discussed later in this chapter under "Modifications in Life-Styles."

Prevalence and Incidence

In the United States it is estimated that there are 42,750,000 cases of heart or blood vessel disease. Of this number 37,330,000 have high blood pressure, 4,600,00 have coronary heart disease, 2,010,000 have rheumatic heart disease, 1,870,000 have had strokes, and 480,000 have congenital heart disease. The incidence of heart disease in 1984 is estimated to be 2,025,000, with 1,500,000 people having coronary heart disease, 500,000 having a stroke and 25,000 people having congenital heart disease. Thus, heart disease is the most prevalent of the life-threatening chronic illnesses.

Although mortality figures for heart disease are declining, they continue to account for the highest number of deaths in each year's U.S. mortality statistics. In 1984 it is estimated that there will be 989,610 deaths from cardiovascular diseases, nearly 50 percent of all deaths.

Association with Other Diseases

Many other diseases affect the heart function either because they invade the tissues of the heart or because they place extra stress on it. Examples are lung disease, blood diseases, thyroid conditions, bacterial infections, toxic conditions, syphilis, kidney disease, and obesity. Lung disease strains the heart because it reduces the oxygen level in the blood and makes the heart work harder. It also increases the possibility of a spread of infection to the heart. Such an infection could inflame the heart muscle and membranes. If clots become lodged in the arteries of the lung, the heart has to work harder. If the lung disease is chronic, a consistently low level of oxygen in the blood can cause one's skin to take on a bluish hue (cyanosis), and eventual heart failure can result.

Diseases of the blood also affect the heart. When people are anemic, they have a shortage of red blood cells, so less oxygenated blood is carried to the rest of the body. If they have polycythemia, an excess of red blood cells makes their blood thicker, and their hearts must pump harder. In the case of leukemia, one's heart may eventually be invaded by the malignant proliferation of white blood cells.

Thyroid disease can also affect the heart. An underactive thyroid can slow the metabolism and the use of oxygen and cause one's blood pressure to fall. An overactive thyroid, on the other hand, can speed metabolism and increase the demand for oxygen to the point where the heart rate must accelerate. Kidney failure also affects the heart. Those with end-stage renal disease who have been maintained on dialysis for a significant period begin to have heart problems. Syphilis, if left untreated, can cause abnormal dilations of the blood vessels (aneurysms) and damage the aortic valve.

Sometimes a bacterial infection can inflame the inner lining of the heart and its valves (endocarditis) or the outer covering of the heart (pericarditis). Occasionally the outer covering of the heart is stiffened through the accumulation of fluid caused by an infection. Another condition, called cardiac tamponade, compresses the heart. It usually occurs as the result of a rupture, a penetrating wound, or an inflammatory process. Alcohol and other drugs can damage the heart. This is true of some drugs used in the treatment of psychiatric difficulties.

General Diagnosis

In developing a diagnosis, the physician uses information gathered about family medical history, occupation, age, life-style, personal habits (especially smoking and drinking), past illnesses, and current complaints in order to look for signs and symptoms associated with heart disease. Sometimes a person presents no obvious symptoms. At other times he can report chest pain, breathlessness, tiredness, a bluish tint to the skin around his mouth or under his nails, swelling of his ankles and feet, a rapid, forceful heartbeat, or blood in the material coughed up from his lungs.

Next, the physician conducts a physical examination. He measures blood pressure, pulse rate, and rate of breathing. Using a stethoscope, he checks the heart rhythm and the sounds made as the heart valves open and close. The physician checks the chest to see if the person's lungs are congested or if there is fluid in the lungs or between the chest wall and the lungs. He also checks the person's pulses; those in his neck to see if blood is circulating properly to his head and those in his groin, legs, and feet to see if blood is circulating properly to his legs. Ankles and feet are also checked for any swelling that might not have been a part of the person's reported symptoms. Palpating the person's abdomen, the physician evaluates the abdominal aorta, the spleen, kidneys, and liver for signs of the disease.

A battery of diagnostic tests contributes valuable information. First, a chest x-ray provides information about the condition of the lungs and the shape and size of the heart, as well as the structure of the entire chest area. Tests are also conducted to determine the level of cholesterol and cardiac enzymes, as well as the clotting attributes of the blood.

Another test that is always used is the electrocardiogram (EKG), which records the electrical activity of the heart and therefore is used to assess the rhythm of the heart, its ability to carry electrical impulses, and any scars on the heart, an indication of damaged heart tissue. In this test no electrical charge is given to a person. Rather, the electrical current produced by the heart's contraction is passed through the machine, which measures that current. With the use of an electromagnetic tape recording, a continuous EKG, called an ambulatory monitor or Holter monitor, records the electrical activity of the heart over a period of usually eight to twenty-four hours. With this device, people can go about almost all of their normal activities, with a few exceptions like bathing. Arrhythmias that might not appear with a routine EKG would appear in this prolonged recording.

An electrocardiogram is also used during and after stress tests, specific levels of exercise used to determine the heart's exercise tolerance. Since the abnormal heart will often function normally at rest with a normal electrocardiogram, the application of stress to increase coronary metabolism and the need for an increase in the blood supply will generally demonstrate heart muscle disease as well as obstruction to blood delivery to the heart. In a stress test a person is instructed to exercise, usually on a treadmill, according to specific protocols that have particular levels for oxygen demands. As the treadmill is made to go faster, the person's heart works harder, demanding increased amounts of oxygen. Both the apprehension about the test and the nature of the test itself are extremely anxiety-provoking. Thus, results are best obtained by letting the person be as much in control of the test as possible through advance explanation, having the person examine and understand the machinery involved, and, to some extent, having the person regulate the level of participation.

An additional technique is an echocardiogram, in which ultrasound waves (mechanical vibrations of very high frequency) are transmitted into the heart and penetrate until they meet various structures and then are reflected back onto a recording device and processed into an image, which allows the physician to view movements of the heart and to examine the state of the tissue. Nuclear imaging is done to document the presence of dead tissue in the myocardial wall, to trace movement of the ventricular wall, and to determine blood flow through arteries and veins. To conduct the test, small amounts of radioactive substances are injected into a vein and then are scanned by nuclear cameras as the circulation passes them through the heart.

In cardiac catheterization, another test, a long, thin, flexible tube is fed through an artery or vein into the heart itself to record pressures, with-draw blood samples, and inject radiopaque dye. The part of the test in which dye is injected into the heart is called cardiac angiography and is used to gather information about deformities and obstructions. When dye is injected into an artery, the test is referred to as an arteriogram; when it is injected into a vein, it is called a venogram. During the procedure, moving x-ray pictures record accurate images of the anatomy of the heart. Although the chances are small, there is risk of a stroke, heart attack, or even death as a result of a cardiac catheterization. Hemodynamic moni-toring is carried out at the same time as cardiac catheterization. Special catheters allow for the measurement of central vein and artery pressure, lung artery and capillary wedge pressure, and the rate of blood put out by the heart. This monitoring can also be done at bedside but requires intensive care facilities. Other tests are specific to particular forms of heart disease (see under "Classification").

General Treatment

General treatment for heart disease includes modification of risk factors, drug therapy, and surgery. Modifiable risk factors are cigarette smoking, hypertension, obesity, physical inactivity, high blood cholesterol and tri-glyceride levels, and poor stress management. Medication is used to relieve symptoms and to impede the progress of the disease process. Drugs gen-erally either improve blood flow or decrease the demand for oxygen. Sur-gery is used largely for symptom relief and for inhibiting or halting the disease process.

Surgery for heart disease can be either closed heart or open heart. In open heart surgery, the heart is opened and a heart-lung machine tem-porarily takes over the functions of the heart by pumping oxygen-rich blood to the rest of the body. Surgery is used to correct heart defects like dam-aged valves, pacemaker disorders, diseased arteries, damaged blood ves-sels, vein abnormalities, or aneurysms, ballooning areas in an artery wall caused by weakness or leakage. In the case of damaged valves, the valve is replaced by an artificial valve or one fashioned of animal tissue. Natural pacemakers that are not functioning properly are aided by the implan-tation of an artificial pacemaker. Varicose veins, veins that have become enlarged or weak, can be excised, and aneurysms can be pinched off and eliminated.

Coronary artery disease is surgically treated through bypass grafting (coronary artery bypass grafting, commonly referred to as CABG, pro-nounced "cabbage"). It is called a bypass because it consists of grafting a vein (usually taken from one's leg) to bypass the obstruction in the artery. The number of grafts (or jumps, as they are sometimes called) ranges from one to as many as four or five. Although this kind of bypass surgery was first reported in 1969 to restore normal blood flow and thus reduce the symptoms of angina, a large proportion of people receive bypass surgery who have severe obstructive multivessel coronary artery disease and are asymptomatic, who have only mild angina, or who have had a heart attack. Some also have bypass surgery on the assumption that they will live longer as a result of the CABG. A random coronary surgery study sponsored by the National Heart, Lung, and Blood Institute reported that in 80 to 90 percent of patients CABG was effective in abolishing or reducing angina that could not be managed medically. With experienced medical teams the death rate for the CABG is 1 to 3 percent. Bypass surgery did not lengthen survival, however, except for people with disease of the left main coronary artery, nor did it affect the patient's employment or recreational status. CABG is the most commonly performed major surgery in the United States. In 1983 about 170,000 of these procedures were performed at a cost of about $20,000 each. Not counted in this estimate is the cost of testing and screening patients for surgery. It is thought that in the future the surgery will be increasingly confined to the treatment of intractable angina.

Nonsurgical interventions will become increasingly effective with the use of beta-adrenergic blockers, calcium channel blockers and cardiac angioplasty (transluminal balloon coronary angioplasty), in which a very thin balloon catheter is inserted into an artery in an arm or leg and then guided into a narrowed coronary artery while its progress is followed on an x-ray monitor. When it reaches the narrowed location, the balloon is inflated with a fluid for a few seconds, compressing the fatty plaques against the walls of the artery, expanding the passage by about 20 percent, and allowing the blood to flow freely again. At present angioplasty is thought to be a useful alternative in less than 5 percent of the patients for whom CAGB might be appropriate. It has a 60 percent success rate. The technique is not yet useful for plaques that are hard or calcified. It also has a high rate (15 to 18 percent) of reclosure or other complications from heart attack, from unstable angina to death. The majority of complications occur at the time of the procedure or just after it. At this time it is thought that angioplasty is most suitable for people whose disease is limited to the left anterior descending branch.

Classification

The principal forms of heart disease are myocardial infarction, angina pectoris, stroke, congestive heart failure, cardiac arrhythmias, hypertension, rheumatic heart disease, congenital heart defects, and peripheral arterial diseases. The first four forms are all part of atherosclerotic cardiovascular disease, in which the insides of parts of the body's system of arteries narrow over a period of years and thus decrease the amount of blood available to the area of the body fed by that part of the system. The most common sites of this disease process are the arteries leading to the heart, to the brain, from the heart, and to the legs. If the situation is not corrected, it will eventually result in a deficient blood supply to an area or to a stoppage and death of the tissue that has been deprived of blood. Narrowing occurs as a result of the development of "fatty streaks" or spots of fatty materials in the intima, the internal coating of the blood vessel; "fibrous plaques" of scar tissue; "atheromata" or plaques made of many different materials; or complicated tissue changes like ulcers, bleeding, blood clots, or calcium deposits.

MYOCARDIAL INFARCTION

The principal form of atherosclerotic coronary heart disease is myocardial infarction or heart attack, which usually results from the formation of a clot in an artery of the heart already narrowed by the disease process. Death occurs to the tissue that would be normally fed by that artery. Heart attack is the leading cause of death in the United States— 559,000 deaths in 1981. Sometimes the attack is preceded by angina pectoris; sometimes it can occur without warning and result in sudden death; and in some cases a heart attack produces no symptoms and is detected only when the person has a routine electrocardiogram.

The symptoms of myocardial infarction include severe crushing pain under the breast bone, which sometimes radiates into the left shoulder and down the left arm or along both arms. The pain usually lasts for two minutes or longer. Many times one also is acutely short of breath. The pain is often accompanied by sweating, nausea, or weakness. When these symptoms occur, a person is helped to sit or lie down in whatever position is most comfortable, and the nearest emergency rescue team should be called. If a person has collapsed, has no pulse, and is not breathing, CPR (cardio-pulmonary resuscitation, also called basic life support) can be used to attempt to revive him. The purpose of CPR is to maintain another person's breathing artificially by keeping airways open, pressing on the chest to compress the heart between the breast bone and the spine, and performing rescue or mouth-to-mouth breathing in order to keep oxygenated blood pumping through the body. Information on CPR training is available through the American Heart Association. In addition to using CPR, emergency rescue units, available in most communities through police or fire departments, also use drugs and electric shock to restore normal heart rhythm. In electric shock (referred to as defibrillation or cardioversion), very brief discharges of direct current are applied across the chest. This approach is generally used in emergencies but can also be used to treat chronic conditions.

When someone is suspected of having a heart attack, she is admitted to an intensive care or a coronary care unit of a hospital. Most heart attacks can be confirmed through the appearance of specific abnormalities on an EKG and the appearance of elevated levels of cardiac cellular enzymes, which have moved from the heart into the blood stream. Coronary care units are specifically designed to provide a protected and closely supervised environment. The patient remains visible to the staff, and the electrical activity of her heart, her heartbeat, respiration, and blood pressure are continuously monitored. A small needle or tube (referred to as an IV) is placed in the patient's vein so that the medical staff can have immediate access in case the patient requires emergency medication. Oxygen delivered by face mask or through small nasal tubes helps decrease the work of the heart. Specific treatment is directed toward repairing and stabilizing complications, reducing risk factors, and preventing additional heart attacks. Complications include pain, electrical problems, and heart failure. Intravenous morphine or demerol, laughing gas (nitrous oxide) mixed with oxygen, or a mild sedative such as Valium is used to reduce pain. Treatments for electrical problems and heart failure are discussed later in this section. Less than 15 percent of people who have a heart attack and reach the hospital die during their hospital stay. Most people recovering from a heart attack that has not been complicated with other medical problems will be able to leave the hospital in two to three weeks after the attack and can resume activity in six weeks to two months. Of the almost 1 million people who have a heart attack each year, about 100,000 will have a fatal heart attack within twelve months.

Four factors have correlated significantly with a subsequent fatal heart attack: accumulation of fluid in the lungs, impaired muscle contraction in the left ventricle of the heart, a history of chest pain while at rest or doing moderate exercise with onset at least a month before the first heart attack, and an abnormal frequency of irregular heart beats. The most powerful predictor is the presence of rales, crackling noises in the chest that can be heard through a stethoscope and are produced by the bubbling of accumulated fluid in the lungs. The bubbling fluid is the result of increased back pressure from the heart, allowing liquid from the blood vessels to leak into the air sacs of the lungs. The increased back pressure is caused by the heart's inability to pump blood effectively.

ANGINA PECTORIS

A second form of coronary heart disease is angina pectoris, recurrent episodes of chest pain usually caused by decreased flow of blood to the heart. Because it describes the kind of discomfort caused by a narrowing of the arteries, the translation of angina pectoris is a "strangling of the breast." The discomfort in the chest is variously described as a constricting feeling, tightness, weight, and a sensation of pressure. It is a radiating pain, felt in the arms, through the back, and up toward the jaw. Sometimes this pain is accompanied by a clammy sweat, shortness of breath, nausea, and/or vomiting.

Episodes can be precipitated by emotional stress, physical exercise, cigarette-smoking, and exposure to cold air, as well as by abnormalities in heart rhythm. Treatment for angina is in three areas: life-style interventions, drugs, and surgery. Changes in life-style will be discussed later in the chapter. Generally, the avoidance of precipitating factors is important for relief. Angina pectoris is treated with vasodilators and propranolal. Vasodilators relax the blood vessels and decrease the resistance to the flow of blood, allowing more blood to reach body tissues without the heart's having to work harder. The two kinds of vasodilators are nitrates and nonnitrates. Nonnitrates are no longer used except in the case of angina caused by heart spasm or where very occasionally heart failure is caused by an overabundance of blood within the heart. They were once used more frequently, until they were found to aggravate rather than relieve angina.

Long-acting and short-acting nitrates, drugs that widen the tubular space in the blood vessels, enhance the flow of oxygen. The most common nitrate is nitroglycerine, a tablet that is dissolved and absorbed under the tongue. Nitroglycerine provides pain relief within three minutes. The drug can also be used prophylactically when one knows she is about to engage in an activity that will probably produce angina. Nitroglycerine also can produce side effects of an increase in heart rate, feelings of warmth and flushing headache, and sometimes lightheadedness and weakness. Other nitrate preparations are longer-acting and are used to prevent angina attacks. They too can be dissolved under the tongue, swallowed, chewed, or applied as a paste to the skin. Side effects of nitrates also result from their dilating action; headache, faintness, and dizziness are caused by lowered blood pressure and dilated blood vessels. Sometimes palpitations are caused by the increase in heart rate and the speed of heart contraction.

Besides the nitrates, propranolol (Inderal) is also used to treat angina, but to prevent rather than to relieve pain. By blocking some of the sympathetic nerves to the heart, it slows the heart rate, decreasing the speed of contraction and lessening the heart's demand for oxygen. When used in combination with nitrates, it prevents the side effects that limit their effectiveness—the increase in heart rate and speed of contraction. Even though propranolol is effective in dealing with the side effects of the nitrates, it has side effects of its own. First, because it reduces the speed and force of the heart's contractions, it can cause congestive heart failure, which can eventually worsen the angina. If congestive heart failure occurs, digitalis alone or with a diuretic is added to the drug regimen. Since the drug's basic function is to block beta-sympathetic nerves, which are found not just in the heart but all over the body, constriction of blood vessels in the skin can cause cold, pale feet and hands. The drug can also aggravate previously existent asthma and can aggravate a low sugar level in a person with diabetes. At times propranolol can cause depression, sleeplessness, and, in rare instances, impotence. When a combination of these approaches does not provide adequate relief, coronary arteriography is indicated to determine the conditions of the person's coronary arteries. When arteriography shows a localized narrowing in a coronary artery, a coronary artery bypass is indicated. Because the disease process continues despite the bypass, it is thought that eventually the symptomatic benefits of the operation will fade and the chance of heart attack and death will again be high.

STROKE

Stroke, a third kind of atherosclerotic heart disease, is the subject of Chapter 9.

CONGESTIVE HEART FAILURE

In congestive heart failure, the heart is unable to pump its required amount of blood, and fluid accumulates in the body tissues of the abdomen, the legs, and the lungs. Fluid in the lungs called pulmonary edema, results from left-sided failure. In left-sided failure an imbalance of excessive pressure in the capillaries of the pulmonary circulation pushes fluid into the lung tissue. Fluid retention in other areas, such as the legs and feet, is a symptom of right-sided failure. The degree of failure can range from mild to severe. Although it can develop suddenly and severely, congestive heart failure usually develops slowly over several years.

The most common symptom of heart failure is initially fatigue, progressing to increasingly severe shortness of breath (dyspnea) caused by pulmonary edema. Dyspnea can be mild, in which case it does not affect a person's functioning to any great degree, or it may be severe enough to awaken a sleeping person. Other common symptoms include swelling of the feet and ankles, tiredness on exertion, weakness, or weight gain.

The following conditions can lead to heart failure. As blood pressure rises, the left ventricle has to strain increasingly to get the blood into the arteries. If the heart valves are damaged or abnormal to the degree that the heart has to pump excessively, heart failure develops. When large areas of the heart muscle have scarred as a result of coronary heart disease, the remaining areas of heart muscle have to compensate. Excessive strain on these areas can cause heart failure. When, as a result of viral infections or the toxic effects of alcohol, enlargement or overstretching of the heart muscle (cardiomyopathy) is caused, failure can occur. Also, severe lung disease can reduce the necessary amount of oxygen, make it harder for the heart to pump, or cause an overproduction of red blood cells, which makes the blood thicker and harder to pump. Failure can also be caused by congenital heart defects, severe anemia, arrhythmias, and an overactive thyroid, which strains the heart by overworking the body.

The body can compensate for heart failure in several ways. To provide added force to the contractions of the heart, the pumping chambers may stretch muscles and thus enlarge their capacity. The ventricle may enlarge and thus provide more muscle for pumping. The sympathetic nervous system can improve the contraction power of healthy heart muscle by elevating the heart rate.

The best way to treat this condition is to correct the conditions that have created it. Coronary artery disease and defective heart valves are treated with medicine and surgery. Advanced or severe congestive heart failure is treated with restriction of activity, bed rest, and drug therapy.

Basically, in congestive heart failure the heart is unable to pump sufficient oxygenated blood. To treat this condition, three types of drugs are used: digitalis, which increases the strength of the heart's contractions and thus brings the rate closer to normal; diuretics, which reduce the swelling characteristic of congestive heart failure by increasing urinary output of salt and water; and vasodilators, which relax the blood vessels and thus weaken the pressure against which the heart must pump.

Digitalis belongs to a group of drugs called cardiac glycosides, of which the most common are digoxin and digitoxin. The danger in these drugs is that because they are eliminated slowly from the body, an excessive amount occasionally accumulates, leading to digitalis toxicity with symptoms that may include irregular heartbeat, nausea, vomiting, headache, drowsiness, and blurred or strangely colored vision. For those also taking a diuretic and for the elderly, there is increased risk of toxicity. For many people the amount of digitalis necessary for strengthening heartbeat is very close to the level that may cause a toxic reaction. Control of the dosage and monitoring for signs of toxicity are important. A discontinuation of the drug usually alleviates the symptoms.

The main problems with diuretics occur with the loss of salt and other minerals, especially potassium. Potassium loss, which can result in feelings of weakness, occurs most commonly with the thiazide class of diuretics: chlorothiazide and hydrochlorothiazide. Potassium replacements or the addition of a second diuretic that does not cause potassium loss usually remedies this problem. However, this second kind of diuretic prevents loss by interfering with the kidneys' ability to excrete potassium and can lead to abnormally high levels of potassium in the body. Thiazides can also reduce the elimination of uric acid, aggravating previously existing gout, but not causing gout. Thus, again, monitoring of the drugs is imperative.

CARDIAC ARRHYTHMIAS

Another manifestation of coronary heart disease is cardiac arrhythmia. Arrhythmias are abnormal rhythms of the heartbeat, which may decrease the total amount of blood pumped by the heart and thus decrease the blood supply to the body. The heart's normal rate at rest is about 60 to 100 beats a minute. The average is about 70. If the heart rate is slow, under 60 beats a minute, the condition is called bradycardia. If it is over 100 beats a minute, it is called tachycardia. Either extreme can be a normal response or a sign of underlying disease. Arrhythmias may be precipated by exertion, emotional stress, stimulants like caffeine, underlying disease, or certain medications. Other symptoms associated with arrhythmias are palpitations, angina, heart failure, and some neurologic signs like fainting, muscle weakness, and speech and visual problems. The kind of arrhythmia that is most often fatal is ventricular fibrillation, an uncoordinated and uncontrolled functioning of the ventricles. The most common kind of nonfatal arrhythmia is auricular fibrillation, an uncoordinated quivering contraction of the atria with the result that beats of the atria are not coordinated with the ventricles.

Drugs to treat arrhythmias are quinidine, procainamide, and disopyramide, which block abnormal conduction of impulses in the heart. Again, their side effects are simply exaggerations of their desired effects. If excessive they can cause the arrhythmias they are meant to treat. Quinidine can also cause bleeding by decreasing the number of platelets in the blood, the cells responsible in part for clotting. It also can cause diarrhea, nausea, or vomiting. Procainamide can cause a decrease in white blood cells, which help fight infection, or an arthritis-like condition. All of these conditions are reversible when the drugs are stopped. Sometimes digitalis is used for preventing certain recurring arrhythmias and to slow the very rapid heart rates caused by certain arrhythmias. Propranolol's ability to slow the pulse is sometimes useful in certain arrhythmias. If the natural pacemaker or the pathways to the conduction system have been damaged, the implantation of an artificial pacemaker may be required.

HYPERTENSIVE DISEASE

In order for the blood to circulate, a constant pressure (diastolic) forces the blood forward. The contraction of the heart adds extra pressure (systolic). Hypertension means that the blood circulates through the arteries at a pressure higher than normal, which can result in degeneration and loss of elasticity within the arteries themselves. That affects the delivery of blood.

Hypertension affects about 37 million people in the United States. Even slight elevations of blood pressure (above 140/90) have been associated with increased risk of premature death. When hypertension is found in people who are already at risk for heart disease, the factors are additive. No one cause for essential hypertension has been found. There are multiple causes for onset, but the basic physiologic mechanisms remain controversial.

Two of the most thoroughly developed attempts to describe the physiology of blood pressure focus on the renin-angiotensin system and the kidneys and fluid balance. The renin-angiotensin system approach argues that arterial pressure is regulated and sodium is balanced through the renin-angiotensin-aldosterone axis. Renin is an enzyme that is stimulated by sodium loss and released into the blood from the kidney cortex. Among other activities, it forms angiotensin, a polypeptide (protein with long chains of amino acids linked together). The renin-angiotensin system regulates the secretion of aldosterone, a steroid that regulates electrolyte metabolism, increases excretion of potassium, and conserves sodium and chloride. Although it does suggest direct interventions, there are many problems with this approach.

The second approach, focusing on blood-volume control in the kidneys holds that only kidney body-fluid control has the capacity to return blood pressure to normal, independent of the pressure abnormality. This approach explains many aspects of hypertension but does not yet suggest clinical recommendations. Activity of the central nervous system also influences blood pressure, although specific mechanisms are not yet clear.

Several studies have suggested a link between hypertension and stress. Salt intake, weight, and exercise also are thought to influence blood pressure. Results of research in these areas are still controversial. Some studies have shown that greatly reduced salt intake, and/or weight loss, and/or an exercise program have reduced blood pressure. Others have failed to demonstrate these relationships. At one time Franz Alexander, a noted psychoanalyst, suggested the existence of a hypertensive personality in which people who have had difficulty asserting aggression and anger become overly compliant and unassertive, overconscientious and too responsible. Although many studies have attempted to test the theory, it has never been confirmed.

Once hypertension has been established, continuous high blood pressure can lead to thickening of the arterioles. Eventually the arteriole walls are weakened and become subject to small clots and hemorrhages. This occurs most often in the brain and the kidney. Because hypertension can cause the insides of the blood vessels to thicken, all blood flow can be affected. Hypertension can thus contribute to atherosclerosis, which can produce widespread vessel disease, to ventricular failure, and to aneurysms or ballooning faults in the walls of the blood vessels.

Blood pressure is generally measured with the aid of a sphygmomanometer, which consists of an inflatable cuff, a rubber bulb used to inflate it, and a gauge to measure the levels of pressure, which are recorded in millimeters of mercury. As the cuff is inflated and then gradually empties, the person taking the measurement listens with a stethoscope for specific characteristic sounds in the artery.

Accurate diagnosis of hypertension requires three elevated blood pressure readings taken at separate times with the person relaxed. The limb use and the body position of the person are also recorded. The systolic pressure is recorded at the point where the heart sound is heard. The diastolic correlates with the disappearance of sound in adults and the muffling of sound in children.

There are actually four terms to summarize diagnostic findings: Hypertensive disease means an elevated blood pressure with no clinically demonstrable disease of the heart and blood vessels; hypertensive heart disease means elevated blood pressure and an accompanying heart abnormality; hypertensive vascular disease means that someone has elevated blood pressure with vessel abnormalities; and hypertensive cardiovascular disease means that someone has high blood pressure with abnormalities of the heart and blood vessels.

Hypertension is also categorized by cause, with hypertension of unknown origin called primary or essential hypertension, and hypertension of known cause being called secondary hypertension. Primary hypertension is further divided into two types, benign and malignant, depending on the severity of the disease in the vessels and the rapidity of development.

Treatment of hypertension combines changes in life-style with drug therapy and, in a limited number of situations, surgery. The common approach to controlling blood pressure through medication is called step-care. Therapy begins with a small dose of an antihypertensive, which is increased gradually. As required, other drugs are added sequentially. The drug is gradually increased until the blood pressure goal is reached, side effects are intolerable, or the maximum safe dose of drug is being used. The first step is generally the use of diuretics, which increase the output of urine. Step two is the use of adrenergic inhibiting agents, which prevent the body from maintaining high blood pressure by inhibiting the instructions sent to the body to tighten the arteries. Examples are alphamethyl-DOPA, clonidine, and reserpine.

Step three employs vasodilators, which relax the blood vessels. Hydralazine is the vasodilator most commonly used for long-term treatment. Its most common side effects are headache and faintness. Occasionally, when used in very high doses, it causes an arthritis-like condition. When used with propranolol and a diuretic it has very few side effects. Most side effects cease when the drug is discontinued. A newer vasodilator called prazosin is thought to block certain kinds of sympathetic nerve responses, so it does not cause the body to compensate as strenuously as does hydralazine.

Step four is the use of an additional, more potent adrenergic inhibiting agent like guanethidine. Because of the many toxicities of these drugs, they are never used alone. Again, the side effects are excesses of the desired effects: faintness or fatigue as a result of too great a drop in pressure, depression, fluid retention requiring a diuretic, and a decrease in the functions of other parts of the sympathetic nervous system. Because the sympathetic nerves act on the bowels, for example, they can cause diarrhea. The drugs can also cause sperm to flow into the bladder and inhibit ejaculation. Antidepressants can inhibit their effectiveness.

Although drug therapy has proved highly effective in controlling hypertension, people tend not to comply with a protracted regimen for the following reasons: The symptoms of hypertension are often silent; the drugs can produce unpleasant side effects; the drugs are expensive; and people are told that since hypertension is a chronic condition, they will have to take drugs for a long time, perhaps for a lifetime. Thus, the question becomes: "Why should I take expensive drugs that make me feel bad, when I feel fine without them?" Besides, sudden cessation of drugs to control hypertension can cause blood pressure to increase to levels that are even higher than the person had before treatment and can even cause strokes. Thus, it is thought that drug therapy must be part of a total treatment plan in order to be effective. A total plan includes drug therapy, relaxation techniques, and a program of weight loss and reduction of salt intake.

Surgical intervention is possible only for a limited number of specific types of hypertension, including coarctation (congenital narrowing of the aorta), renovascular hypertension (elevated blood pressure due to narrowing in the vessels to the kidneys), and tumors of the adrenal medulla, the adrenal gland that secretes noradrenaline, which in turn has a powerful ability to constrict the blood vessels.

RHEUMATIC HEART DISEASE

In rheumatic heart disease, an untreated streptoccocal infection (strep throat) has developed into rheumatic fever, which has then damaged the heart valves. The goal is to diagnose and treat the infection before it develops into rheumatic fever. If the diagnosis is not made before rheumatic fever has developed, the goal is to treat the fever before it damages the heart valves. If the valves have already been damaged, the goal becomes symptom alleviation, eventually through the replacement of damaged valves.

The American Heart Association reports that in 1981 deaths from rheumatic fever and rheumatic heart disease combined numbered 7,700. In the same year more than 2 million people were estimated to have rheumatic heart disease. Common symptoms of strep throat are sudden onset with pain on swallowing, fever, swollen glands under the angle of the jaw, headache, nausea, and vomiting. A microscopic examination of the mucus in the throat can determine the presence of a streptoccocal infection. On detection, the infection is treated with penicillin or another antibiotic. If the infection is untreated, the person may develop rheumatic fever, a reaction to one of the streptoccocal bacteria, Group A streptococcus.

Rheumatic fever generally occurs in children and adolescents between the ages of five and fifteen. Symptoms include high fever, which may last as long as two weeks, and joint tenderness and pain, which can move from one joint to another. Sometimes joints become warm, swollen, or red. A rash may appear; often a child is tired and pale and has a poor appetite. Occasionally a person experiences chorea, involuntary movements of the extremities. Heart involvement may also produce shortness of breath or chest pain, an enlarged heart, or other damage to the heart muscle, valves, and/or pericardium.

There is no specific laboratory test for rheumatic fever, but the presence of infection can be detected by measuring how fast red blood cells settle out or by detecting the presence in the blood of an abnormal protein. In addition, chest x-ray, electrocardiogram, fluoroscopy, echocardiography, and cardiac catheterization can be used to assess functioning as well as damage.

People who have had episodes of rheumatic fever are more susceptible to futher attacks. Thus prevention of a second attack becomes paramount. Some physicians think that an extended program of antibiotic treatment is necessary, and others believe that a person should follow such a regimen for life. Another precautionary measure is to prescribe a course of antibiotic whenever a person who has had rheumatic fever must undergo a surgical procedure. Such procedures place one at greater risk for bacterial endocarditis, another kind of inflammation, which may affect the heart valves.

Rheumatic fever, in turn, can cause chronic rheumatic heart disease, of which an important feature is scarring of the valves of the heart. Scarring can cause stenosis or insufficiency. In stenosis, the valve cannot open fully. Often symptoms do not develop for many years until the valve opening has become markedly narrowed. Because stenosis creates resistance to emptying the chamber behind the narrowed valve, blood pressure must rise in order to pump enough blood through a smaller space. In the case of insufficiency an improperly closing valve allows blood to leak back into the chamber from which it has been pumped. The volume of blood the chamber must pump is increased, because some of it is pumped back through the valve that did not close. This condition is also called leakage or regurgitation, because each time the heart beats, both the regurgitated blood and the normally flowing blood must flow through the valve. The heart is already working harder because of the leakage. Any additional work—walking, recreational activity, or stress—causes the heart to work even harder, and people with insufficiency can feel their hearts being overactive. Gradually the left ventricle increases in size to try to keep up with the extra need, and it is eventually unable to pump adequately. The increased pressure in the ventricle causes shortness of breath (as a result of affecting the lung's blood vessels), fatigue (since there is a lessened supply of blood to the body), and fluid retention (since there is a decrease in blood flow to the kidneys).

The degree and range of symptoms vary, but problems with heart valves can eventually be disabling, depending on which heart valve is affected and the extent of the damage. The principal valve problems resulting from rheumatic heart disease are mitral stenosis, mitral regurgitation, aortic stenosis, and aortic regurgitation. Because blood pressures are higher on the left side of the heart, abnormalities of the mitral and aortic valves, both located on the left side of the heart, develop symptoms earlier. On the other hand, the tricuspid and pulmonary valves, which are located on the right side, develop symptoms later and much less often.

Mitral stenosis occurs primarily in women. The age of onset for symptoms is generally from thirty to fifty. In mitral stenosis one develops symptoms related to blood being backed up in the left atrium and the lungs. Symptoms include abnormal heart rhythm, failure of the right ventricle, low output of blood pumped from the heart, and the formation of clots inside the enlarged left atrium, which can break off into the circulatory system. If they lodge in the brain, these clots (emboli) can cause a stroke; if they lodge in the legs or arms, they can stop circulation and cause a gangrenous infection and eventually require a limb to be amputated. They can lodge in other organs as well, particularly the kidney. Mitral stenosis is treated surgically by opening the scarred valve in a procedure called mitral commissurotomy. It is not unusual for the valve to narrow again, but the operation can be repeated.

Mitral regurgitation places a volume load on the left ventricle and left atrium because it allows blood back into the left atrium in addition to the normal flow. It thereby creates the conditions for heart failure and concomitant symptoms of shortness of breath, swelling of the ankles and feet, fatigue on exertion, general weakness, and/or weight gain.

Aortic stenosis requires the left ventricle to work harder, increasing pressure in the left ventricle. Because of diminished cardiac output, systemic blood pressure falls. Its symptoms include fainting or lightheadedness, low output, and, in the case of severe stenosis, angina pectoris. Aortic regurgitation produces symptoms of pump failure by increasing the blood volume load on the left ventricle. The treatment for each of these major valve problems is valve replacement surgery. In the surgery the diseased valve is replaced with an artificial valve made of metal and plastic or a valve taken from an animal, most often a pig. Replacement surgery is generally very successful in alleviating symptoms. Most people who have had valve replacements are also on a permanent regimen of anticoagulant drugs to prevent clots from forming on the new valve. An artificial valve may be a focus for serious infections like bacterial endocarditis, inflammation of the inner lining of the heart.

CONGENITAL HEART DEFECTS

Occurring in approximately one out of one hundred births, congenital heart defects are abnormalities in the heart's structure existing at the time of birth that impair blood flow. Symptoms include cyanosis (a bluish tint to the nails, lips, and skin caused by an undersupply of oxygen), fatigue, rapid breathing, eating difficulties, and failure to thrive. Further diagnostic information can be gathered through the detection of a heart murmur; the use of chest x-ray, which would depict an enlarged heart or congested lungs; echocardiography to check the structure of the heart; and, if surgery is being considered, cardiac catheterization.

Some defects are very mild, causing no apparent damage. Generally their cause is unknown. However, one known cause is rubella (German measles), which, if contracted by a woman during her first three months of pregnancy, can interfere with several aspects of the fetus's development, including the normal structure of the heart.

The most common congenital defects that obstruct the flow of blood are narrowing of a heart valve (stenosis) and constriction of the aorta (coarctation). Both cause the heart to pump harder to try to attain normal pressure. The most common defects that reroute the blood from the left to the right side of the heart instead of into the arterial system are holes in the dividing wall between the lower chambers of the heart (ventricular septal defect) and in the wall separating the upper chambers (atrial spetal defect) or the continued opening of a tube between the aorta and the pulmonary artery which would normally close before birth (patent ductus arteriosus). The ventricular septal defect overloads the heart and lungs because blood from the left side of the heart flows into the ventricle of the right side of the heart, and this greater volume of blood is pumped to the lungs. As a result the ventricles enlarge and the lung vessels thicken. Sometimes these defects affect growth. An atrial septal defect sometimes causes heart enlargement because too great a quantity of oxygen-rich blood is coming into the right side of the heart. Patent ductus arteriosus causes some blood to circulate uselessly between the heart and the lungs, requiring the heart to work harder.

The three most common congenital defects that deny the body its necessary supply of oxygen-rich blood by rerouting the blood from the right to the left side of the heart are tetralogy of Fallot, transposition of the aorta and the pulmonary artery, and hypoplastic left heart syndrome. Tetralogy of Fallot is a combination of a large hole between the ventricles, a constriction beneath the pulmonary valve, an overly muscular right ventricle, and the placement of the aorta directly over the hole between the ventricles. In the transposition of the aorta and the pulmonary artery, blood is not routed back to the lungs for additional oxygen and the blood within the lungs is recycled back to the lungs rather than circulated to the rest of the body. In the case of hypoplastic left heart syndrome, the left side of the infant's heart is underdeveloped and therefore can neither receive nor pump oxygen-rich blood. Some defects repair themselves. Others are treated with drugs. Drug treatment is prescribed sometimes to relieve symptoms until the infant is ready for surgery, to prevent complications, or to relieve symptoms later in life. However, drugs cannot repair the underlying defects. Surgery is directed to the repair of defects in order to normalize the flow of blood. Stenosis, a patent ductus arteriosus, septal defects, transposition of the pulmonary artery and the aorta, and coarctation of the aorta, as well as many other less common defects, can generally be repaired through surgery. If the surgery is fully corrective, a child will be able to assume normal activity. Even a partial correction means the assumption of limited activity.

PERIPHERAL VASCULAR DISEASES

Peripheral vascular diseases are those affecting the blood vessels that carry blood from the heart: vasospastic, in which small arteries constrict or go into spasm; aneurysm, in which a weakness causes the wall of an artery to bulge; and occlusive, in which blood flow is blocked.

Vasospastic. The two most important disorders in the vasospastic category are Raynaud's disease and livedo reticularis. Raynaud's Disease is characterized by the sequence of paleness, blueness, and then redness of both hands in response to cold or stress. Usually beginning in women in their late teens, it is generally benign. If it is secondary to another disease, it is usually a serious symptom.

Livedo reticularis is a benign condition that gives the skin a "fishnet" appearance through a bluish mottling of the skin. Basically people with these conditions are told to avoid exposure to the cold. In their primary forms the conditions are sometimes treated through medication. In their secondary forms they are managed through treatment of the underlying disease.

Aneurysm. An aneurysm is a ballooning fault in the wall of an artery due to weakness caused by arteriosclerosis, syphilis, or some other infection. If an artery bursts, sudden loss of a great deal of blood can cause a person to die. A common site is the abdominal aorta.

Occlusive. The most important disorder in the occlusive category is arteriosclerosis obliterans, a slowly progressive disease in which the buildup of plaque in the arterial walls interferes with blood flow and especially affects the legs and feet. The process is the one which causes coronary heart disease. Symptoms may occur at rest or with exercise. At rest, symptoms include numbness, tingling, and continuous pain, generally in one's toes or feet. On exertion, one experiences claudication, in which blocked blood flow causes severe calf, thigh, or buttock pain and limping. If the disease blocks blood flow to the point where tissues are denied adequate nutrition, gangrene and ulcers (open sores) can result. At that point amputation of the diseased portion of the leg is required.

Buerger's disease is a less common form of obliterative arterial disease that occurs in men between twenty and forty years old who smoke cigarettes. In contrast to arteriosclerosis obliterans, which involves medium and large arteries, Buerger's disease involves small arteries in the hands and feet. Symptoms include visual disturbances, severe pain in hands and feet, and fingertip ulcers, which may necessitate amputation.

Management of occlusive disease includes meticulous care of one's feet and all cuts and bruises, exercise to improve blood flow, and weight reduction. Surgical therapy is rarely required. Occasionally lumbar sympathectomy (interruption of the sympathetic nerve supply) or vein grafts to bypass obstructed arteries are indicated.

Several medications are used to treat occlusive disease. Clofibrate lowers the level of cholesterol and other fats in the blood but can cause side effects of nausea, drowsiness, and occasionally cramps and stiff muscles. Nicotinic acid, another drug, lowers fats and also dilates the blood vessels. In addition to achieving its desired effects, it can also dilate the blood vessels of the skin, causing one's face to flush. Cholestyramine lowers fats by changing absorption and promoting elimination because it binds bile in the bowel. The body needs bile in order to absorb fat. Since the drug keeps bile unavailable, fat is less readily absorbed. Side effects of this drug include nausea, stomach upset, constipation, and an unpleasant taste.

Anticoagulants are used to prevent the formation of clots by decreasing the amount of proteins or inhibiting the clotting tendency of the platelets needed for formation. Those that act on proteins, such as Warfarin and bishydroxycoumarin, are of value in treating clots in the veins but are of questionable value in treating those in the arteries. The danger in using these drugs is that they could cause serious bleeding by interfering with the normal clotting function. The anticoagulating effect is also often increased when other drugs are taken. This effect can be reversed with an excess of vitamin K, which is necessary in the production of the clotting proteins. Thus anticoagulants are carefully monitored to maintain normal clotting functions.

Other drugs, like aspirin, dipyridimole (also a vasodilator), and anturane (for the treatment of gout), rarely cause bleeding and thus are less dangerous than the previously described drugs, but their effectiveness has not yet been proved. In the past vasodilators were used to treat arterial disease, but it was discovered that diseased vessels cannot dilate and that healthy vessels, which did respond to the drug, in effect lowered the supply to diseased vessels, diminishing their already low flow. When decreased blood supply is due to spasm rather than clots or arteriosclerosis, vasodilators are sometimes useful. Because the degree of damage may be lessened if blood supply can be restored quickly after a stroke or heart attack, some drugs have been developed to dissolve blood clots in these circumstances. Such drugs can cause severe bleeding, and thus people have to be hospitalized and carefully monitored while receiving them. To date there is no conclusive evidence that such drugs minimize the damage from stroke or heart attack.

Psychosocial Information

The primary focus of this section will be coronary heart disease and primarily heart attack rather than congenital heart defects, hypertension, rheumatic heart disease, or peripheral vascular disease. Most heart disease is not incapacitating. The most severe forms can render one an invalid, but milder, less damaging forms allow one to live in much the same way as she has always lived. Because many aspects of life-style are risk factors in heart disease, modifications in life-style can be preventative. Overall, those who do not have a hereditary pattern of heart disease, who exercise regularly, whose diet is high in complex carbohydrates and low in salt and fat, who do not smoke, are not obese, and do not live with excessive stress are less at risk for heart disease than those who do not exercise and are obese, whose diet is high in salt and fats, and who smoke and live with excessive stress.

Once someone has experienced a heart attack or an episode of angina, his view of life and that of his immediate family are affected to the degree that it can happen again without warning and can be fatal. All the while, the person with heart disease can look well and be leading a normal life. One informant whose father eventually died of a third heart attack said it was like going about your business while holding your breath.

Modifications in Life-Style

DIET

A high-fat, high-salt diet and obesity place one at greater risk for heart disease. For obese people the death rate for heart disease and hypertension is three times as high as it is for those of normal weight. High-fat diets are linked to the fatty deposits in the arteries that are the primary sign of arteriosclerosis. High salt intake, mainly in the form of table salt, is linked to hypertension. People with heart disease, as well as those who want to prevent heart disease, are therefore cautioned to maintain normal weight and to lower their intake of fats and salt. Part of the attention to diet means an increase in the amounts of complex carbohydrates (found in fresh fruits and vegetables) one eats. Chemically simple sugars like those found in soft drinks, desserts, and snack food are to be avoided, because they have very little nutritive value and are high in calories. Alcohol also contributes to obesity, because it too is high in calories and low in nutrients. Dramatic reductions in cholesterol levels can be achieved through drug therapy. A study at the National Institutes of Health demonstrated that use of the drug cholestyramine accounted for a 25 percent reduction in blood cholesterol levels and 50 percent fewer heart attacks in the test group by reducing the levels of low-density lipoprotein (LDL), a type of fat/protein that is thought to deliver cholesterol to the cells or to fail to remove it. Low-density lipoprotein should be differentiated from high-density lipoprotein (HDL), which is thought to help metabolize or remove cholesterol from cells.

There are also special dietary concerns for people with congestive heart failure. First, when many people are in failure, they make themselves a soothing bowl of soup in order to feel better. Often the soup is very salty, and the salt contributes to the failure. Some people with congestive heart failure also have a condition called pica, in which they have an unusual desire to eat ice. The excess fluid often goes unmentioned by the ill person and his family, but it too contributes to recurrent heart failure. Thus, it is critical for family members and the ill person to monitor the amount of liquid, ice, and salt consumed.

SMOKING

Smoking is clearly linked to heart disease for both men and women. It is considered the greatest risk factor after family history. The more one smokes, the greater is one's risk of heart disease. Smoking one pack of cigarettes a day will produce an increased incidence of premature heart attack. Smoking four packs a day increases the risk for premature heart attack and sudden death two hundred times. After a total abstinence from smoking for a ten-year period, one's risk for heart disease is almost the same as that of a nonsmoker.

EXERCISE

The lack of regular exercise is a risk factor in heart disease. A vigorous, physician-monitered exercise program can improve cardiovascular fitness, the ability of the heart and blood vessels to supply the oxygen needs of body tissue by increasing the maximal oxygen uptake, the maximum amount of oxygen that can be transported from the lungs. Body tissues consume more than 75 percent of the oxygen delivered through heavy exercise. This high level of oxygen extraction requires much less work by the heart. As the heart muscle becomes stronger, it requires fewer beats to deliver the same amount of blood and oxygen.

Three forms of muscular activity—aerobic, isometric, and isotonic— each produce a special cardiac response. Aerobic exercise includes movements that are continuous and rhythmic like those involved in walking, cycling, swimming, and jogging. Each increases oxygen consumption, heart rate, and systolic blood pressure while maintaining or slightly lowering diastolic pressure. Thus, the heart pumps out more blood per minute. Aerobic exercise has been demonstrated to be beneficial for people with coronary artery disease.

Isometric exercise, sometimes called static exercise, is muscular activity against a fixed, unmoving resistance. This type of exercise rapidly increases blood pressure with very little increase in heart rate, cardiac output, or oxygen consumption irrespective of the area or part of the body involved. Thus the demands on the heart and blood requirements increase. Coronary heart disease obstruction may prevent an adequate supply of blood for meeting the demand, and symptoms such as angina will occur.

Isotonic exercise is activity that maintains equal tension in a muscle through a full or partial range of joint motion. Cardiovascular response is related to the resistance provided by the object moved. Low resistance provides a response like aerobics; high resistance, like isometrics. Thus, it is helpful to find the means for lowering the resistance of objects and turning what might have been detrimental into beneficial exercise. Thus, lifting and carrying a 50-pound bag of potatoes would be isometric, but quickly transferring the bag to a cart and pushing the cart would lessen the resistance and may be beneficial. It is recommended that exercise be part of a regular routine in which one begins gradually with a warmup, moves into the workout phase, and then cools down adequately to avoid a rapid drop in blood pressure. Sporadic, exhaustive effort is antiproductive.

Treatment for recovery from a heart attack also involves exercise. Soon after a person is admitted to a coronary care or intensive care unit, he is given passive range of motion exercises in which his limbs are moved for him. As he becomes stronger, he carries out range of motion exercises himself. Early physical mobility is considered critical to recovery. The ill person sits up as soon as he is able, then walks with support, then is urged to walk regularly on his own. Exercise is systematic, graduated, and educative.

WORK

Generally people who have had heart attacks begin soon after their attacks to plan to return to work. Studies report different rates of return depending on the kinds of jobs people held previously, the severity of the illness, and other factors, often related to the studies themselves. Overall, about two-thirds of the people who survive heart attacks eventually return to work.

Blue-collar workers, the less educated, and those with lasting emotional distress or serious medical problems have the greatest occupational problems. Excessive and continuous stresses on heart muscle and the cardiovascular system, such as heavy lifting, chemical hazards, and noxious environmental conditions, are suggested to be associated with heart disease. Psychosocial work stresses like long working hours, role conflict, heavy work load, status incongruity, multiple responsibilities, and lack of rewards and gratification are also associated with heart disease.

Often jobs are classified as sedentary, light, medium heavy, or very heavy. Sedentary requires lifting a maximum of 10 pounds, modest walking and standing, and sitting. Light work requires lifting up to 20 pounds with substantial walking and standing. Medium work requires lifting up to 50 pounds with a usual requirement of 25 pounds and substantial walking and sitting. Heavy work requires lifting a maximum of 100 pounds with a usual requirement of 50 pounds, and very heavy work requires a lifting maximum of greater than 100 pounds. As routine job activities, the heavy and very heavy classifications should be avoided by people with heart disease. In the same way, people with heart disease should avoid working conditions that involve extreme temperatures, which increase the stress on the heart, or high levels of carbon dioxide, which adversely affect the transport of oxygen to the tissues.

Approximately one-third of people with heart disease have to modify their daily job activities. Many work situations can be improved through work-simplification techniques, identifying and minimizing isometric stress and optimizing aerobic and low-level isotonic activity. Members of cardiac rehabilitation services, especially occupational therapists and rehabilitation counselors, are able to improve work situations by using these techniques.

RELAXATION TECHNIQUES

Relaxation techniques have proved effective in reducing blood pressure. Biofeedback has been used in three ways. In the first blood pressure is measured with a blood pressure cuff (a sphygmomanometer), and the person is informed what his pressure is. In the second the person wears a cuff that has been inflated to about the average diastolic pressure and is held constant. Whenever the person's pressure rises, a sound alerts him, and he is told to eliminate the sound. The third approach uses blood pressure velocity to measure pressure indirectly. This is accomplished by using two pulses separated in space or by using the ECG wave and the peripheral pulse (the pulse in one of the limbs). Usually blood pressure increases as the pulse wave velocity increases. These methods have not proved more effective at six months than relaxation procedures that people can incorporate into their lives. One such method, the relaxation response, is a conscious meditation-like mental effort over bodily characteristics like blood pressure, heart rate, and blood flow. Relaxation techniques are also briefly discussed in the Chapter 5 on diabetes, under "Impact of the Disease on Social Life."

Legal Issues

Legal issues in heart disease are the right to work and, very occasionally, legal guardianship when severe heart failure and a low cardiac output have caused an inadequate supply of oxygenated blood to the brain. Again, as with other diseases, the National Rehabilitation Act of 1973 prohibits discrimination on the basis of a physical or mental handicap in a job for which a person is qualified. Thus a person cannot be discriminated against simply because he has heart disease. For an explanation of the ability of the state to protect the rights and property of people who can no longer manage their own affairs, see under "Legal Issues" in chapter 4 on the dementias.

Insurance

Once someone has been diagnosed with heart disease, it is very difficult to obtain health, life, or disability insurance coverage. In the case of congenital heart defects, some progress has been made to differentiate relative risks presented by different kinds of defects. State laws and insurance companies vary in the coverage provided for each kind of heart illness.

Social Security Disability Payments can be obtained if a person can demonstrate that he has severe cardiac impairment resulting from congestive heart failure, a deficient blood supply to the heart (ischemia), or fainting episodes as a result of conduction disturbances and/or arrhythmias (cardiac syncope). The criteria for evaluation are based on symptoms, physical signs, and pertinent laboratory findings. For example, severe cardiac impairment as a result of congestive heart failure can be demonstrated through evidence of vascular congestion such as an accumulation of fluid in the lungs and extremities. All findings besides vascular congestion must be persistent. Clinical examination must demonstrate physical signs consistent with shortness of breath, fatigue, and rhythm disturbance. The clinical findings must be confirmed by objective studies like electrocardiograms obtained by themselves or in conjunction with exercise tests, echocardiography, or cardiac catheterization. Criteria for ischemia (deficient blood supply) spell out the kind of pain the person must experience. Included is pain, which can be described as crushing, squeezing, burning, or oppressive. Excluded is pain that can be described as sharp, sticking, or rhythmic. Basically, the standard is that a person must be severely impaired to qualify for Disability Payments. He and his physician must be able to document with precise clinical and laboratory findings the exact nature of the impairment and its fit with the Social Security Disability criteria. Certain occupational groups, such as police or firemen, sometimes assume heart disease to be a consequence of their work.

Relationships with Family Members

Because heart disease is thought by many to be exacerbated by stress, troubled relationships at work and at home are sometimes cited as contributing to the illness, particularly to angina and heart attack. Both ill people and their spouses make these claims at times. Family members, especially wives, may think their husbands have had attacks because they themselves pushed them to ask for promotions at work or even to take a second job. People with heart conditions and their spouses point to marital conflict or conflict between parent and child as a reason for the illness. None of these associations of various aspects of relationships and heart disease has been significantly demonstrated in research at this time.

The death rate of heart disease is associated with certain aspects of relationships with others. For example, the death rate is lower for those who live in company (even with a pet) than for those who live alone. The death rate for all groups except white females is higher for those who are single than for those who are married.

Relationships with others are important not only in terms of stressors in heart disease but in the postonset phases of the disease process as well. The relationship between spouses is thought to be most affected. Wives are often anxious and concerned. They may become overprotective and oversolicitous in their desire to help their ill husbands. One informant, a nurse whose husband had had a heart attack a few months earlier, said that she had learned in nursing courses that wives sometimes smothered their recovering husbands in their determination to prevent another heart attack. They monitored eating and drinking, forbade smoking, hounded their husbands about proper amounts and kinds of exercise, and would barely let their husbands watch television for fear that they would become "overexcited" and have another attack. What she could not believe was that she was doing all the same things and enraging her husband with her intrusiveness.

Soon after a heart attack couples generally tend to be very careful of each other's feelings and to avoid conflict. Wives often strive to have their husbands comply precisely with every suggestion made by the physician. They try to restrict their husbands' activities and to protect them from almost all stress. On the other hand men who have had heart attacks generally want to get back to their lives and back to work. They do not see the point of absolute compliance.

The ill person and his spouse rarely think the disease is affecting the children in the family. The social and psychological burden is thought to remain with the parents. This is thought to be partly a reflection of the denial that accompanies heart disease. Because the ill parent often does not appear ill, children see little to worry about. One informant whose father had a heart attack when the informant was fourteen years old remembers clearly being told to go see his father in the hospital and then leaving to play basketball. Another whose father had his first heart attack when she was eleven remembers being told that her father was fine, seeing him look fine, and going out in the backyard to play with friends. Each informant, however, remembers the day very clearly. Thus they were made aware that the day was significant but also that they had little responsibility in it.

Family relationships are different in the case of children with correctable heart defects. Family dynamics are often directed toward protecting the child until he can have an operation that will repair the problem. The future looks different for such youngsters than for adults with coronary heart disease. Often families equate repair of the defect with a cure for the illness. Many times it is a cure. The dynamic in the case of children with rheumatic fever seems generally to be different. Because the possibility of future problems resulting from the original illness continues, families sometimes remain cautious even when there is no evidence of heart damage. One twenty-five-year-old informant who has no known heart damage from childhood rheumatic fever says that her mother remains overprotective of her. She worries that her daughter might place too great a strain on her heart or catch a chill, but she is not protective of her other grown children.

The services of extended kin and quasi-kin are important in a family's dealing with heart disease. Such services include emotional support, helping with transportation and house chores, and financial assistance. One informant, an elderly woman whose husband has severe congestive heart failure, says it is her neighbors who have kept her husband home with her. They not only shop, visit, and take him to the doctor, but they helped rearrange the furniture in the house so that her husband would never have to climb the stairs.

Sexual Activity

After a heart attack sexual activity frequently does not return to former levels. Problems are thought to be more psychological than physiological. If a man has experienced no complications, he may be told that it is all right to have intercourse by about the fifth week after leaving the hospital or about ten weeks after the heart attack. At first it is suggested that the person who has had the heart attack be relatively passive, with the spouse doing most of the work. In time people can resume their former activity. Often, because ill people know that intercourse does increase blood pressure, pulse rate, and the work of the heart, they are afraid intercourse will cause a heart attack. Many times the spouses are fearful too. An informant, concerned that her husband was experiencing discomfort during intercourse, whispered to him that it was all right with her if he wanted to wait a little longer before trying. He lost his erection and turned away from her. Her husband then waited several weeks before trying again. No research has demonstrated that intercourse can cause a heart attack. The occasional person who experiences angina during intercourse will be instructed to take a nitroglycerine tablet just before intercourse.

Relationships with Strangers

Most people with heart disease do not appear to be sick. Even after coronary bypass surgery, when many people feel as if they have been hit by a truck, they look good. Thus relationships with strangers are affected only in so far as a person with heart disease might restrict himself from certain activities. One informant was asked by a neighbor to help him carry a sofa down a flight of stairs. When he said he could not do that kind of lifting because of his heart condition, the neighbor pointed out that he looked as fit as anyone else.

Psychological Issues

Psychological issues in coronary heart disease relate both to etiology and to the phases of the process of treatment and convalescence. In relation to etiology, most discussion and research have focused on the type A personality—people who are chronically struggling to gain an unlimited number of ill-defined objectives from their environment as quickly as possible, if necessary over the opposition of other people or obstacles. Type A is not considered a character trait or a personality type but a reaction of a characterologically predisposed person to a situation that challenges him. It is a style of behavior with which some people respond to challenging situations. A Type A person feels and acts pressured and shows tense facial musculature, explosiveness of speech, and a chronically hyperarousable anger. A positive correlation has been demonstrated between aggressive, impatient, competitive (type A) behavior and stressful life events before a heart attack. For example, an informant said that a forty-seven-year-old professional friend of his who has had two heart attacks was notified that the building in which he had his office was being sold and he would have to move. When he decided that the rent for a new office was excessive, he had a temper tantrum, screaming at his staff, his family, and the rental agent. That night he was admitted to the hospital with chest pain. An overlay of disappointment, hopelessness, and helplessness further exacerbates the situation. Symptoms include anxiety, sadness, exhaustion, and lack of interest in sex. Type A people are generally unconcerned about contracting a serious illness.

Type A is clearly and independently associated with increased risk of coronary heart disease. Type A men under fifty years old have twice the rate of coronary artery disease as those who are not type A. They are also at least at that level of increased risk for recurrent or fatal myocardial infarction. However, while type A status doubles the risk of new coronary artery disease, only 1 percent of type A subjects develop coronary artery disease each year. Thus, although there is a clear association, the relationship is not causal.

STAGES OF PSYCHOLOGICAL RESPONSE

Certain psychological issues are related to the stages of treatment for and convalescence from heart disease. After a heart attack, people's levels of anxiety and depression remain high. Depression usually peaks three to five days after admission. Most people report that the coronary care unit is depersonalized and timeless, but not traumatic. Although they are anxious for the first couple of days after admission, they are generally reassured by the visibility of the equipment and the number of physicians and nurses in the unit. While they are in intensive care, they are also separated from their families. Visiting times are short, perhaps only ten-minute periods, and all visitors but one's immediate family are discouraged. While in intensive care people tend to be passive and present-oriented. The structure of the unit and the threat of the illness restrict, define, and control the person's behavior. Because patients and families are afraid of getting bad news, they do not ask questions. A cardiologist stressed that asking questions is critical. He thinks people who force themselves to ask questions manage their illness better simply because more information makes one feel as if he has more control of his situation.

People feel anxious and frightened again when they are transferred from the coronary care unit to a stepdown unit or to a general medical floor. There are no monitors and few restrictions. An informant said that this move was traumatic for him. Although he knew better intellectually, he felt that the monitors were somehow keeping him alive. Once they were disconnected, he was afraid he would die. A designated nurse or physician responsible for overseeing the move can ease this difficult transition.

Once someone is transferred from an intensive care unit, he gradually becomes more active and future-oriented. He is rejoined with his family after a traumatic and stressful period in which each member defined the situation and his expectations about the future without an awareness of what the other was thinking. Often couples hold discrepant views. Both patient and family are uncertain and fearful. Many times, families want the ill person to be less active.

Homecoming usually occurs in an atmosphere of worried concern. At first home and one's daily routine are made to resemble the hospital as closely as possible. Sometimes people are less active than they were at the end of their hospital stay. Wives often see their recovering husbands as fragile and continuing to need protection. When husbands begin to assert themselves, wives remind them of their fragility and insist on compliance. This is a difficult time for families, because people want to resume their former roles, and everybody is uncertain about the convalescing person's fitness. Generally, once the ill person is out of the hospital, he and his family make most of the decisions about the individual's level of activity.

PARTICULAR PSYCHOLOGICAL ISSUES

Ongoing psychological issues are depression, a long-lasting emotional distress, fear, and denial. Depression almost always accompanies the acute stages of heart disease. As a person recovers physically, his depression usually lifts. Occasionally, especially after a heart attack, an individual experiences severe and extended depression with accompanying feelings of worthlessness and guilt. After bypass surgery, some people, more often those who were not experiencing severe pain beforehand, experience some depression. Because of the nature of the surgery—opening the chest, cutting the sternum, and removing veins from the leg—a person does not feel well for several months after the operation. The presence of the scar sometimes makes people feel as if they have been damaged, especially if they had no noticeable symptoms before surgery. The scar, a large "T" that runs from just under the collar bone to the bottom of the sternum (the xyphoid tip), becomes a focus for many people who have had open heart surgery. The peer support groups organized through the American Heart Association for people who have had open heart surgery, for example, are called Zipper Clubs. One informant, a twenty-three-year-old woman who had had an aortic valve replacement when she was seventeen, said that whenever someone threw a ball at her or even began to give her a bear hug, her hand instinctively went to her chest to protect her scar. It hurts sometimes, and she sees it and not her heart as the site of her vulnerability.

Fear is a pervasive issue. Severe angina or shortness of breath resulting from heart failure make one feel out of control and sometimes on the verge of death. A woman who has severe angina said that she became so afraid of the pain that it became more important to her than the disease. She would sit immobile and retreat inside herself to avoid bringing on the pain. A man who had severe congestive heart failure described an incident in which he awoke short of breath in the middle of the night. Desperate to get more air, he leaned so far out of his bedroom window that he almost fell. Rather than be alone with his fear again, he chose to live in a nursing home. An informant who had bypass surgery was worried about life at home during her convalescence. Her husband was so eager to believe that everything would be fine when she went home that he could not bear to hear her talk about her fears. She finally had to enlist the help of the social worker in the coronary care unit to help her talk to her husband.

Denial can be characterized as aggressive, regressive, or constructive. To deny aggressively the illness itself or any disability can interfere with treatment for complications or with the reduction of risk factors. Aggressive deniers may recover from an acute episode, then quickly resume smoking, high-fat diets, and highly stressful activities. An informant whose husband died as a result of a second heart attack said that he simply refused to believe he had had the first. It was simply indigestion, he said, and he had always had trouble after eating short ribs, the meal he had had just before the attack. When released from the hospital, he refused to follow any medical regimen or modify his life-style.

To deny regressively means that one is so distraught with the knowledge of his illness that he is unable to function. An informant said he had become so aware of his damaged heart and so terrified that he would have a second attack that he could think of nothing else. He was self-employed and had to go back to work, but he did so with one eye on his heart and one eye on his cash register. Laughing, he added that he is a very sociable fellow and that eventually he became sufficiently involved with his sales and his customers that he was able to forget about his heart. Later his home life became equally absorbing, but he looks back at that time and sees that he could have become an emotional cripple.

People who deny constructively have a realistic attitude toward their illness. Their denial helps them to cope with the fear, anxiety, and depression that often accompany heart disease. They can take care of themselves and live as normally as possible. A forty-three-year-old informant said that when he had a heart attack at thirty-five, he and his wife saw his convalescence as a chance to review their life. They thought about their lifestyle, discarded what they no longer wanted, reviewed their financial situation, reduced as many risk factors as possible, and went on with their lives.

How to be Helpful to Someone with Heart Disease

First, try to avoid being overprotective. It is important for the person with heart disease to find his own comfortable level of activity. Also, allow yourself to listen gently to the fears a person may have about his illness and its meaning. Do not be so reassuring that the person is unable to express her fears openly.

Without being overbearing, acquaint yourself with the modifications in life-style that could best help the person to manage his disease. Become knowledgeable about the salt and fat content in foods and find ways to help the person exercise routinely and stop or reduce smoking. Finding ways to reduce excessive stress can also be helpful. Above all, it is important to be positive. Most people with heart disease lead full, productive lives. Although heart disease is the most prevalent of all the life-threatening chronic diseases, great strides have been made not only in the treatment of the illness but in its prevention.

8

Respiratory Disease

IN NORMAL BREATHING, air high in oxygen content is taken in through the nose or mouth, a process termed inhalation or inspiration. The air passes throught the throat (pharynx and larynx) into the trachea or windpipe. The trachea divides into two branches called bronchi or bronchial tubes, one to each lung. The bronchi divide into a system of progressively smaller branches called bronchioles. The breathing system from nose and mouth to bronchioles is called the airway.

The inspired air finally enters through alveolar ducts into alveolar sacs, which have many pockets called alveoli. The bulk of the lung substance consists of about 600 million alveoli, within whose walls oxygen and carbon monoxide are exchanged with capillary blood. Air high in carbon dioxide content is expired or exhaled through the same airway system. The process of respiration is aided by the action of the respiratory system in the brain stem, and the muscles of the chest, abdomen, and diaphragm.

The nasal alveola and pharynx warm and humidify the inhaled air and protect the lungs from irritants such as dust, pollen, and bacteria. The mucosa of most of the airway contain cilia, special cells with hairlike projections, which "beat" rhythmically, driving mucus and the entrapped particles toward the throat and the digestive system. Each respiratory disease interrupts some part of this process.

Medical Information

Symptomatology

The most common symptom in respiratory disease is dyspnea, difficulty with breathing, which may be experienced as labored breathing, shortness of breath, or breathlessness. Dyspnea occurs most commonly in nondisease conditions when a person engages in more strenuous work or exercise than usual. The characteristic experience under such conditions is panting or heavy breathing, pounding of the heart, a sense of weakness in the limbs, and light-headedness. In cases of chronic respiratory disease in adults, these symptoms occur at progressively less strenuous activity levels. In advanced stages, walking across the room or engaging in simple activities of daily living such as preparing a simple meal, bathing, or even eating can cause breathing difficulties. Coughing, another prominent symptom of respiratory disease, often occurs in conjunction with breathing difficulty and contributes to the feeling of asphyxiation. Another common symptom, a feeling of weakness and fatigue, is a result of hypoxemia, diminished amounts of oxygen in the arterial blood.

Prevalence

In the course of this century prevalence of respiratory diseases has shifted. Earlier in the century tuberculosis, also known as consumption, was a much more prevalent and feared disease. Improvements in public health, prevention, and treatment have greatly reduced the prevalence of tuberculosis; the estimated number of cases of active tuberculosis in the United States in 1981 was only 181,716. In that same year there were estimated totals of 7,942,815 cases of chronic bronchitis, 2,088,592 of emphysema, and 7,244,481 of asthma. In 1983 approximately 62,000 people died of chronic lung disease. Between 80 and 90 percent of the deaths are attributable to smoking.

Diseases increasing in prevalence are those associated with industrialization and the use of tobacco. the rate of chronic obstructive lung disease, including bronchitis and emphysema, is increasing in all industrialized countries. Also increasing are tumors of the lung and diseases that occur in special conditions such as asbestosis, which primarily affects those who have worked with asbestos, and black lung, or coal miner's disease.

Classification

Respiratory disease is classified by cause and symptomatology. The principal chronic respiratory diseases are asthma, emphysema, and chronic bronchitis. Chronic obstructive pulmonary disease (COPD) is the term used when emphysema and chronic bronchitis occur in the same person. Those diseases will be the focus of this chapter. However, it is important to mention several other chronic respiratory diseases: cystic fibrosis, pneumonia, pulmonary embolism, lung abscess, and occupational lung disease.

CYSTIC FIBROSIS

Cystic fibrosis, like asthma, bronchitis, and chronic obstructive pulmonary disease, obstructs the airway. An inherited disease beginning in infancy, it affects one child in every 1,500 to 2,500 live births and is largely an abnormality of the mucus-secreting glands. An excess of mucus, thicker and more tenacious than normal, blocks the digestive juices and halts the digestion of food. The mucus-secreting glands are replaced by fibroid tissues and cysts as the illness progresses. Diagnosis is established by a positive family history and the finding of sweat sodium and chloride concentration of greater than 60 mg per liter in children, in addition to sputum examination, pulmonary function studies, arterial blood gases, chest x-ray, immunoglobins, and blood and stool examinations to demonstrate failures in the absorption of nutrients and digestion. The disease is characterized by chronic respiratory infection, pancreatic insufficiency, and susceptibility to heat. With good treatment, many children with cystic fibrosis are living to adulthood.

PNEUMONIA

Pneumonia is an acute infection of the alveolar spaces of the lung. It is usually classified as bacterial or nonbacterial, or by specific cause. Viral pneumonias are most common. Involvement of an entire lobe is called lobar pneumonia; of parts of the lobe, segmental or lobular pneumonia; and of alveoli contiguous to bronchi, bronchopneumonia. Predisposing factors are the common cold, alcoholism, malnutrition, exposure, coma, bronchial tumor, treatment with drugs that suppress the immune system, foreign matter in the respiratory tract, and the congestion of blood due to impaired circulation in the case of debilitated, immobile patients. Treatment consists of antimicrobial drug therapy. Each kind of pneumonia varies as to specific treatment as well as prognosis.

PULMONARY EMBOLISM

Pulmonary embolism is the lodging of a blood clot in a pulmonary vein with subsequent obstruction of the blood supply to the lung. Pulmonary infarction, an infrequent consequence (10 percent) of pulmonary embolism, is death of a part of the lung. Symptoms range from mild chest discomfort to fever, shock, coughing up of blood (hymoptysis), and heart failure. Diagnosis is difficult and involves the use of several kinds of scans to detect the clot. Treatment consists of drug therapy to inhibit clotting and occasionally to dissolve existing clots.

LUNG ABSCESS

Lung abscess is a localized area of some dead and some inflamed tissue. Generally it occurs when an unconscious or inebriated person breathes infected material from the upper airway. It is diagnosed through chest x-ray, sputum examination, and clinical evaluation. Penicillin is usually used to eradicate the infection, and postural drainage, in which the throat is lower than the lungs, is used to drain the infected area.

OCCUPATIONAL LUNG DISEASES

Occupational lung diseases are directly related to the inhalation of dust, fumes, vapors, and gases in the workplace. These are especially irritating to the nasal and respiratory membranes of smokers and people with COPD. Some compounds such as oxides of nitrogen, cadmium, beryllium, and other metals, as well as chemicals used in the rubber and plastics industries, can cause scarring and inflammation in the lungs of people who are continuously exposed.

Occupational lung diseases can be classified according to the responsible inhalants; inorganic (mineral) dust, organic dust, and irritant gases and chemicals. Silicosis, the oldest known occupational disease, is caused by inhalation of particles from industries such as mining, foundries, potteries, and stone cutting. Asbestosis, probably the most publicized of the occupational diseases in the United States, results from the inhalation of asbestos dust and causes the formation of excessive fibrous tissue in the lungs. It is preventable through the effective suppression of dust in the workplace. No specific therapy is available, and treatment is symptomatic. Mesothelioma, a rapidly fatal tumor that spreads over the pleural covering of the lung, is also associated with asbestos. It is thought, too, that chronic, low-level exposure to irritants may initiate or accelerate other lung diseases such as chronic bronchitis or emphysema. Cigarette smoking compounds the risks.

ASTHMA

In asthma a chemical response in the body stimulates constricting spasms of the muscular walls of the bronchi, and excessive mucus production interferes with the normal flow of air. As air moves through the partially obstructed channels, wheezing occurs. As the spasms abate, coughing occurs in an effort to remove mucus.

Asthma can be classified as extrinsic or intrinsic. In extrinsic asthma the chemical response that triggers an attack is due primarily to an allergen such as pollen, dust, or animal dander. Although it has not been proved

conclusively, it is thought that extrinsic factors account for the large percentage of asthma in childhood and that this type of asthma is more frequently outgrown in adolescence. Intrinsic asthma is nonallergenic.
Attacks may be triggered by infection, environmental conditions such as
temperature and humidity, physical and emotional stress, or an uniden-
tified factor. While psychological factors can exacerbate asthma attacks,
they are not considered causative.

While the most prevalent chronic respiratory diseases are most often
associated with older age, asthma affects large numbers of children as well
as adults. An estimated total of 7,244,481 Americans have asthma, including 2 million to 3 million children. An estimated 5 to 10 percent of
all children under fifteen have had at least one episode of asthma. Boys
are affected two to three times as frequently as girls. Age at onset is usually
after three years old. Although the frequency and severity of attacks may
vary, a large percentage of children outgrow the symptoms. Still, asthma
accounts for a large proportion of the disability caused by childhood
chronic disease. Deaths from asthma are considered rare, but 2,000 to
4,000 people die of the disease each year.

The most frequently affected adults are men over forty-five. In adults
asthma may be a continuation of childhood asthma, a response to environmental or occupational conditions, associated with other diseases of the
lungs or heart, or the result of unknown factors. The first acute episode
often occurs in conjunction with another disease or acute infection. The
onset of the attack may be gradual, with a sense of tightness in the chest
or a dry cough, or the symptoms may appear suddenly with wheezing,
coughing, heart pounding, and difficulty breathing. Although an attack
may occur at any time, night attacks are most frequent. For a person with
extrinsic asthma, an attack may be triggered by a particular type of allergen, by more widespread allergens or irritants, physical or emotional
stress, or a combination of these and unknown factors. Many people with
extrinsic asthma can identify patterns of attacks associated with various
activities, events, or conditions.

During an attack resistance to air moving out of the alveoli and bronchioles because of the constricting spasms of the bronchi make breathing
difficult. Resistance to air moving into the lungs is compounded by the
presence of partially trapped air. In a prolonged attack the lungs may
become hyperinflated. Wheezing sounds develop as the air moves through
the narrow airways, which are also being blocked by excess mucus secretion. The perception of the breathing difficulty and fear of asphyxiation
cause a feeling of panic. The person tries to compensate by breathing more
rapidly but ineffectively moves air primarily in and out of the upper airway. The feeling of panic and breathing adjustments also have a physiological basis. If the ability to breath in oxygen is ineffective, the
concentration of oxygen in the lungs is lowered and the level of oxygen in

the blood will fall. In the case of severe respiratory insufficiency, the level of carbon dioxide in the blood may rise. In order to compensate for the lower blood oxygen level, the heart rate increases to deliver more blood to the lungs, and the breathing rate is adjusted to increase the air supply. Too little oxygen delivered to the brain can increase the feeling of anxiety and even lead to confusion. Insufficient oxygen in the muscle tissue can lead to feelings of weakness.

In an effort to move air in and out of the lungs, accessory chest and abdominal muscles may be used. Ineffective breathing may be complicated by the antagonistic action of these muscle groups. Other symptoms include pallor, profuse perspiration, a gasping voice, and a bluish color in the fingernail beds or earlobes. If the airway is so constricted that almost no air is being moved through, wheezing may be absent.

Asthma attacks are classified according to the degree of breathing effectiveness. People with asthma may have different stages of severity at different times. A stage I attack is considered mild, as adequate air exchange is maintained, wheezing sounds occur only occasionally, and there is little shortness of breath. Stage II is considered moderate, as the individual experiences respiratory distress at rest, breathing is rapid, and wheezing sounds occur regularly; however, the air exchange may be normal. A stage III attack is severe; the ability to inhale and exhale may be only 25 percent of normal capacity, blood carbon dioxide levels may be increased, and wheezing sounds may be absent due to extreme constriction of the bronchi. If a stage III attack persists, stage IV or respiratory failure may result in which blood carbon dioxide levels are very high and confusion and lethargy ensue. Death will result without treatment.

Once an asthma attack begins, it will not necessarily progress to the next stage. Some individuals have only mild symptoms with occasional wheezes and mild coughing that may last for a period of a few minutes, hours, or days. Untreated symptoms may persist or abate spontaneously or abate and recur. The rate of progression may be slow.

As the person recovers from an acute attack, coughing changes from dry to productive in an effort to rid the airways of the excess mucus. The predominant experience following an attack is soreness of the chest muscles and a feeling of tiredness. Some dehydration is also common due to the loss of fluid through perspiration. Even though symptoms may be absent, some changes in respiratory function measures may persist for several weeks. Although asthma attacks are often unpredictable, medical treatment, education, and attention to those factors frequently associated with attacks lead to greater control. Lack of follow-up treatment enhances the chances for recurrence.

The natural history of asthma over the course of a lifetime varies according to the individual. While the disease does not generally cause permanent lung deterioration, some few people experience increasingly severe attacks. If asthma occurs in a person whose underlying respiratory disease has already compromised breathing effectiveness, the attacks may appear to be more severe. For some adults attacks vary in frequency and intensity without a clear pattern, while for others attacks rarely occur.

CHRONIC OBSTRUCTIVE PULMONARY DISEASE

The two principal chronic obstructive pulmonary diseases are chronic bronchitis and emphysema. Chronic bronchitis and emphysema often occur together. For that reason it is customary to use the term chronic obstructive pulmonary disease to refer to both, although bronchitis usually has reversible features, and emphysema does not. Not all of the literature conforms to this usage; some researchers use emphysema and COPD interchangeably, while others use the term to refer to all categories of obstructive lung disease, including asthma. Since COPD as a diagnostic group is associated with greater disability and mortality than emphysema or bronchitis alone, most of the discussion regarding disability and adaptation will refer to the combined category of COPD. COPD also occurs in a small number of people who have neither bronchitis nor emphysema. COPD is described as an irreversible airway obstruction due to varying degrees of chronic bronchitis and emphysema. It combines the alveolar damage of emphysema with the bronchiole damage, mucus hypersecretion, and coughing associated with bronchitis.

COPD is thought to begin early in life, although the symptoms are often insignificant until later. It affects an estimated 15 percent of older men, who are symptomatic eight to ten times as frequently as women. A major cause of disability and death, its mortality statistics increased 500 percent between 1955 and 1980. Some of this dramatic increase may be attributable to greater diagnostic accuracy and greater survival rates for patients with infectious diseases than occurred before the COPD was recognized. In addition to infections, heart disease is strongly associated with COPD because of the great demand placed on the heart to pump more blood to compensate for the diminished capacity of the lungs to oxygenate the blood effectively. As a result, death often occurs from heart failure.

CHRONIC BRONCHITIS

In chronic bronchitis, chronic inflammation of the bronchial tubes cause increased quantities of mucus and mucus-secreting cells. These secretions cause obstructions of the bronchioles. The obstruction traps air and thus interferes with expiration. In an effort to clear the mucus, a productive cough develops. Shortness of breath occurs with exertion. Each new respiratory infection, such as a cold or pneumonia, causes further deterioration of the bronchioles.

Populations at risk are cigarette smokers and those who work and live in highly industrialized areas where pollution, dust, and toxic fumes are heavy. A combination of these factors increases the risk. Those at greatest risk are males in their middle years. An estimated 7,942,815 people in the United States have chronic bronchitis. It is the cause of death for approximately 4,500 people each year.

EMPHYSEMA

Emphysema is a destructive process involving breakdown of the alveolar walls with enlargement of the alveoli. With chronic inflammatory reactions in the alveoli, the air sacs are damaged, and they begin to balloon and rupture. The rupture of a few or even a few hundred alveoli would not be noticed, but as increasing numbers of balloonings and ruptures occur, dead air spaces develop and trap stale air, thus preventing fresh air from coming into those spaces. The interface between the capillaries and the alveoli is lost, and the oxygen–carbon dioxide exchange cannot occur. As the ballooning, ruptures, and creation of dead air space continue, the lungs lose their elasticity, and exhaling air becomes increasingly difficult.

An estimated 2,088,592 people in the United States have emphysema. Increased incidence is associated with urban living, industrial pollution, and smoking. Men are affected seven times more often than women, and there is a ten to fifteen times greater incidence in people with a history of cigarette smoking. It is thought that one of every fourteen workers over the age of forty-five is affected. At greatest risk are males between the ages of fifty and seventy. Occasionally emphysema occurs at an earlier age because of the absence of a body enzyme (alpha-one antitrypsin). Emphysema is the primary cause of death for approximately 20,000 people each year. It is commonly associated with heart disease.

Natural History of Chronic Obstructive Pulmonary Disease

Warning symptoms for COPD are shortness of breath and a cough not related to an infection. The most striking symptom of progressive obstructive lung disease is the occurrence of dyspnea at progressively less strenuous activity levels. For example, someone who regularly walks two flights of stairs will gradually experience shortness of breath before he reaches the top. The difference between dypsnea occurring three steps from the top or six is not likely to be noticed. Eventually the person may be short of breath by the time he reaches the top of the first flight. He may alter his habits by using an elevator or using the stairs less frequently and still avoid recognition of increased shortness of breath as a symptom of disease.

Even if he seeks medical attention, it is generally because he perceives that he has less energy or tires more easily rather than that he is short of breath. Most often a person goes to the doctor because of cold or infection has lingered for months. Each respiratory infection results in a cough that persists longer than the previous one. Again, although early recognition is possible, the difference is gradual and easily ignored.

A person with emphysema will have a dry cough, and someone with chronic bronchitis as a disease alone or as an element of COPD will have a cough productive of mucus. Coughing early in the morning is common because of need to clear mucus that accumulates overnight and is not necessarily indicative of respiratory disease. Also, most long-term smokers cough without having bronchitis. If the person does smoke cigarettes, he may not seek medical attention even when he recognizes symptoms, because he knows the first thing the doctor will tell him is to stop smoking. He may avoid a return visit if he has not stopped as the doctor requested. When respiratory deterioration is advanced, coughing causes sleep disturbance, persists through the day, or results in the coughing up of a large amount of mucus.

The progression of the obstructive respiratory diseases is not rapid. Even when symptoms are discernable, the progress may extend over a period of many years. Because the onset is insidious, deterioration is often quite marked by the time a diagnosis is made. If diagnosis is delayed until late stages, the progression may appear to be rapid. The prognosis for long-term survival is based on the results of measures of lung function. Even if the person's breathing capacity is one-third normal, his chances for surviving for five years are two out of three, and for surviving for ten years or longer are one out the three.

Although deterioration is progressive, the survival time will depend on lung functioning. The rate of deterioration can sometimes be slowed if a person is able to avoid chronic irritants such as smoking and working in a polluted environment. If the disease progresses without rehabilitative treatment, progression is often cyclical. As a person becomes more short of breath and fatigued, he may become increasingly inactive, leading to deconditioning of the muscles and increased energy requirements with the resumption of activity. When activities such as walking across the room are difficult, the individual may stay in bed to avoid exertion and associated distress. Within a short time he may lose the ability to walk. This cycle of limitation of activity and deconditioning of the muscles followed by further limitation, often precedes the limitations imposed by the disease process.

The effect of chronic inefficient oxygenation is the same in progressive respiratory diseases as it is in asthma, even though the obstruction is not due primarily to bronchospasms. Inadequate levels of oxygen cause fatigue, irritability, anxiety, and lethargy. To raise blood oxygen levels, the body develops compensatory mechanisms such as increased heart and breathing rates.

Coughing occurs more frequently as the disease progresses, leading to or exacerbating shortness of breath in bronchitis or following shortness of breath in emphysema. When the disease has a large bronchitis component, the person may wheeze on exertion or when lying down. Increased demands on the heart add to increased pressure or hypertension in the pulmonary artery, which brings blood from the heart to the lungs. This increased pressure can lead to the characteristic late complication, cor pulmonale, an enlargment of the right ventricle of the heart resulting from the constant need to pump against the pressure in the pulmonary artery. Edema or swelling caused by fluid retention and enlargement of the liver are frequently associated with right ventricle enlargement.

In the early and middle stages of the disease the body is able to compensate for the development of high levels of carbon dioxide in the blood. As the diseases advance, however, the compensatory mechanisms are inadequate and hypercapnia, excessive carbon dioxide in the blood, develops. High levels of carbon dioxide lead to further constriction and increase pressure in the pulmonary artery. Loss of coordination, confusion, and lethargy may result. The body's attempt to compensate for the low level of oxygen and the rising level of carbon dioxide appears as huffing and puffing.

Another way in which the body compensates for pulmonary insufficiency is through the increased development of red blood cells. High concentrations of these cells require more effort to move through the circulatory system. This condition, known as polycythemia, increases the blood pressure in the pulmonary artery and thus contributes to the development of heart failure. Bronchospasms similar to those of asthma may occur periodically or chronically.

Chronic hypercapnia and cor pulmonale are serious late complications that will result in death if not treated. Even with treatment these complications, coupled with extreme expiratory slowing, have a prognosis for survival of less than two years. Infections occur with greater frequency, severity, and impact. Each new infection causes further deterioration. Failure to have infections treated not only adds to the deterioration but can result in death as well.

Diagnosis of Asthma

The diagnosis of asthma is complicated by the fact that onset is often associated with other diseases. In diagnosing asthma, the physician looks to family history; half of those with asthma have a close relative with the disease. Family history can also reveal a pattern associated with attacks such as symptoms that occur during or following a particular activity, environmental condition, or other event. While wheezing is characteristic of asthma, the symptom alone is not diagnostic as it may be associated with other conditions or obstruction by a foreign object in the airway.

Chest x-rays are commonly used but may not reveal any changes, particularly in the absence of symptoms. During or immediately following an attack, an x-ray may reveal hyperinflation of the lungs or small areas of lung collapse. Tests of blood and sputum may reveal unusually high levels of a blood cell called an esosinophil, indicating the likelihood of an attack. The sputum of someone with asthma has a characteristic color and consistency. Blood tests can also reveal elevated levels of antibodies in people with asthma. Findings may be followed by a panel of skin tests with various common allergens to identify potential triggering factors. Once possible allergen triggers are identified, tests of pulmonary function are carried out before and after the substance is sprayed into the airway. If the allergen being tested is actually involved in precipitating an attack, the person may experience symptoms during the test.

Pulmonary function tests are used in the diagnosis of all respiratory diseases. In simplest form a spirometer, an instrument for measuring the capacity of the lungs, measures the amount of air that can be expelled. The person breathes into a tube attached to a flexible reservoir according to instructions given for the specific test. The volume of air in the reservoir is measured in liters, and this volume is recorded graphically on a rotating cylinder. The recording is a tracing of the volume and flow of air by time.

The most frequently used spirometric measures are forced vital capacity (FVC) and forced expiratory volume (FEV). To obtain these measures, the patient is asked to breathe in as much air as possible and then forcibly to breathe out as much as possible into the spirometer. The FVC is the maximum volume of air that can be exhaled with effort. This volume and the time required to exhale it are recorded. The FEV is the volume of air that is exhaled in the first second of forced expiration. Normally, a person who forcibly exhales will exhale 75 percent of the total amount of air in the first second of the effort. A decrease in FEV is associated with obstructive diseases and may be less than 40 percent of the FVC in severe impairment. For the person with asthma the FEV is usually within normal limits when the person is symptom-free and decreases as an attack progresses.

Usually the tests are repeated three times and then given periodically to monitor the course of the disease. Sometimes the tests may be given before someone has inhaled a substance to dilate the airways or before and after exercise. These tests are not harmful, but they may be frightening if they leave the person short of breath. A number of more sophisticated tests of lung function are designed to measure different aspects of the breathing process, but the basic principle of breathing in and out of a tube is similar.

The graphic tracing in lines, curves, or loops have characteristic shapes, which can be used to differentiate the degrees of impairment associated with different respiratory diseases.

The next most frequently administered tests are arterial blood gas measurements. These are carried out in order to gather a combination of metabolic and respiratory parameters. The level of carbon dioxide in the blood, which determines the acid-alkaline balance, is a function of ventilation—how much air is moved in and out. Oxygen measurements are a function of the oxygen content that is breathed, the adequacy of ventilation, and, primarily, the relationship of ventilation to blood perfusion of the lungs. If, as one breathes, the circulated blood is normally exposed to the inhaled gases, there is the proper exchange of gases between the blood and the alveoli. However, if there are ventilation perfusion abnormalities, the oxygen is not properly absorbed, the blood oxygen levels diminish, and there is a V/Q or ventilation/perfusion abnormality in the arterial blood.

Diagnosis of COPD or Chronic Bronchitis

A history of smoking, chronic exposure to irritants, shortness of breath increasingly associated with exertion, and a chronic cough that lasts for three months are important diagnostic factors in chronic bronchitis or COPD. Chest x-rays are normally used. Isotope scans following an injection with radioisotopic material are sometimes ordered to better define areas of diminished lung function. Bronchoscopy allows the physician to view the interior of the bronchi or to extract a tissue sample for microscopic examination. The instrument has a curving flexible tube containing glass fibers with special optical properties that carry light down and that return a clear magnified image from the end of the tube to the viewer. The tube is inserted through the nose or mouth, using local anesthesia. Although the test is brief, shortness of breath and diminished amount of oxygen in the tissues may result. Oxygen, drugs, and equipment for resuscitation therefore should always be available in the bronchoscopy room.

Other tests, more invasive, may be used when attacks are severe or a disease is in advanced stages. For example, in the diagnosis of pulmonary hypertension, cardiac catheterization involves threading a flexible tube through a vein in the arm and the heart into the pulmonary artery.

Treatment for Asthma

Treatment for asthma primarily comprises drug therapy, exercise programs, and stress management. Asthma medication is used to treat an acute attack, to prevent further episodes, or as an aftermath to an attack. Drugs are arranged hierarchically, with more potent drugs being saved for more severe attacks or for symptoms that remain unresponsive to drugs lower in the hierarchy. During an attack a group of drugs called bronchodilators are administered to alter the body chemical response that triggers and maintains the bronchospasms and thus to relax the bronchial walls.

The most frequently used class of these drugs are adrenergic agents, of which the most prescribed are epinephrine and isoproteronol. During a mild or moderate attack an injection of epinephrine may provide relief within minutes. In the early stages of an attack, before the bronchi become so constricted that the spray cannot pass the narrowed tubes, inhalant forms of these drugs may be effective. People who suffer frequent attacks have aerosols prescribed for home use. For those whose symptoms are associated with specific activities, the use of an inhalant just before might prevent an episode.

These drugs cannot be used by people whose heart activity they stimulate. Also, if they are abused, their effectiveness may be diminished; side effects, including, paradoxically, the lowering of blood oxygen levels, and even death may result. Because the potential for abuse is great, education about proper use is vital.

A second class of drugs, used alone or in conjunction with the first group if symptoms are difficult to reverse, are bronchodilators with a different chemical mechanism from the first group. These drugs, an example of which is aminophylline, are effective when an optimum level of theophylline, a diuretic related to caffeine but stronger, is maintained in the blood plasma. If the level is exceeded, side effects that may develop include nausea and vomiting, nervousness, and irritability. Toxic levels may induce abnormal heart rhythm and convulsions (involuntary muscle contractions).

A third group of drugs, the corticosteroids, may enhance the effectiveness of the other groups and reduce swelling and inflammation in severe attacks characterized by marked impairment of breathing and lowered oxygen levels. Prednisone is one example of a corticosteriod. This group of drugs is best used for the short term with frequent medical evaluation. There are many side effects associated with long-term use, among which are fluid retention, Cushing's syndrome (a moon-shaped face and central body obesity), hypertension, gastrointestinal disorders, destructive bone changes, glaucoma, cataracts, and susceptibility to other infections. Some control of these side effects is achieved through prescribing these drugs on an alternate-day basis. Patients who have attacks severe enough to warrant the use of steroids may require hospitalization. In the hospital oxygen is administered to raise blood oxygen levels, and intravenous fluids replace lost fluids and correct body chemical imbalances. Intensive care may be necessary for those threatened with respiratory failure.

Following an acute attack, excess mucus is removed from the lungs through a combination of extra fluid intake, coughing, and sometimes medication. Even after symptoms have abated, some pulmonary function abnormalities persist for two to four weeks after an attack. During this period medication is given to prevent the recurrence of symptoms. Cromolyn is an example of a drug used only after acute episodes are fully resolved in order to prevent further attacks.

For people with extrinsic asthma, immunotherapy or desensitizing drugs may be injected on a seasonal or yearly basis if a specific allergen can be identified. Antihistamines may be prescribed during allergy seasons, but many of them promote drying of the respiratory tract.

Additional therapies include exercise to improve the tolerance for activity and stress management and psychotherapy to learn to reduce anxiety, identify stressors that may trigger an attack, and find ways in which the family can live more comfortably with the disease. (These therapies will be discussed later under the heading "Modifications in Life-Style.")

Progressive Respiratory Diseases

For the progressive respiratory diseases treatment involves drug therapy, breathing retraining, physical and respiratory therapy, exercise programs, programs to help people stop smoking, education, and oxygen therapy. Drug therapy is directed toward reducing bronchospasms and treating exacerbations due to infection and heart complications. Although some therapies may slow the rate of deterioration, lung function does not generally improve.

Patients with COPD and bronchitis may have bronchospasms periodically in asthma-like episodes or on a chronic basis. To reduce the obstruction, asthma-type drugs are used, although the regimen may vary. These drugs are also used to reduce resistence to air flow in some patients who do not have bronchospasms. Although effectiveness and indications vary, some patients have bronchodilators prescribed on a regular basis, and others are maintained on steroids for extended periods. Because of the potential of cardiac involvement in the progressive diseases, some drugs that might otherwise be effective cannot be used, and others are used only with close monitoring.

Other agents such as humidification and aerosol agents are sometimes used to promote removal of excess secretions. Intermittent positive pressure breathing (IPPB) treatment machines may be used to deliver aerosol medication into the lungs under pressure, and some patients regularly use these treatments at home. There is lack of consensus regarding the value of this treatment.

Respiratory infections are often treated with antimicrobial medications. If prescribed early, they can prevent the infections that can cause those with severe insufficiency to suffer dangerously reduced blood oxygen levels. For this reason, vaccinations against viral infections are often recommended.

Taught by a physical or respiratory therapist, breathing retraining has as its goal the reduction of the amount of energy it takes to breathe, thus making more energy available for other activities. With COPD, breathing is difficult because clogged, narrow airways and/or damaged air sacs trap stale air in the lungs, thus preventing fresh air from entering. Being taught to breathe out slowly through pursed lips increases the pressure in the airway as the individual breathes out against the resistance of the lips. The increased pressure assists in preventing partial airway collapse, which contributes to airway resistance. Many people do this intuitively. Learning to cough in a way that clears the airways is another technique. One sits with his head slightly forward, feet on the floor; breathes in deeply, holds his breath, coughs once to loosen mucus and a second time to bring it up, breathes in again by sniffing gently, and gets rid of the mucus, never swallowing it. Strength-building exercises include knee raises, head and shoulder raising, arm raising, forward bending, and trunk turning.

Other breathing retraining techniques include the teaching of deep breathing with the aid of the diaphragm and abdominal muscles. This type of breathing is both more effective and energy efficient than the use of accessory chest muscles, which are commonly used by those who have breathing difficulty. A typical exercise may involve having the individual lie on his back with a weight such as a bag of flour on his stomach. This weight promotes an awareness of areas of the body that need to be involved and the type of breathing necessary to move the weight up and down.

Awareness of habits that increase breathlessness can be promoted, such as the awareness of breath-holding while concentrating. A number of informants cited breathing training as the most important aspect of therapy in helping them remain active. There is no evidence that this training alters lung function, although it can reduce the occurence of shortness of breath and allow someone to remain more active.

Postural drainage and chest percussion may be recommended for those who have difficulty removing secretions by coughing. Postural drainage is accomplished by assuming various positions that promote draining of mucus from the lungs by lying with the throat lower than the lungs. Lying on one's side, back, or stomach allows the various areas of the lungs that are uppermost to drain. This is not appropriate for everyone and should be done only with medical supervision.

Percussion is accomplished by gentle pounding or claps on the back at different sites with the use of a percussor or vibrator. It is sometimes combined with postural drainage and may be helpful in breaking up the mucus. These techniques may be recommended for use four or more times a day. If they are carried out first thing in the morning and last thing at night, some of the congestion that increases during sleep can be more easily relieved.

Exercise training programs are designed to increase a person's tolerance for exercise, to promote and maintain general conditioning, and to break the cycle of inactivity and deconditioning. Although some people are able to remain active without formal training, this type of program is effective even when a person is severely debilitated. Generally exercise is most effective when it is activity-specific. For example, if the goal is to improve walking tolerance, the exercise is walking increasing distances. Bike pedaling will increase tolerance for that activity but will have little effect on walking.

For some individuals tolerance is increased with the aid of oxygen. After the training, the person can maintain the achieved activity level while breathing room air. This type of training decreases the amount of energy required for physical activity so that oxygen is used more efficiently by the body. Oxygen therapy has also been used to reduce the distress of shortness of breath in certain activities of daily living that would otherwise be very uncomfortable. For its use in reducing pulmonary artery hypertension and exacerbations of cor pulmonae, it is sometimes prescribed for as much as fifteen to twenty hours a day. Oxygen has also been associated with reduction of depression, anxiety, and the confusion and coordination problems that are associated with increasing blood carbon dioxide levels. Units are available for home and portable use. Oxygen can have toxic effects and it is not prescribed until the blood oxygen falls below a certain level. For some people this level falls only at night as congestion increases. In those situations oxygen may be prescribed for use during sleep.

Anticipated Course of the Treated Disease

For people with asthma it is generally possible to reverse attacks and control the disease process sufficiently for participation in most activities. While many people with asthma continue to have attacks even when treated, control can be optimized if the factors that trigger the attacks can be identified, and permanent lung damage is rare. For people with progressive respiratory disease, treatment does not improve lung function or slow the progress of the disease. Instead, medical treatment can ease the distress associated with bronchospasms, infection, and other exacerbating factors. Respiratory rehabilitation programs are effective in maintaining and increasing activity tolerance through conditioning; reducing energy requirements for activity; increasing breathing efficiency and effectiveness; and promoting wellbeing. Unfortunately, comprehensive programs are not available consistently throughout the country, and they are not consistently used as a resource even when they are available. The diseases progress slowly. In some cases diseases progress to the point of total debilitation. However, because these diseases are most common in old age, death may result from another cause or from an associated condition such as heart disease before a person can become debilitated.

Psychosocial Information

The response to respiratory disease is based on people's understanding of the disease process and symptoms. Because progressive obstructive respiratory illness is insidious, people often do not realize that they are affected. Many are smokers who have been coughing and short of breath for years. The gradual increase in those symptoms is not cause for alarm until the disease begins to hamper their activities. Often the ill person and his family see symptoms as a sign that the disease is advancing and they had better become less active. The result is that people become weak, depressed, and often isolated. In fact symptoms do not affect the disease process, but avoiding exercise in order to avoid symptoms will hasten debilitation.

Modifications in Life-Style

Those who have mild symptoms need make only minimum modifications in life-style. One's activity level should always be the maximum possible within the limitations of the disease. Activities should be modified rather than eliminated unless they are harmful. For those who are impaired, many modifications can help to maintain the maximum level of activity and independence.

SMOKING

One of the four new warnings on cigarette packages and all forms of advertising reads, "SURGEON GENERAL'S WARNING: Smoking cigarettes causes lung cancer, heart disease, emphysema and may complicate pregnancy." The risk of getting COPD, for example, is six times greater for smokers than for nonsmokers. Smoking does not cause asthma but exacerbates it. Smoking added to other respiratory irritants like poor air quality has a cumulative effect. The risks involved with passive smoking, while not yet proved as conclusively, are also significant. Of the 183 million adults in the United States, 53 million smoke. The year 1983 saw a 7 percent decline in cigarette smoking. While in 1977, 30 percent of high school students smoked, in 1983, 21 percent smoked. A massive antismoking campaign on the part of the Surgeon General's Office, American Lung Association, American Cancer Society, American Heart Association, and many other interested groups is attempting to achieve a smoke-free society by the year 2000. By the spring of 1984 thirty states had approved antismoking restrictions in public places. Supporting this "war against smoking" is a tremendous research effort, much of which is reported in the annual *Bibliography on Smoking and Health*, published by the Public Health Service.

Still, many people with respiratory disease continue to smoke. It is difficult for families and friends to watch an impaired person smoke while struggling for breath, but it is also difficult for that person to quit smoking. Several informants recount seeing respiratory patients turn off their oxygen to smoke a cigarette. Many people stop smoking when a physician tells them that their lungs have been affected. Others avoid treatment because they are not prepared to stop. When neither scare tactics nor information is successful, other approaches, including forms of individual and group therapy, medication, communication techniques, and hypnosis are often introduced. No program has been more than 35 percent effective, however, and many people who do stop smoking resume after a period of abstinence. Most important to remember, especially for nonsmokers, is that smoking is an addiction, which many people can control only with a great deal of support from concerned loved ones.

DIET

A well-balanced diet is an important consideration in respiratory illness. Calories are expended by the effort to breathe as well as in activities that require increased effort. High protein is necessary for the rebuilding of muscles and for functioning following illness. A poorly nourished person will have more difficulty recovering from infection and will become disabled more rapidly because of muscle atrophy. An obese person will require more energy to move and increased oxygen to supply body tissues.

The cost of high-protein foods and the lack of energy for grocery shopping are often cited as reasons for poor diet by low-income elderly people. Many people regard reduced intake and requirements as a natural part of the aging process, while others think they need only as much as they feel like eating. Poor appetite can lead to poor nutrition, and dietary problems tend to cycle in a downward direction, contributing to loss of energy, muscle atrophy, and deconditioning, which contribute to depression and further loss of interest in eating.

People with asthma must determine if food products or additives are contributing factors in triggering attacks. Particularly following an attack, people should increase fluid intake to aid in rehydration and to thin mucus secretions. In addition there is some evidence that foods and beverages may play a role in preventing bronchospasms.

Substantial modifications in eating patterns may be required for people with progressive obstructive diseases as well. When hypersecretion of mucus is a problem, 2 to 3 liters of fluid a day are often required to aid in the thinning of mucus. One informant with a high daily fluid intake requirement commented that the need to get up during the night to go to the bathroom was more troublesome to his sleep than the symptoms of the disease itself. For people who retain too much fluid or who have heart failure, fluid intake and salt intake may be restricted, and in some cases diuretics, agents that increase the production of urine, are required. As the use of diuretics is associated with depletion of body potassium (which can cause a range of symptoms from nausea to muscle weakness to heart rhythm inequalities), foods containing potassium such as bananas and orange juice are often recommended.

A number of factors associated with progressive obstructive diseases create difficulties with diet. Depression, lethargy, and lack of energy to prepare meals contribute to the loss of interest in eating. Chewing and digestion require energy, and holding one's breath while eating and drinking can contribute to shortness of breath. A feeling of fullness in the stomach or abdomen can contribute to breathing difficulty at the time when energy requirements for digestion are at their highest. Some medications may cause nausea or contribute to loss of appetite.

Modifications can help someone to minimize breathlessness while eating. These include eating and chewingly slowly, eating six small meals daily rather than three large ones, and saving uncooked foods such as breads and desserts to be eaten between cooked meals. Gas-forming foods such as onions, cauliflower, and melons, which bloat the abdomen, limit the movement of the diaphragm, and make breathing more difficult, should be avoided. Medication and treatment may ease eating difficulties. Using bronchodilators or treatments such as percussion an hour before eating can reduce shortness of breath. Mealtimes may be adjusted to avoid times when breathing is difficult, such as early morning.

Although these recommendations are simple, they often require changing lifelong habits. For example, in people who also have heart involvement, salt intake is frequently restricted. People accustomed to salting food complain that nothing tastes right any more, and they are just not interested in eating. Changing dietary habits involves both the ill person and his family. If a person experiences paroxysmal coughing, meals are disrupted for everyone. If the family pattern is to rush through meals, it is difficult for the ill person to eat slowly. In many homes mealtime is the only occasion for the family to assemble. Opportunities for discord are therefore heightened. While this can be unpleasant for everyone, it is of particular concern for the ill person, who must eat well to maintain himself and avoid emotional distress, which exacerbates breathing difficulty.

Modifications can be made alone or with the help of family and friends, but community resource people can also be helpful. Dieticians can suggest substitutes for restricted foods and spices, as well as ways to simplify meal preparation. Occupational therapists can teach energy conservation during meal preparation. One elderly woman, who had always enjoyed cooking but increasingly converted her diet to toast and food brought in by family and friends, was thrilled to learn how to cook while seated. Neither she nor her family had considered this simple adaptation.

EXERCISE

People with respiratory disease often avoid exercise because they fear shortness of breath. Those who remain active often have fewer complications and a better attitude with less depression. Basically, if muscles are used, they will use oxygen more efficiently. If they are not used, more effort will be required when the person attempts to resume activity. This principle is true for people who are healthy or ill, young or old. Deconditioning occurs much more rapidly in those who are sedentary. Even an otherwise healthy young person who has been confined for several weeks to recover from an accident will find himself weak and tired. For those who must be confined, proper exercise keeps deconditioning at a minimum.

Exercise or fatigue associated with exercise may be a factor in triggering attacks, but progressive conditioning can be effective in increasing tolerance for people with asthma and progressive obstructive diseases. For those who tend to have bronchospasms during exertion, the use of bronchodilators before exercise is sometimes recommended. This may not be necessary after the body is conditioned. Swimming has been considered an excellent activity for those with asthma because of the humidity. For those with extrinsic asthma, certain outdoor activities may be restricted during allergy seasons or in the presence of dust or animal dander. Children with asthma may be restricted by anxious adults or by their own fear of precipitating an attack. For children, nonparticipation in active pursuits with peers can have a negative effect on social development.

CLIMATIC CONDITIONS

Climatic and environmental conditions such as elevated pollen counts, dry air, poor air quality, extremes of temperature, and high altitude exacerbate respiratory disease. Pollen is harmful only to someone allergic to it. Some people must try to avoid areas with high pollen counts. For some people it is possible to desensitize the body's response with immunotherapy or injections. For others antihistamines are sometimes prescribed.

Generally the dry air produced by steam heating systems or air conditioning lowers humidity. Home humidifiers are the safest and most effective methods of adding humidity, but vaporizers and even a receptacle of water on the stove or radiator top will help in a limited way. High pollution or poor air quality is an irritant in asthma and progressive obstructive diseases. Those with mild impairment should therefore avoid outdoor work when pollution is high, while those with greater impairment should stay indoors.

Air quality is a particular problem for urban dwellers in the summer months. The usual solution is to stay indoors with air conditioning. Air purifiers and fans that do not reduce humidity or the use of air conditioning during the day, while opening the windows at night, may be more appropriate for improving air quality even if they are less effective for cooling. In winter, dressing appropriately saves energy by avoiding the need to shiver or use other bodily means for maintaining body temperature. Adaptation to cold air may be as simple as placing a muffler over the nose and mouth and breathing the warmed and humidified air this creates. In order to reduce exposure to infections, it is best to avoid crowded conditions during cold and flu season. Poor air quality is intensified in rush hour traffic. Travel by train or bus reduces the exposure to pollution while increasing exposure to infections. The use of car air conditioning or adjusting work and driving schedules to avoid peak traffic hours helps lessen the exposure.

Many people see moving to a more favorable environment as the solution to poor air conditions. For some moving to a lower altitude will result in improved breathing ability; for others climatic change means only an avoidance of exacerbating conditions. More than altering air conditions, moving means leaving one's social support system. For example, a couple moved from an urban setting to a retirement community a considerable distance away in an attempt to find a more comfortable environment for the husband, who had COPD. Shortly after the move the man developed heart failure. The couple had not had time to make new friends, and the people that they could usually rely on were too far away to respond. His wife said that the feeling of being alone was the most difficult part of the process for her. Even a move to live with or near one's children, though less isolating, involves the loss of old friends and peers, extended family, and medical network.

One solution might be planning a vacation during the very cold months or during high pollution or pollen seasons, if the person can afford it. Another might be developing new interests that can be carried out in more favorable conditions. For example, one informant, too disabled to work, found that he was most comfortable near the water. He had always been interested in boating and fishing, and he was able to remain active in those pursuits.

Air travel is often a concern, because high altitudes often make breathing more difficult. The airline should be notified in advance about people's needs and fears regarding inadequate pressurization in the cabin, the possible need for oxygen—which many airlines will supply in flight—the identity and seat of the person with respiratory difficulty, and the importance of seating the person as far from the smoking section as possible. The altitude of the destination may also be of concern. Even healthy athletes need extra time for conditioning in high-altitude locations such as Mexico City. For a person with breathing difficulty at sea level the altitude of most United States coastal cities, high altitudes can cause great difficulty, and activity may need to be severely restricted.

SLEEP

Sleep is often difficult for people with respiratory illness. Not only do asthma attacks occur more frequently at night, but anxiety about the possibility of an attack disturbs sleep. Especially in the weeks following a child's attack parents find it difficult to sleep, because they are listening for sounds of the child's distress. Sometimes, bronchodilators are prescribed to be kept at bedside. One young girl said she often had symptoms at night that could be successfully treated with a bronchodilator. Even though the symptoms were usually mild, her fear that they would escalate, leaving her unable to shout, made her awaken her mother each time. When a bell was placed next to her bed for summoning her mother, she was assured that she could be heard even if she wasn't able to call out. As a result she and her mother could rest more comfortably.

During sleep congestion often increases for people with obstructive diseases. Increased congestion restricts air flow and can result in muscle weakness, fatigue, and restlessness. For those whose blood oxygen levels fall below recommended limits, oxygen is prescribed. People who feel well during the day say they are often awakened at night by coughing or breathing difficulties. Others sleep sitting up in an easy chair because they are fearful that they will suffocate if they lie down. Using bronchodilators, drinking liquids without filling the stomach, coughing, postural drainage, and/or breathing exercises before bedtime may aid sleep. People who sleep too much and are lethargic may have elevated carbon dioxide levels, which may be altered with oxygen. Interrupted sleep and napping often disrupt the schedule of the ill person and his family. Finding ways to make sleep comfortable and avoiding naps help the ill person to stay in step with his family.

RELAXATION AND STRESS MANAGEMENT

Relaxation techniques, often taught as part of pulmonary rehabilitation programs, can be very effective in controlling the escalation of asthma attacks that are triggered by emotional stressors. Conscious relaxation slows the breathing rate and promotes deep breathing. Any relaxation technique can be effective, and there are a wide range of techniques available, including biofeedback, progressively tensing and relaxing muscles, and self-hypnosis. These techniques are preferable to drug therapies for stress reduction, because sedatives depress the respiratory system and are generally contraindicated.

DAILY SCHEDULE

People often become acutely aware of the need to change routine when they are hospitalized or acutely ill. At that time they are also feeling most overwhelmed and need family members, occupational and physical therapist, nurse, and social worker to help them think through the necessary modifications. The main considerations are to reduce oxygen requirements and to identify times of the day when breathing is most and least difficult.

Breathing is usually most difficult in the early morning, when the body works to relieve the congestion that worsens during sleep, and often after meals, when a full stomach limits the movement of the diaphragm and additional energy is required for digestion. Thus, beginning the day with juice or other liquids and eating the rest of breakfast later in the morning may be more satisfactory. In the same way reading or resting in a chair after eating is more comfortable than taking a nap or undertaking strenuous activity. Because extremes of temperature and dry air also are difficult for people with respiratory illness, it is best to arrange one's schedule according to the season. In winter midday is often warmest, and in summer early morning and evening are often coolest.

Most people become comfortable doing things the same way and in the same order. However, modifying one's schedule to meet the demands of the illness requires flexibility. One woman who was neglecting her diet said she just didn't feel like eating in the morning. When she reviewed her morning, she realized that she was making her bed as soon as she arose and using valuable energy just because she had always made her bed first thing in the morning. By delaying and simplifying her bed-making, she was able to have the energy for a small breakfast.

Bending, stooping, and reaching are activities that require a good deal of energy. Although it is important to retain these physical skills, energy requirements for certain tasks may be reduced by substitution. An independent elderly man with obstructive respiratory disease managed quite well with household activities such as light cleaning, food preparation, and supervision of his disabled wife. He was able to walk to the store and do his own shopping, but carrying the groceries home was too difficult. Although his son was willing to shop for him, the need to accommodate to each other's schedule was frustrating. After a few weeks the son bought a grocery cart for his father, who had the grocery clerk put the groceries in the cart and a neighbor carry them into the house. This simple solution allowed the man his independence and reduced family friction.

The bulk of meal preparation can be adjusted to midday, with only the actual cooking or baking left until evening or after a nap. Food and cooking utensils can be stored for easy access. For those who live in multistory houses, the day's activities have to be planned to minimize use of the stairs. Once the ill person comes downstairs in the morning, he should probably avoid using the stairs again until it is time for bed.

For some people even walking is restricted. With the use of crutches, a seventy-three-year-old widow had managed to live independently for twenty years following the amputation of her leg resulting from an accident. As acute episodes of hypoxemia, diminished amounts of oxygen in the arterial blood, occurred more frequently, requiring emergency care, her doctors determined that the energy required to support her body weight was too great, and she was restricted to wheelchair use.

Legal Aspects

Legal restrictions pertain to respiratory disease only when the symptoms of the illness make it impossible for the individual to carry out a state-monitored activity. There is no driving restriction for respiratory illness *per se*. However, someone with hypoxemia, who may be confused or have poor judgment at certain times of the day, should not drive. Although the process varies from state to state, where there is no provision for periodic testing the motor vehicle bureau ought to be notified of the impairment so that the person's driver's license will be revoked. Such notification in some ways compromises the relationship of the ill person to the person who has notified the authority. (A similar situation occurs in epilepsy and is dealt with more extensively in Chapter 6.)

Schools usually require that a child with asthma bring a note from his physician stating that he is allowed to participate in field trips, physical education classes, and team sports. Often adults will have to supply similar certification about their capacity to do specific kinds of work. There may be restrictions relating to the use of oxygen in certain situations. For example, although the risk of fire from low-flow oxygen is very low, certification of safety is required before oxygen can be used in the home.

Social Aspects

INSURANCE

Group health insurance is available for those who work or are children of workers. Limited life insurance plans that require no physical examination are sometimes available through groups such as unions and veterans' associations. Because many people with pulmonary obstructive disease are smokers, some insurance companies now deny policies to smokers or charge them higher premiums.

A history of frequent hospitalization makes health insurance almost impossible to obtain. Since most of the severely impaired are over age sixty-five, they are covered by Medicare. Medicare Part B covers 80 percent of the cost of home oxygen. Skilled home health care, occupational and respiratory therapy, social work, and certain other related services are covered after the payment of an annual deductible fee. Medication can be very expensive, and coverage is available only through high-option supplemental plans, which are themselves expensive, or through state-administered Pharmacy Assistance plans for people with low incomes. Medicare will not pay for nursing home custodial care for a person who is debilitated but on stable levels of oxygen. It will sometimes cover nursing home costs if oxygen needs vary and frequent evaluations are required.

Some nursing homes that do not have multiple levels of care, that is, parts of the home that have been certified for skilled care and others certified for intermediate or custodial care, will not accept a person who needs continuous oxygen, a skilled service. Because of this, among other reasons, it is critical that people assess all available services a nursing home has to offer when selecting a facility. Beginning this process in advance of emergent need is important. Otherwise the decision is made when someone has been hospitalized and the person cannot return home. One elderly woman who had been in an intermediate-level facility for seven years was managed quite well when her need for oxygen was limited to occasional emergencies. However, when her doctor determined that she required continuous oxygen, she had to move to another facility. For this alert and oriented woman, the experience of moving was devastating. Another elderly woman chose to enter a nursing home when she became wheelchair-dependent, only to discover that the facility did not have wheelchairs. Her insurance, which covered the cost of rental at home, did not provide the same coverage for institutional use.

State Medical Assistance plans are available for those with very low incomes. In some states medical expenses are considered in reducing income limits for eligibility so that someone whose income might exceed the limits for medical assistance may become eligible because of large medical bills. For children with asthma, Crippled Children's Services available through state health departments can assist with the costs of therapy. The financial criteria for these services are less stringent, making the services available to some middle-income families as well as the poor.

The greatest financial burden falls on those who are uninsured or underinsured. All of these diseases involve regular visits to a physician, medication, diagnostic tests, and emergency care. Some will eventually involve home care and oxygen. Many policies do not cover these kinds of expenses.

SOCIAL SECURITY DISABILITY

Obstructive respiratory diseases are the second most frequently represented condition for Social Security Disability. Most chronic pulmonary disorders may be adequately evaluated on the basis of history, physical examination, chest x-ray, and ventilatory function tests. Determination of disability is based on documentation of a specific degree of irreversible loss of pulmonary function capacity (ventilatory impairment, gas exchange impairment, or a combination of both) in three successive pulmonary function tests. Shortness of breath on exertion must be present. Direct assessment of gas exchange by exercise arterial blood gas determination or diffusing capacity is required only in specific relatively rare circumstances, depending on the clinical features and specific diagnosis. For asthma, criteria are based on the frequency of severe attacks and the presence of symptoms between attacks. There must be evidence of recent, recurrent intense asthmatic attacks requiring medication that could not be taken by mouth or persistent, prolonged expiration with wheezing between acute attacks and x-ray findings of disease around the bronchial tubes.

Convincing a company that a disability is work-related is very difficult. A forty-five-year-old man who had worked for twenty years in the coke oven section of a steel mill had frequent asthma attacks and severe respiratory insufficiency due to emphysema. Unable to work and considered disabled by his physician, he exhausted his sick leave and much of his savings in a unsuccessful effort to obtain either company disability pay or transfer to a cleaner branch of the company in another state.

RELATIONSHIP WITH OTHERS

The episodic nature of the attacks makes asthma both disruptive and unpredictable. The fear, panic, and helplessness that the child feels are generally relieved through the parents' calming response, administration of medicine, and/or providing access to emergency care. Thus family members must quell their own anxiety in order to be helpful to the ill child. The parent–child relationship is also a factor in exacerbating episodes. Emotional stress or excitement can trigger an attack. Thus an attack can occur the night before a long-planned family vacation or during a parental argument. The more frequent the attacks or the more attention the child receives, the more the disease can control family life. Siblings and parents can begin to resent the ill child, ignore his symptoms, or even blame him for attacks. At times the stress within the parent–child relationship fosters the attacks. Separation of the child from his parents has resulted in the improvement of symptoms in some children, even when exposures to allergens and other identified triggering factors has remained the same. When this occurs, families must learn to restructure their relationships and the role that asthma plays in the family so that the child can return to his family. It is more common for parents to overprotect their ill child, who may become fearful, anxious, and slow to seek independence. Education, family counseling, and support groups help families put asthma in proper perspective.

Not only the family but the school must adjust to a child's asthma. Other children and teachers are often frightened by the attacks. In response to frequent attacks some teachers tend to restrict a child's activities or treat him in a special way that sets him apart from his peers. The other children begin to see him as a curiosity, and a sibling-like resentment can develop. The fact that infections often cause the child with asthma to miss more school than his peers adds to the distance. When asked how they would like their classmates to act, children often respond that they just want them to play. Education programs that provide information and relieve anxiety are available for children and school personnel in many communities.

For adults with progressive respiratory disease, as the disease progresses, the ill person becomes more dependent. In many situations it is less the disease than the associated anger, depression, or demanding behavior that becomes the controlling factor in the family. As with children, family response runs the gamut from overprotection to resentment. If the ill person is a man, his wife may have to assume more responsibility for family income and household chores. A young man who was unable to continue his work as a painter because of emphysema and asthma assumed responsibility for the care of his young children and for household chores, while his wife returned to work outside the home. Even though the wife's income was less than the husband's work had provided, the family made the necessary adjustments without complaint. The husband's asthma attacks became increasingly frequent, however, and his wife had to assume responsibility for some of the household duties as well. In seeking to control the asthma attacks further, the man's doctor asked him to list the circumstances and possible triggering factors. The man listed the hair spray that his wife used when getting ready for work, his wife's perfume, the dishwashing liquid, and rushing to the telephone when one of the children fell and cut his lip. Although irritants or excitement were involved in all of the factors, the man recognized a pattern of helplessness and resentment related to his wife's working and his being placed in a role that he felt was inappropriate for a man.

Although his wife did not acknowledge any feelings she may have had about the situation, she agreed to be supportive of his attempts to take responsibility for changing his response to the altered family situation. He arranged for his mother to care for the children and enrolled in a job training program, and the frequency of his attacks decreased.

Family members must remember that even a bedridden person can make decisions and be involved in family activities. Respiratory illness does not affect mental abilities other than in some cases of severe hypoxemia or carbon dioxide retention. Assuming that the person's activity level cannot be higher or taking responsibilities away from a person that he is quite able to manage is promoting inactivity and isolation. The children of those with progressive diseases are most often adults. Like the ill person and his spouse, they begin to assume that things cannot be otherwise. Because the development of the disease is so insidious, there is no critical event to rally the family as there might be in a sudden crisis like a stroke. If an activity causes coughing and shortness of breath, people assume that it is affecting the disease process, so ill people are cautioned to stop.

One elderly man gradually limited his activity to his second-floor bedroom leaving his bed only with assistance to go to the bathroom. He tapped on the floor when he wanted his wife to come upstairs. His wife, who also had respiratory insufficiency, was unable to differentiate among his need for help due to physical distress, his demand for lunch, and his desire to have the television channel changed. Although frequent use of the stairs was very fatiguing for her, she always responded. Without discussing the matter with her husband, she asked his doctor to help her place him in a nursing home because of her own deteriorating health. Rather than undertake this drastic solution, the physician suggested a home health aid could assist the man with bathing and some other aspects of personal care. Even an inexpensive intercom could have helped. However, both the patient and his wife expressed their displeasure with a new arrangement because it interfered with their daily routine. Through counseling they recognized their responsibility in this mounting crisis. By continually responding to her husband's demands, the woman was endangering her own health and growing increasingly resentful and despairing. By failing to differentiate his needs, the husband was both alienating his wife and increasing the risk that she would be unable to care for him. The man had never considered the effect on his wife, nor had either of them considered the possibility that anything could be different. With home nursing and physical therapy the man was able to develop the confidence necessary to overcome his fear of exertion, to walk unassisted, to take up more of his personal care, and occasionally to go downstairs. Family and friends were amazed at his improved functioning and outlook.

Seeing a person gasp for breath and sometimes develop a cyanotic appearance during uncontrollable outbursts of coughing evokes fear and helplessness. Sometimes the person appears to be dying before your eyes. The wife of a seriously ill elderly man reported that she could no longer sleep with her husband, because his coughing disturbed her sleep. She moved to another air-conditioned bedroom, from which she could not hear him, but her sleep did not improve because she got up several times each night to check on him. Oddly enough, hearing him cough reassured her that he was at least alive.

A productive cough is also isolating. Although respiratory diseases are not communicable, people associate a productive cough with contagious diseases. Coughing up mucus is unpleasant for the ill person and for his family and friends. People tend to keep a coughing person at a distance; they may stop inviting him to dinner or avoid sitting too close to him. Often the person is embarrassed by his coughing and further isolates himself.

SEXUAL ACTIVITY

Although respiratory illness does not alter a person's ability to respond sexually or his need for closeness, many people with respiratory disease avoid sexual activity because they fear it will make them short of breath. Fatigue and depression contribute to a loss of interest. Some individuals feel as if they are suffocating during intercourse. Diminished sexual interest and activity are often attributed to the aging process, and helpful adaptations are never negotiated. However, many couples remain sexually active, simply slowing their pace or taking more frequent breaks.

Modifications of sexual activity must conserve energy and locate the time of day when breathing is easiest. Positions that require supporting oneself on the arms or pressure on the chest and abdomen are often contraindicated. A side-by-side position is less energy consuming, and more attention to caressing allows satisfaction of sexual needs with less consumption of energy. For couples who have considered sex a nighttime activity, changing the time to midday or another comfortable time requires communication and negotiation. For some people the use of bronchodilators before intercourse is recommended to prevent bronchospasm.

DEPENDENCE, CONFINEMENT, AND ISOLATION

At any stage in any respiratory illness increasing dependence, confinement, and social isolation can contribute to feelings of helplessness and depression. To battle these feelings and keep a positive outlook helps people to remain active and included. For children with asthma the continuing task is to strike a balance between the need for independence and control of the disease. Sometimes, by the time a child reaches adolescence, he is either denying his illness and neglecting his symptoms or remaining fearful, anxious, overly concerned with his disease, and overly dependent on his parents. Similarly, older people must find ways to remain as independent as possible within the limits imposed by their disease. Patients who ignore symptoms until a crisis develops, who continue to smoke, ignore their diet, and generally fail to take responsibility for their health needs are often referred to by members of the health team as noncompliant. Other people remain fearful, demanding, dependent, preoccupied with their symptoms, and increasingly isolated and inactive. With optimal adaptation it remains necessary to rely increasingly on others as the illness progresses. However, even people who require continuous oxygen are often able to live alone. When a person is unable to care for himself with continuous oxygen, a more to the home of a relative or a nursing care facility becomes necessary.

Still, it is most important to retain control of the decisions that affect one's life. A woman who was hospitalized with an acute exacerbation of COPD was told by her doctor that she would have to limit her use of stairs. Since her only bathroom was on the second floor, her adult daughter immediately planned to move her mother to her home, where she could have a room next to the bathroom. The woman, however, was very clear that she wanted to remain in her own home. She arranged to have a plumber construct a bathroom on the first floor of her home while she was still in the hospital and stayed with her daughter only until the construction was completed.

The need to use the stairs presents a considerable barrier. Even those who are able to walk considerable distances on level surfaces may experience a dangerous increase in heart rate when using the stairs. For those living in older urban homes, the decision becomes whether to stay on the second floor where the bathroom is or on the first floor near the kitchen and living areas. Choosing the second floor means isolation from the outdoors and the activities of the family. Visitors will stop by to say hello and then proceed on to other family members in the kitchen or living room. Another option, which prevents this kind of isolation, is to convert a little-used dining room, for example, to a bedroom with a portable commode available for use on the same floor.

The most confining time in the course of the disease occurs when the person suffers from severe shortness of breath and diminished amounts of oxygen in the arterial blood that are just above the level at which oxygen is indicated. During this time activity is associated with distress, and the person often feels increasingly lethargic.

Like other activities, social interaction is possible through planned adaptation. If a person can walk only short distances, a wheelchair can be rented to enable him to participate in long outings. A meal in a restaurant can be scheduled for the lunch hour or in the early, less crowded evening hours if those are times when breathing is easier. Certain sports such as fishing require less exertion than others. Card playing and table games require little more energy than sitting in a chair. Portable oxygen units can be carried on a shoulder or in small wheeled units. With the use of oxygen, lethargy often lifts, and the person feels more like participating in activities.

WORK

The ability to work depends on the symptoms of the illness, the nature of the work, and the flexibility of the work environment. A large group of people who develop manifestations of progressive respiratory disease are past retirement age and work in the house or as volunteers. Among those who are gainfully employed, the people who are self-employed or are highly valued in their business or profession will be more likely to have work adapt to the demands of the illness. Such modifications may be a later arrival time, rest periods during the day, and absences when the person feels ill.

Certain types of work that are physically demanding or in a polluted environment may be intolerable for a person with respiratory illness. If there are no less demanding positions available for which the person has the necessary skills or education, the choices are a new job, retraining, or retirement. If the disease is diagnosed early, retraining is usually available through vocational rehabilitation agencies, which do the necessary testing to determine if it is safe for a person to continue in his present job. This is often necessary both to reassure the worker and to serve as documentation for an employer who is encouraging early retirement. Even in a sedentary job the ill person may be subject to discrimination when an employer feels uncomfortable with the illness and the necessary modification in work routine. Through vocational rehabilitation a former steelworker with limited skill and education was able to enter a job training program and become an electrician. Many of those who retire and remain inactive have more physical complications and depression. The difference is not in gainful employment, but rather in finding something to hold one's interest. Another man who had worked successfully in a fast-paced sales postion could afford to retire and chose to spend his time restoring his boat rather than change to a job he would like less well. A fifty-year-old woman with severe respiratory impairment complicated by extreme obesity was totally disabled for work. She was able to walk only very short distances before she needed to sit and rest until she could stop gasping for breath. When she was not in the hospital, she was confined to her home. When her doctor determined that she needed continuous oxygen, she enrolled in a physical conditioning program, which taught her to walk with oxygen. She loved children and became one of the most popular volunteers on a pedatric inpatient unit. It was a common sight to see this woman walking down the long hospital corridor, pushing a stroller or holding a small child on her shoulder and wheeling her small oxygen unit with her other hand.

Psychological Issues

Again, as with some other chronic diseases, there has been discussion about an asthmatic personality. For many years psychoanalysts focused on the child's dependency and fear of separation from his mother as contributing to the development of the disease. According to the group, wheezing was a supressed cry for mother. However, this theory has never been proved. It is now recognized that people with asthma are a heterogeneous group whose variations cannot be accounted for in a single relationship theory. At this point, common psychological factors are thought to be a response to the disease rather than the cause of it.

Frequently recognized psychological symptoms in progressive pulmonary diseases are fear, anxiety, hypochondriasis, and irritability. Each is tied to physical symptoms. Fear of shortness of breath and coughing is a common cause of self-imposed inactivity. Depression, which can be self-perpetuating, can also lead to loss of interest in eating, social interaction, and activity. It may have a somewhat contagious quality, emotionally draining friends and relatives, who further isolate the ill person as a way to give themselves a rest.

People who believe they have some control over what happens to them are able to recover from periods of depression. An emaciated elderly woman in the hospital awaiting admission to a nursing home was noticeably short of breath even with the use of oxygen. Striking about this woman were her neatly polished bright red fingernails. She described herself as a glamorous person in her younger years and explained that red nail polish had always been a special trademark. Because it was important for her doctor to be able to observe her nailbeds for the bluish color associated with insufficient oxygenation, she had negotiated with him over the one nail she would leave unpolished.

Although all of these people had smoked heavily, they did not blame themselves for their illness but placed all blame outside. The projection of anger and the denial of responsibility contribute to psychological problems. People who understand their part in the disease process and feel they have some control over their lives do best. As one informant commented, the disease might slow him down, but he was determined that it was not going to get him down.

How to Be Helpful to Someone with Respiratory Disease

First educate yourself about the disease process and its limiting factors. Learn not to be terrified of watching someone gasp for breath or cough up large amounts of mucus. Encourage the person to participate in respiratory rehabilitation programs so that he will learn to function to his maximum ability. Help the person and his family to maintain a positive outlook in the face of flagging physical abilities by seeing days made up of times when the person will feel quite well and other times when he will feel terrible. Pay consistent attention to activity, setting priorities and planning adaptations. Rather than give up activites, the ill person must learn to use less energy in doing them.

Stroke

STROKE IS the common term for cerebrovascular accident, death to some part of the brain caused by bleeding, a clot, or some other means of obstruction. Oxygen, glucose, and other necessary nutrients are carried to the nerve cells in the brain by the blood. When the blood supply to a part of the brain is reduced or curtailed, nerve cells in that part of the brain cannot function, and a stroke occurs, leaving that portion of the brain tissue which has not been supplied dead or infarcted. Although its onset is sudden, a stroke is often the result of the aging process and can be thirty to forty years in the making. The stroke itself may progress over a few hours or a few days. The illness is not generally progressive, although the underlying (usually atherosclerotic) process may be progressive. Once a stroke has occurred, the disease has reached its lowest point for the time being.

Most people suffer a combination of symptoms as a result of a stroke, and few have full recovery. Symptoms can be slight or severe, temporary or permanent, visible or invisible. The most common as well as the most obvious effect of stroke may be pronounced weakness on one side of the body. However, loss of sensation, speech disturbance, intellectual disorder, visual difficulty, and other symptoms are also regularly occurring symptoms.

Medical Information

Classification and Etiology

Strokes can be classified according to symptom complex or cause. Symptom complex refers to the parts of the body affected and the state in which they are left after the stroke. This kind of classification derives from what the person with the stroke and her family bring to the attention of a physician: Someone may complain that her arm is weak or that she has lost her side vision. Classification by etiology describes the agents that caused the stroke and, in turn, the conditions under which these particular agents developed. This classification system relates directly to the treatment plan, especially the drugs or surgery prescribed.

In terms of etiology there are three types of stroke: thrombosis, embolism, and hemorrhage. Thrombosis and embolus are kinds of clots. A thrombosis forms in the artery through which the blood is supplied to the brain. It can occur as a result of atherosclerosis, excessive platelets in the blood, or excessive blood viscosity. Excessive blood viscosity may be the result of elevated hemoglobin, abnormal proteins in the blood, or hemoglobinopathy (diseases like sickle cell anemia in which there is an abnormality in the hemoglobin molecule, resulting in abnormal red blood cells). Another cause of thrombosis is disseminated intravascular coagulation (DIC) in which the blood "just clots," often resulting in death. Many terminal illnesses end with DIC.

An embolus is a piece of clot that has formed elsewhere in the body, broken off, traveled to the brain, and then plugged a blood vessel in the brain. Many strokes of this type are of primarily cardiac origin, a result of a clot within the heart, a clot from a diseased valve, or an arrhythmia (an irregular heart rhythm). Heart problems that can lead to a stroke of this type include rheumatic heart disease, atrial fibrillation, infected heart valves, and congenital anomalies. For explanation of these terms, see Chapter 7, "Heart Disease."

Embolus and thrombosis are more common than the third cause of stroke, hemorrhage. In a hemorrhage, the wall of an artery has burst and caused bleeding and local compression in some part of the brain. A hemorrhage is usually more severe than a thrombosis or an embolus. Causes of hemorrhage include hypertension (elevated blood pressure), aneurysms (local dilation of a blood vessel at a weak point in the wall), malformations of blood vessels, blood dyscrasias such as leukemia, resulting in impaired coagulation and abnormal formation of blood, and malignant brain tumors. Stroke can also be caused by low-flow states (low blood pressure with coincidental blood vessel problems); by inflammation of the blood vessels (vasculitis), including such systemic illnesses as lupus erythematosus (see Chapter 2, "Arthritis"); and by amphetamine abuse and the use of oral contraceptives.

Prevalence and Incidence

There are approximately 400,000 new strokes each year. *The National Survey of Stroke*, published in 1983 by the National Institute of Neurological and Communication Disorders and Stroke, report that 31 percent of all people treated for stroke in a United States hospital die during that hospitalization. The risk of fatality during hospitalization varies from 25.8 percent for people with thrombotic strokes to 67.9 percent for people with intraparenchymal hemmorhages. In 1982 about 159,630 people died as a result of an acute stroke or later complications, a drop from 214,333 deaths in 1973. At present there are approximately 1.9 million disabled stroke survivors in the United States.

The risk of stroke increases with age. In the past decade, with advances in prevention and treatment of heart disease and hypertension, the average age of the stroke victim has risen by ten years. In children, there is thought to be an annual incidence of 2.52 cases per 100,000. Strokes in children differ from those in adults in three ways: predisposing factors, clinical evolution, and anatomical site of pathology. While atherosclerosis and hypertension predispose adults to stroke, predisposing factors in children are cyanotic heart disease and leukemia.

For adults under thirty-five the annual incidence of initial strokes is about 3.5 per 100,000. It increases to 30 per 100,000 between ages forty-five and fifty-five and doubles in each succeeding decade. Before age thirty women are more likely to have a stroke than men, possibly because of complications of pregnancy or oral contraceptives. After thirty more men than women have strokes. Heavy smoking increases the incidence of stroke. Young men who smoke heavily have a six times greater chance of atherosclerotic brain infarction than nonsmokers. Cigarette smoking also increases the risk of subarachnoid hemorrhage (bleeding into the space of the brain that contains cerebrospinal fluid) four to six times in men and women. The prognosis for young adults with stroke caused by insufficient blood supply is better than it is for older people: Almost 75 percent of young survivors improve or recover completely. The recurrence rate is 0.5 percent, as against 5 or 6 percent in older people. The most common cause of subarachnoid hemorrhage is head trauma. Approximately 26,000 subarachnoid hemorrhages each year cause about 10 percent of all stroke deaths, and more than half affect people under forty-five years old.

Populations at Risk

The risk of incurring a stroke is greater for men than for women and greater for blacks and Orientals than it is for caucasians. It is highest in the Southwestern United States and lowest in the mountains; higher in rural areas than in metropolitan areas. Incidence is greater among diabetics, those with heart disease, and those with elevated hematocrits. People who have transient ischemic attacks—reversible short-lasting symptoms resulting from interference with cerebral blood supply—are at great risk for having a stroke within five years of their initial TIA. Finally, it has been suggested that stroke may be exacerbated by stress, particularly by stressful changes in role and status such as divorce.

Natural History

A stroke can occur through an extraordinary range of brain lesions. Although the onset is usually sudden, a person sometimes has some kind of warning sign like a temporary loss of some part of her vision, a transitory weakness of some part of her body, unusual irritability, dizzy spells, or speech difficulty. Because attacks generally last only ten to thirty minutes, they are sometimes brushed off and forgotten. Such occurrences are called transient ischemic attacks (TIAs), and they result from temporary interruption of the blood flow to the part of the brain that controls the affected area. Because the interruption is temporary, people often pay little attention to it. However, prompt attention is critical, because a person untreated after a TIA runs a high risk of having a stroke within five years. Treatment for a TIA may include anticoagulation and/or antiplatelet therapy, which prevents and retards the formation of clots.

Strokes are usually marked by localizing signs, which relate directly to the part of the brain damaged by the stroke. Sometimes they can be limited to the face, one limb, or part of one limb, but the most frequent result of stroke is a degree of paralysis on one side of the body. The symptoms can be purely motor, affecting only the ability of the person to move, but they are usually associated with visual, speech, sensory, or coordination problems. Also, after a stroke a person almost always appears psychologically different because of changes in either personality or temperament. The person with a stroke is unusually subject to disturbances of the cardiovascular system, infections of the respiratory and urinary tract, and various musculoskeletal problems. Most people with hemiplegia remain considerably handicapped.

Because a stroke is a fixed structural lesion rather than a disease process, it will not progress in the way that, say, cancer would if left untreated. The underlying vascular disease that created the conditions under which the stroke occurred, however, might progress and possibly result in another stroke. Problems would occur also if the symptoms of the stroke remained unattended and no attempt were made to rehabilitate paralyzed limbs or reeducate the person to walk, speak, or use her hands. If unattended, the paralyzed limb or limbs may contract as unused muscle fibers shorten and thus may produce increased pain and be rendered useless.

Symptoms

One group of symptoms often precedes a stroke, while another relates to the effects of the stroke. Many prestroke symptoms are caused by other conditions. Prestroke symptoms are dizziness; weakness of the arm, hand, or leg on one or both sides of the body; weakness of the facial muscles with sagging on one side or the other; feelings of numbness or tingling in an arm or leg; inability to feel painful or warm things; coldness or pain in the fingers; cramps in an arm on exercise; and a mild balance problem. People sometimes think these symptoms are related to something else. For example, someone might say she felt dizzy because it was a hot day or because she had gotten up too quickly; she might say she was forgetful because she was getting on in years.

One informant said she had several bouts of facial sagging, which she attributed to tiredness. Another attributed weakness in an arm to the fact that he always leaned on his desk with that arm while he wrote with his opposite hand. Other prestroke symptoms include clumsiness in the use of a hand, problems with speech like slurring, loss of vision in one eye, loss of peripheral vision, or increased forgetfulness. An informant who developed slurred speech was accused of being drunk by his family and told to stop talking like that.

Poststroke symptoms are related directly to the part of the brain affected. Most strokes are serious enough to impair the function of the brain cells in the motor area and to cause some paralysis but not so damaging as to cause death. The paralyzed side or limb is at first limp and then develops stiffness or spasticity. The majority of strokes are of middle cerebral artery distribution and primarily effect the face and arm. Anterior cerebral artery strokes, on the other hand, can spare the arm and face and primarily effect the leg.

RIGHT BRAIN INJURY—LEFT HEMIPLEGIA

Each side of the brain controls the opposite side of the body as well as certain specific abilities. Damage to the right side of the brain can produce paralysis on the left side of the body (left hemiplegia). Someone with right brain damage can often have difficulty with spatial–perceptual tasks like judging distance, direction, size, rate of movement, form, and the relation of parts to the whole. Insides and outsides may be confused, as well as right and left. Someone may have difficulty placing her cup on the table or steering a wheelchair through a doorway. Even if her spatial–perceptual difficulties are considered slight, she may have great difficulty driving a car. She may have trouble reading or adding because she loses her place on the page or in the column. Even with the help of rulers, these activities can be difficult and extraordinarily frustrating.

People with right brain strokes behave in ways that promote overestimation of their capacities. They may sound and look all right. They tend to talk a lot and to use flowery language. They tend to move impulsively and fast and to act unaware of their deficits. In this regard, it is thought that what has been damaged is their ability to judge their own capacities. Because people with right brain injury often look well; their difficulty with simple activities can be misunderstood by others, and they can be adjudged confused or uncooperative. Sometimes people with right brain injury are left with slurred speech. They also may cry without knowing why. An informant said that this symptom was more upsetting to her than any of the other deficits with which she was left. She had always been proud of her self-control. Crying among her friends as well as strangers with no advance warning or ready explanation was horrifying.

LEFT BRAIN INJURY—RIGHT HEMIPLEGIA

Someone with left brain injury may have a paralysis of the right side of her body (right hemiplegia). In addition, she is likely to have aphasia, a reduction or disruption in the ability to use words or other symbols in any form. That may mean difficulty in speaking, understanding speech, reading, writing, arithmetic, or all of these aspects of language. The obvious part of aphasia is speech disturbance. Sometimes the symptom is automatic speech in which certain simple words like "hi," "no," and "yes" or swearing is used without relation to the content of the other person's message. Sometimes aphasia takes the form of word substitution in which the person intends to say one word and says another. Aphasia can be inconsistent, so that one minute the person is speaking well, and the next minute she is not. People rarely have arm or leg paralysis along with aphasia.

It is not unusual for the person with a left brain stroke to have altered behavior and affect. For example, she may be angry, frustrated, irritable, demanding, depressed, and less inhibited than she had been before her stroke. Her attention span will be shorter. She may cry or laugh inappropriately, knowing full well that she is doing so but unable to control herself. Compared with her prestroke relationships, she may have less interest in people and events. The husband of a woman with a left brain injury said he could not believe the change in his wife's attitude about their grandchildren. Before her stroke they had been the light of her life. Now she did not care if she saw them or not, and she got angry with them no matter how hard they tried to please her.

VISUAL FIELD DEFECTS

The visual field is the area within which objects can be seen. With normal vision an individual can look straight ahead and see an area of about 360°, almost a complete circle of vision above, below, and to the sides, without moving her eyes or her head. After a stroke many people are left with defective visual fields or what is commonly called field cuts. If someone with a visual field cut looks straight ahead, she will see what is in front of her and on her unaffected side but not what is on her affected side. It is as if someone were wearing goggles with either the left or the right halves of the lenses blacked out.

For example, a left field defect would mean that looking straight ahead she could not see left, only straight ahead or right. In order to see left, she would have to turn her head to the left. She sees with both eyes, but her field of vision is restricted to the center and right in each eye. A left field defect may cause one to ignore objects and space on one's left side. A man may not shave the left side of his face or comb the left side of his hair. A right defect would mean that there would be no right field of vision with either eye.

ONE-SIDED NEGLECT

Most people learn to compensate for field defects by turning their heads to face what they want to see. Sometimes people do not quickly make this adjustment and have what is referred to as one-sided neglect. This condition involves much more than hearing loss or field defects. Those with right brain strokes have more problems with neglect than those with left brain strokes. At times someone may not only neglect input from one side but divide what she sees at midline, reading only half a word or eating only from one side of her plate or only looking at one side of her room. A person may not realize that a limb is her own, actually asking why someone else has been put to bed with her, or she may ignore someone who approaches her on her impaired side. She may become isolated if her unaffected side faces the wall and her impaired side faces a room full of activity. Finally, she may become confused when going back and forth, thinking that she has followed one route leaving and returned by another, because she has seen one side of her route coming and another going.

GENERAL SYMPTOMS

One poststroke generalized symptom is fatigue. Almost all people who have suffered strokes complain for months of excessive fatigue. Everything is more tiring than it used to be. Watching patients in rehabilitation centers, one can see fatigue spread over their faces after short periods of exercise. People who have had strokes also say they can do only one thing at a time and that it takes much more concentration than it would have before the stroke. Although someone who has had a stroke may seem to have had no residual intellectual deficits, even minor damage can interfere with complicated functions of intelligence. An activity such as keeping a checkbook becomes enormously difficult. Even carrying on a conversation with many issues or making plans to do several things in one day becomes frustrating. Some symptoms relate to knowing how to conduct oneself in a particular situation. At times people may say the wrong thing at the wrong time, become sloppy, change from mild-mannered to aggressive behavior, or repeat themselves often.

Those who have had strokes also say that they can retain less information and that their memory is not as good as it was before their stroke. New or poststroke learning is also more difficult than prestroke learning. A person's ability to generalize, to derive a general conception from a particular event, is also often impaired. Transferring learning from one setting to another becomes more difficult, and changes in routine are not welcomed. Those who have had strokes say that, to a much greater degree than before their strokes, they depend on notes to themselves, appointment books, and calendars to act as artificial or prosthetic memories. Although prosthetic is a strong word to use for a memory aid, it does underscore the kind of memory deficit felt by many individuals who have had strokes and the degree to which they depend on any helpful aid.

Another symptom is emotional lability, excessive crying or laughter not appropriate to the occasion. People laugh or cry and do not known why. They say that their crying depresses them rather than that they are crying because they are depressed. Sensory loss is also a problem. Significant sensory loss contributes to the isolation of the person with a stroke. She literally feels cut off from what is going on around her. She may hear and see, touch and speak less well than she did before her stroke. Everything is muted.

Diagnostic Procedures

There are two objectives in evaluating a person who is thought to have had a stroke. The first is to decide if the person has in fact had a stroke. Other illnesses can produce strokelike symptoms, and differentiation is important for treatment plan development. The second purpose is to determine the extent of the effects of the stroke. The diagnosis is made from the results of the individual's personal and family medical history, the physical examination, and a series of laboratory tests.

The history is generally obtained from the patient. In the event that the patient may not be able to speak or her memory is impaired, a family member is consulted. The evolution of the symptoms, the onset of the stroke, the course of the illness, and past personal and family medical history are all described. In this way the symptoms are put into context.

The physical examination comprises evaluation of the person's motor abilities, mental status, cranial nerves, and sensory system. Motor function is examined in order to determine muscle strength, reflexes, freedom of movement, and locomotion. The mental status evaluation checks cognitive function, most particularly language. The examination of the cranial nerves evaluates the functioning of the nerves in the head, face, and eyes. The sensory system is examined to evaluate the person's perception of pain, light touch, and direction. This is the most difficult area to evaluate, because it relies so completely on the person's subjective response. However, a person's consistent inability to sense stimuli on one side or one part of the body indicates a major sensory deficit.

Next, the person's vascular system is checked. Blood pressure is measured in both arms to be certain that the pressure is equal. The heart is examined for the presence of abnormal rhythms (arrythmias) or sounds (murmurs). The carotid arteries, the principal arteries on either side of the neck through which blood is carried to the brain, are examined for abnormalities. Finally, the ways in which a person walks, speaks, and understands are observed.

LABORATORY TESTS

Several laboratory tests are carried out with all people who are suspected of having had a stroke in order to screen for underlying illnesses and risk factors. Analyses of the blood and urine, chest x-rays, and electrocardiagrams are routine. Computerized cranial tomography (CCT) is used to demonstrate the presence, the location, and, to some extent, the cause and age of a stroke. For example, in people with infarction, brain swelling may be visible in the brain for the first three to ten days after onset. Several weeks later the infarction will appear on the CCT as a well-outlined, translucent defect. CCT will demonstrate whether the cause is a hemorrhage or a clot. The kind and age of the hemorrhage are also indicated on a scan taken before the hemorrhage is reabsorbed and its x-ray density decreases.

In order to examine the spinal fluid for cellular content and chemical constituents, a lumbar puncture or spinal tap may be carried out. Blood in the spinal fluid is an indication of a hemorrhage in or around the brain. Intracranial pressure may also be measured at the time of the lumbar puncture. Arteriography outlines the blood vessels in the brain. Digital subtraction angiography (DSA) gives direct visualization of arteries in the neck and head by means of an intravenous injection with less potential hazard than arteriography.

There are also several noninvasive ways of looking at cerebral circulation. Ophthalmonynamometry, oculoplethysmography, and directional Doppler carotid circulation analysis and ultrasonography measure the patency of the carotid arteries, the degree to which they are open. Electroencephalography (EEG) measures electrical impulses from the brain.

Laboratory tests, then, serve three purposes. First, they confirm the diagnosis made from the history and the physical examination. Second, they rule out other illnesses. Third, they confirm the cause of the stroke.

Therapies

The primary therapies for stroke are a specific drug regimen directed toward the cause of the stroke in an attempt to prevent a recurrence and a specific rehabilitation program designed to reeducate the person to compensate for the deficits created by the stroke. Basically drugs and surgery are used to try to prevent another stroke or a first stroke if there has been sufficient warning. Often the cause of the stroke relates to heart disease, which is described in Chapter 7. Neither therapy can rectify the cardiovascular accident. There is no cure for a stroke.

DRUGS

Drugs are prescribed to treat the underlying illness that caused the stroke, to relieve some of the effects of the stroke, and to prevent recurrence. For example, steroids are given to people with inflammation of the blood vessels (vasculitis) in order to diminish the inflammation. Antihypertensive drugs, antifibrinolytic medications to prevent clots from breaking off, and steroids to decrease brain swelling are used for treatment of aneurysmal bleeding.

Treatment of acute stroke may include anticoagulants to retard additional clotting of blood, steroids to decrease the swelling of the brain tissue, volume expanders to increase blood volume, antihypertensives to lower the blood pressure, osmotic agents to decrease brain swelling, and antiplatelet medications like aspirin. The object of most of these drugs is to keep blood flowing normally to the brain and to keep the brain in a state that will allow it to receive normally the oxygen and nutrients that the blood carries. For long-term treatment of stroke, antihypertensive, anticoagulant, and antiplatelet medications may be used.

SURGERY

Surgery is both therapeutic and preventive. To evacuate a hematoma (a swelling filled with blood), a craniotomy or surgical opening of the skull is performed. The clipping of an aneurysm to prevent a recurrence of its rupturing is also a surgical procedure. Preventive surgery includes carotid endarterectomy (removal of an atheromatous core from an artery) and a variety of bypass procedures including connecting an extracranial to an intracranial artery. However, the most effective therapy is prevention, most particularly control of hypertension, diet, and avoidance of smoking.

REHABILITATION

Treatment also includes bed rest and means for reducing the complications of immobility. To reeducate the mind and the muscles to compensate for the damage done to the brain and to prevent additional wasting, contractures, and pain which come to unused and atrophying muscles, rehabilitation services are introduced. They help the person to maintain the highest level of mobility and motility she can reach after her stroke, and to restore confidence after the individual has sustained this devastating loss.

For the first several weeks after a stroke it is difficult to predict how long symptoms will last and which will remain. A recent study of a group of patients suffering from what was called "the middle band of strokes of intermediate prognosis" says that the best predictor for rehabilitation is the return of upper limb motor function in four weeks. That plus proprioceptive abilities (position sense) and postural function (the ability to keep oneself erect and to right oneself after leaning over) were the only clinical tests the study found useful in predicting the rehabilitative potential for those with strokes. At present rehabilitation is considered important for every poststroke person to keep muscles limber and to reeducate all people who have had strokes to reach the limits of their poststroke capacity.

Many people who have had strokes go to rehabilitation centers for their post–acute care therapy. These centers are staffed by physiatrists (physicians who are trained in the specialty of physical medicine and rehabilitation), nurses, physical therapists, occupational therapists, speech therapists, social workers, and psychologists. Many centers also have music and art therapists.

The hallmark of rehabilitation is a positive, reasonably demanding approach that understands and yet counteracts the person's despair with firm, kind, hopeful support. Rehabilitation centers look like spas, with many exercise mats on low platforms, weight machines, and other equipment for the retraining of muscles.

Most centers have clear criteria for admission relating to the patient's capacity to be retrained, as well as her having a home and family to which to return. Being selected for a rehabilitation center is cause for elation. This step means that no one has given up. When people begin active therapy, however, they again find progress slow. At that point family, friends, and staff must help them to sustain themselves.

Obviously a great deal of what is accomplished in a rehabilitation center is mental as well as physical. Companionship and mutual aid develop among patients and between patients and staff. Space is open, and everyone sees what everyone else is doing. The lack of privacy may hinder some people, but on the whole it helps to build group spirit and cameraderie and to motivate individuals and their families to work harder.

Rehabilitation means the retraining of body parts affected by the stroke. Because parts of the brain have been damaged, the person with a stroke must reeducate her body to do things she has taken for granted since she was a small child. In essence, through rehabilitation she must learn to compensate for the deficits in thinking and in action that have occurred as a result of her stroke. The goal in rehabilitation is for each person to live as independently and as productively as possible.

To reach this goal the person must have the ability to respond, and she must actively cooperate in the rehabilitative process. Limbs often feel as if they cannot be relied upon. Sometimes they feel as if they belong to someone else. Weakness, fatigue, and often depression are part of the after-stroke process. For these reasons people need a lot of encouragement from family, friends, and rehabilitation personnel in order to persevere.

Rehabilitation begins quickly in the process of recovery from a stroke. It is said that the main recovery takes place within the first two months after the stroke has occurred, but improvement goes on for six months to a year, as the affected parts of the body are exercised and used. If a person is hemiplegic, the first step, which begins as soon as the physician indicates that the person is ready, is passive range of motion exercise. In passive exercise the person's muscles are exercised for her. If passive exercise is not begun, spasticity of the muscles can pull the arm toward the body, rotate the leg outward, and pull the foot downward. Carried out by a nurse, physical therapist, or a family member who has been trained to do it, passive exercise works to prevent these postural changes from becoming fixed.

When the physician indicates that the patient is ready, active exercises can begin. These strengthen and retrain the legs, arms, hands, and torso. Walking is the most important function for the legs to relearn, and it is estimated that at least 80 percent of people whose legs have become paralyzed as the result of a stroke can resume walking with or without an aid of some kind. If necessary a person can be taught to use a cane, walker, or brace to facilitate her ability to walk.

Return of the use of paralyzed hand or arm is more difficult, since both are used in extremely complicated movements requiring precise coordination. Even actions like combing hair, eating, writing, or brushing teeth require large motions of the arm plus fine movements of the fingers. The first movements to be restored are large movements, which involve the entire arm, such as slipping one's arm into the sleeve of a jacket. The movement of wrist and fingers is extremely difficult, so that one might be able to pull her blouse onto her arms, but she might not be able to button the sleeves or the front of the blouse. For the affected limbs, all of these motions have to be relearned through dogged practice.

Some speech problems, such as slurring, may recover spontaneously or improve with simple exercises. Others, such as aphasia, require more than the kind of learning it takes to learn a new language. Most language defects require specific exercises as well as a great deal of practice on the part of the person who has had the stroke and patience on the part of her friends and relatives.

Many problems are addressed by teaching a person with a stroke how to perform activities that will allow her to care for herself. Rehabilitation personnel refer to these tasks as activities of daily living (ADL). They include bed activities, rising and sitting, transfer from bed to chair and back, standing transfer, bath transfer, locomotion, dressing, personal hygiene, care of bowel and bladder activities, and feeding. Most of the activities fall into the areas of eating, dressing, moving around, and hygiene, but some miscellaneous activities include using the telephone, turning on a faucet or a light, and opening a drawer.

There are many appliances available that can help the person with a stroke. These range from complicated electronic gadgetry to simple tools like a combination fork, knife, and spoon to aid someone who can use only one hand to eat; velcro fastenings for the clothing of someone who has the use of only one hand; or elastic shoelaces enabling one to slip her foot into tie shoes. There are also many devices that can be installed in the home in order to make it safe and manageable for someone who has had a stroke. For example, grab bars can be installed next to bathtubs and toilets to facilitate use. The home can be evaluated by an occupational or physical therapist in order to make it as safe and as free of barriers as possible.

The greatest step is not from the hospital to the rehabilitation center but from the rehabilitation center to the community. One moves from an accepting, supportive, barrier-free, and ordered existence to all the contradictions and exigencies of home. The person with a stroke and her family are elated at the prospect of homecoming, only to find that being home is physically harder and that the work toward reaching an optimal level of functioning continues.

Psychosocial Information

Modifications in Life-Style

People who have had strokes alter their life-styles in order to compensate for resultant deficits. Activities that were once taken for granted are often impossible. New activities or new levels of old activities, suitable for the person's current abilities, have to be found. One has only to imagine oneself hemiplegic to see how restrictive that state might be without extraordinary will power and support. For those whose sight has been affected, other kinds of restrictions exist. A diminished ability to speak, to reason, to handle several complex ideas, or to do arithmetic can also drastically limit activity. Diet, exercise, sleep, rest, and activity have to be reconsidered and often restructured by the person who has had the stroke as well as her family. Diet above all is geared toward the control of hypertension through weight control and the decreased intake of salt. Food should be nutritious and energy-giving. Regular exercise commensurate with the person's abilities is critical for retraining muscles and regaining strength. Effective exercises are taught by physical therapists and can be found in many publications. None should be attempted until the person has been cleared medically. Two excellent pamphlets published by the American Heart Association are called *Strike Back at Stroke* and *Up and Around: A Booklet to Aid the Stroke Patient in Activities of Daily Living*. Often a person's sleep pattern is altered by her stroke, and she must learn to adjust her sleep to conform reasonably to her home schedule. Fatigue is a common symptom for people poststroke, and they need frequent naps or rest periods. Fatigue lessens over time but remains a problem.

Most people who have had strokes say that a regular, predictable daily schedule is important. With a daily pattern, there is less to remember, less to try to sort out, and more opportunity to schedule rest periods. Memory aids, notes, and reminders can lessen a person's anxiety about memory difficulties and help her to manage with more confidence.

Impact of the Disease on Social Life

There are times when a stroke leaves one unaffected, but those times are relatively rare. In those cases the stroke, like a TIA, is a warning to control hypertension and other conditions that might cause a recurrence. However, most people who have strokes are left with significant damage to which they must adjust in order to live as productively as possible.

Legal Issues

A stroke affects someone legally in regard to her capacity to drive and to manage her own affairs. Even if she appears able, she probably should not resume driving until she has passed a state driving examination after having recovered from her stroke. Physical ability and judgment are integral to operating a motor vehicle.

Rehabilitation centers offer special driving programs, which involve testing by psychologists as well as driver education. Psychologists can test a person's perceptual ability as well as her ability to understand signs and signals. When a person enters a rehabilitation center, her state department of motor vehicles is notified that she is disabled, and she must be requalified before receiving a new license. Many people are never sent to rehabilitation centers either because there are none available, they are not considered good candidates, or their physicians do not refer them. Many physicians do not address the driving question, preferring to leave the decision up to the patient and family. For safety's sake, the rehabilitation center solution seems the wise one.

The other situation in which a person who has had a stroke might be restricted is when she is found to be *non compos mentis* or not of sound mind. Hemiplegia and visual field defects are not indicative of unsound mind, nor are many other symptoms of stroke. If the person is married or has children who willingly assume responsibility, the family begins to handle the decisions. However, many old people with strokes do not have a close relative who can assume responsibility. Thus this situation involves the law only if the person's thinking is affected to the point where she is unable to make sound decisions, and no one else is in a position to take responsibility. If this situation exists, the court must be petitioned to declare the person of unsound mind and appoint a guardian to take care of her financial matters.

Insurance

Most people who have strokes are adequately covered for their acute care through private insurance plans, Medicare or Medicaid. Rehabilitation services are also covered by most major insurance plans. Automobile insurance would have to be reissued after the patient is deemed fit to resume driving by her state department of motor vehicles.

Many people who have had strokes are already receiving payments from Social Security, having become eligible through retirement or age. If people are younger than the age required for retirement or old age status, they can only receive Social Security Disability payments only if they can prove they are no longer capable of any sort of gainful activity. Generally it is easier to plead the case of those with gross motor disabilities than those with poor vision or defective judgment. The latter disabilities are invisible and difficult to evaluate but they may interfere more with the ability to work than gross disabilities. A young woman who had worked as a secretary had recovered from an aneurysm with no visible symptoms. Yet she was unable to organize her time, become overwhelmed when asked to do anything but the simplest tasks, and was a poor judge of her own abilities. Because she was unable to prove her incapacity to work, she was refused disability payments. The burden is on the patient, family, and physician to document the disability. When a person is refused, she has the right to appeal. At that juncture it is necessary to discern what documentation was missing. Applying or appealing without documentation of the inability to work will probably result in refusal.

Relationship to Others

Unless she can manage a great deal of self-care, the person who has had the stroke is quite dependent on her family and particularly on her spouse. Once the person is home, she may improve slowly in some areas, but she probably will never be as capable as she was before the stroke. One may learn to cope, but one does not become well. An informant said of her debilitated husband. "All of a sudden, I realized that he was badly crippled and going to be around for years." Although it sounds harsh and unsympathetic, that remark probably captures the despair of many spouses. Grown children are often part of this scenario, especially as they might be more physically capable of participating in the care of the disabled person than the spouse. Problems often arise because of this unanticipated role reversal in which the child has to assume some caretaking responsibilities. A proud Italian immigrant man of fifty-one had worked as a highly skilled carpenter. A strict father, he had always belittled his intelligent, accomplished son, who also worked as a carpenter. When the man suffered a stroke that left him hemiplegic, he was no longer able to work and had to depend on his son even for grooming. It was an excruciating experience for both men. Eventually the son was able to make peace with the situation, but the experience was so terribly upsetting to the father that the family had to hire help to assist him.

Such role reversals are even more poignant because of the swiftness with which they occur. The loss is devastating. It is different from the normal experience of adult children watching their parents grow old. One day a wife or husband, mother or father, is healthy and strong, and the next she can be frail, angry, confused, or unable to speak. She is certainly changed. It is almost as if a different person is returning home from the hospital or rehabilitation center. Yet the most important factor in the person's continued recovery is the companionship of loved ones and the sharing of their motivation and courage.

Sexual Activity

Intercourse will not cause a stroke, but lack of interest and the generalized fatigue that accompanies most strokes can interfere with one's sex life. One informant said that in addition to feeling tired all of the time, she felt less attractive and did not believe her husband when he said he wanted to make love. Because abstinence was a problem for him, she forced herself to go along with him, but it was never good for her because she felt ugly. Most people can find ways to accommodate to their fatigue and their disability to continue a degree of sexual activity that is satisfying for both partners. A couple said that they considered the continuation of sexual activity part of the challenge of life after a stroke.

Relationships with Strangers

The way a person looks generally determines the response of a stranger. Visible signs of disability often elicit an exaggerated response. Often people react to a person who drags her leg or is wheelchair-bound as if that person's mind were affected as well as her body. Slurred speech reminds strangers of drunk talk. In response to aphasia, people speak as if the person were retarded or holler as if she were deaf.

Just as inappropriately, strangers react to someone who appears to be intact as if she were well. It can be as much of a problem for someone to have her capabilities overestimated because her difficulties in thinking or seeing or computing do not show, as it can be for capabilities to be underestimated because someone needs assistance in order to walk. A very dignified informant in her middle sixties who has no visible impairment was soundly berated by a brash, young bank manager for making a mistake in a withdrawal. When she explained that a stroke had affected her vision, making it difficult for her to place information on the correct line, he began to talk to her as if she were retarded. Neither response was helpful.

Ability to Work

In this society, where earning power is so critical to adult status, the inability to work deals a heavy blow. Of course, many people have mild strokes that do not affect their ability to work. However, many others find their former jobs too difficult. If their work was physically taxing or required a great deal of coordination, they may not be able to return to it, because they are neither sufficiently strong nor sufficiently dextrous. If they had a job that required a great deal of hand–eye coordination or memory for many details, that might be overly taxing because it was too pressured, fast-moving or complicated. The movements and mental capacity necessary to answer a phone and take a message, lay bricks, operate a cash register, or sell a box of cookies are complicated. Those tasks, which are only parts of relatively low-pressure occupations, are very difficult for someone who is hemiplegic, who has visual field cuts, or whose memory has been affected. The hope is painstakingly to relearn lost skills and to compensate for what one cannot do with something else that one can do.

Psychological Issues

SELF-CONCEPT

A stroke is an enormous blow to an individual's self-concept. One informant, trying to explain the loss she felt as a result of her stroke, said that it is literally a death of a part of oneself that one still has to carry around. Loss of one's physical and/or cognitive abilities, as well as independence, are damaging to self-concept. Often, one's body is changed, roles that were hers can no longer be carried out, and her abilities are in some ways diminished. It takes an extraordinarily strong self-concept to face a stroke squarely and learn to cope.

PARTICULAR PSYCHOLOGICAL RESPONSES

It is said that people initially respond to a stroke with great anger or great passivity. As they become used to their condition, these emotional states wane to some degree, and people are able to participate more fully in their rehabilitation. Some rage remains. Patients find that it comes to the fore when they are particularly tired, discouraged, or mistreated by someone around them. When life goes better, the rage generally abates.

STAGES OF PSYCHOLOGICAL RESPONSE

Psychological stages seem to match phases of treatment. When the person who has had the stroke first comes to the hospital, she and her family initially despair at the loss and then seem more hopeful because she has survived the stroke. People generally believe that medicine can effect change. For the rest of the acute phase people seem more passive, waiting to see what is going to happen and which capacities will be spontaneously recovered. At the next phase, when everyone is told that the person has been accepted for rehabilitation, there is euphoria in the anticipation that rehabilitation will recover lost abilities. Euphoria soon gives way to dogged determination when the person realizes that rehabilitation is a long, hard process marked by small incremental changes.

A similar euphoria occurs when someone is told that she is ready for discharge from a rehabilitation center. The feeling is accompanied by fear of what will happen when one loses the safety and support of the rehabilitation facility. Still, most people go home with great expectations. Everyone must be forewarned that nothing magical happens on the way home to make the person the same as she was before the stroke occurred. Some people say that home is the hardest place to be, but with adequate preparation and realistic expectations this can be joyful time. People must be helped to maintain their courage and motivation, because life will be harder. People who make an extraordinary effort at readjustment generally do best.

CHANGES IN APPEARANCE, MOOD, AND AFFECT

With most people who have had strokes, there will be some change in appearance. The change might be a slight drooping on one side of the face or a dragging of one side of the body. Part of the change may also come from one-sided neglect, explained earlier, or from a kind of sloppiness or inattention to dress that seems to accompany some kinds of strokes. People can be taught to dress differently and to attend to all parts of themselves.

Some changes in mood and affect such as crying or laughing for no apparent reason usually get better over time. Some major personality changes, obvious soon after the stroke occurs, get better in time. Others are the result of brain damage and become a permanent part of the person. Generally a person's prestroke strengths will support her in her effort to rehabilitate herself.

How to Be Helpful to Someone Who Has Had a Stroke

A stroke is a blow, a quick sharp injury whose aftermath is carried by the person for her lifetime. Depending on the part of the brain affected, a stroke can be expressed through myriad symptoms. Knowing the person well enough to understand how she is affected is critical to your being helpful. She will become tired and overwhelmed more easily than before her stroke. Thus the rehabilitation effort must be sustained even when progress is slow. Once the person is finished with most medical treatment and rehabilitation, she and her family will continue living with the results of the stroke. Helping the person to maintain an interest in life and a willingness to join in company is most important.

10

Substance Abuse

A drug is a substance that, when ingested, may modify one or more functions of a living organism. In contemporary society millions of people have taken or are taking drugs solely to alter their mood, affect, or state of consciousness. Use can be casual, as when an individual tries drugs a few times and stops; it can be experimental, when someone terminates use before becoming dependent on the substance; or it can be continuous, in which case the person becomes dependent on the drug. Not all drug dependency is necessarily harmful. Excessive use of substances like coffee, tea, or cola does not produce the same magnitude of social and health problems as excessive use of alcohol, heroin, or barbiturates.

Alcohol dependency is the most prevalent abuse problem in the United States. Unlike the abuse of other substances, which can be confined to one age group or related to criminal activities, the abuse of alcohol is found all across American society. Its cost to our economy is estimated to be about $49 billion a year. It also plays a role in 10 percent of all the deaths in the United States and is the principal cause of death through accidents for those aged 15–24. The abuse of alcohol is implicated in a wide range of other illnesses, including some discussed in this volume. People who abuse other drugs also often abuse alcohol. For these reasons, the chapter will treat alcohol abuse as the prototype for all addictive problems. The abuse of other drugs will be discussed at the end of the chapter.

Substance abuse is a chronic, progressive, and potentially fatal disease characterized by tolerance, physical dependency, and/or pathological organ changes, all of which are the consequence of the drug ingestion. Tolerance means that the drug dosage must be increased over time in order

239

to maintain the same effect. Physical dependency refers to the intense physical disturbance or withdrawal syndrome experienced when the drug is discontinued. Pathological organ changes means that the drug will have damaged at least one of the individual's organs.

The course of the disease depends largely on whether the individual stops using the drug and how much irreversible damage has occurred. If the person stops using the drugs before he has badly damaged organs, the disease need not be progressive. If he continues to abuse the substances, becoming increasingly tolerant and dependent, the disease will progress. Crises are related to the particular drug ingested and the response each individual has to the drug.

Substance abuse, with alcoholism as its prototype, differs from the other eight disease categories included in this book, not in kind or degree of physical damage it causes or in terms of its social or psychological impact, but in the way in which society views the illness and its victims. Many people continue to believe that everyone should know when to stop drinking, that if people really wanted to, they would. This case of "blame the victim" is woven deep into American culture from Prohibition and the Women's Christian Temperance Union to parents who teach teenage children how to hold their liquor. We do not look with distain at the people who have lung cancer or emphysema largely as a result of smoking cigarettes, nor do we laugh at the man who has suffered a massive heart attack while pushing and lifting heavy shovels of snow after months of sedentary life. We do not even sneer at the person who has for years ignored medical advice about treatment of hypertension and who has a stroke that leaves him paraplegic. However, despite legal and professional recognition of alcoholism as a disease, many people continue to see all drinking as intentional. These examples relate to several issues about the definitions of acceptable behavior and responsibility in our society that, to some degree, make it difficult to let substance abuse take its place alongside the other chronic diseases in this volume. The issues are (1) the distinction among use, misuse, and abuse; (2) the distinction between physical and psychological dependence; (3) substance abuse as disease, deviation, or criminal act; (4) legal issues concerning the abuse of alcohol and other drugs; and (5) the definition of responsibility.

The use of alcohol is considered normal for most groups in the United States. In fact, there are times when it is almost expected that people will get drunk. The time and place for this behavior is acceptable to most of the people involved. When people drink beyond those parameters, they are generally considered to be misusing alcohol. The issue is less clear for marijuana and, perhaps, cocaine. The popularity of both drugs is growing, and many groups, particularly young adults, artists, and entertainers view these drugs as recreational in the same way that other groups view alcohol. The law is clear, however, that involvement with drugs other than alcohol is illegal. Physical dependency along with disruption of health, family life, friendships, or work distinguishes misuse from abuse.

The second issue concerns the definition of dependency. In physical dependency, the person's body adapts to the substance, and withdrawal of the drug creates a physical reaction. In psychological dependency, the drug helps an individual to avoid discomfort or produces a feeling of great pleasure, awareness, or energy. The person takes the drug regularly in order to produce these feelings. After a time the physical dependence supersedes the psychological. The person no longer finds the great high. Avoiding withdrawal symptoms becomes the motivation.

Judging substance abuse to be disease, deviation, or criminal act also remains an issue. Until recently alcoholism was viewed as an individual failing, a sign of debauchery, malingering, or sometimes criminal behavior. Then alcoholism was declared a disease, entitled to the same forms of respect and treatment accorded to other illnesses. Although the legal definition of alcoholism has changed, many continue to view it in the old way.

Certain parts of the drug enterprise are clearly illegal, but laws regarding possession or ingestion vary. For example, the legal possession of alcohol is determined by age. If people damage the persons or property of others while drinking, their behavior is considered criminal. If they drink to the point of damaging themselves, their behavior is considered sick. For drugs that are created or procured illegally, the distinction is even less clear.

The last issue concerns the parameters of responsibility. Our society believes that people generally are not responsible for their illnesses, that it is not an individual's fault that he has contracted a disease. However, society also says that an individual is responsible for his own behavior. Thus, although it is not someone's fault that he is an alcoholic, he is still responsible for ingesting the drug, and he is responsible for his behavior when he is under the influence of the drug. Although questions of definition and responsibility are important in several of the illnesses discussed in this volume, nowhere are they as obfuscated or important.

Medical Information

Demographic Characteristics

About 100 million people in this country over the age of fifteen consume alcohol. In 1981 the equivalent of 2.77 gallons of pure alcohol was sold for each person in this country over fourteen. Translated into alcoholic beverages, this is about 115 bottles of wine, 35 fifths of 80 proof whiskey, or 591 12-ounce cans of beer. About one-third Americans do not drink at all, one-third have about two drinks a week, and the remaining one-third report fourteen drinks a week. Approximately 10 percent of the drinking population consumes half of the alcoholic beverages sold. Between 5 and 10 percent, or 5 million to 10 million, of the people who consume alcoholic beverages are alcoholic. Populations who are at risk for alcoholism are changing. One-third of alcoholics are women, with the number of known women alcoholics having doubled since World War II. The Metropolitan Life Insurance Study, which was reported in the mid-1970s, said that alcohol-related deaths rose 36 percent for white women and 71 percent for nonwhite women. The National Center for Health Statistics reported in 1975 that American Indian women were more likely to die of cirrhosis of the liver at a younger age than either white or black women. The gay and lesbian population in the United States is also at greater risk for alcoholism.

The National Council on Alcoholism estimates that 6 to 10 percent of all employees are alcoholics. Most alcoholics are functioning to some degree with jobs and families. Black and Puerto Rican alcoholics are more likely to be unskilled or unemployed than their white counterparts. Black alcoholics are also more likely to be single or separated, while whites are more likely to be currently married and living with a spouse. Certain occupations are also at increased risk for alcoholism. According to *Occupations and Alcoholisms: 1982* (NIAAA Research Monograph #8), the ten occupations associated with highest standardized mortality rates for cirrhosis of the liver in the United States were (1) waiters, bartenders, and counter workers; (2) longshoremen and stevedores; (3) transportation workers with the exception of railroad workers; (4) cooks: (5) laborers in manufacturing and transportation equipment; (6) musicians; (7) authors, editors, and reporters; (8) bakers; (9) other categories of laborers, and (10) shoemakers and shoe repairers.

Certain demographic differences may also influence prognosis. For example, regular employment in skilled or white-collar occupations and the availability of economic resources have been associated with greater improvement following treatment. Married patients and those who live with their families persist in treatment longer and have a better prognosis.

Because of easy access to drugs and alcohol and the power of the peer group, teens and preteens are also at increased risk. About 6 percent of high school seniors (more than 250,000) reported drinking daily in 1981, and 56 percent of these students said that they had begun drinking before they entered high school. Generally, drinking problems occur for women when they are in their thirties and forties. Among men, drinking problems most often begin when they are in their twenties. Although women begin drinking later, they often telescope their drinking, moving rapidly to later stages, so that they often require first hospital treatment in relation to alcohol around age forty, the same time as men who have been drinking longer. The elderly are also at risk for alcohol abuse. Some are survivors who have been drinking heavily for a long time, some are intermittent drinkers who have drunk heavily at other times in their lives and stopped, and some are reactors who begin drinking heavily late in life because of bereavement, retirement, or loneliness.

Skid row alcoholics make up only 3 to 5 percent of the alcoholic population. Only 10 percent of this group are women. Because of the public nature of their drinking and their concentration in a close geographical area, they often receive an inordinate share of attention. They are people who have lost most of their social anchorages. The skid row alcoholic used to be typically white, male, and forty-five or older. Now, skid row is made up increasingly of Chicanos, blacks, drug users, and deinstitutionalized mental patients making the circuit of agencies and facilities that have grown up around them.

Alcohol is involved in two-thirds of all accidents. Half of the auto fatalities (25,000) and permanent disabilities (75,000) each year are alcohol-related. According to the National Council on Alcoholism, 80 percent of fire deaths, 65 percent of drownings, 77 percent of falls, 55 percent of arrests, 36 percent of pedestrian accidents, and 22 percent of home accidents are linked to the use of alcohol.

Natural History

The natural history of alcoholism and the abuse of other substances is different from that of the other diseases in this book, because much of what happens to an individual's health depends on his continuing or stopping the ingestion. If one abstains from use and permanent organ damage has not occurred, some symptoms may continue to progress, some may remain the same, but many disappear sooner or later.

Some who posit stages of alcoholism say that in the early stages of alcohol dependency one drinks increasing amounts in order to feel a glow, sneaks or gulps drinks, looks for occasions to drink, and begins to lie about the amounts consumed. He begins to look for social groups that drink more and are more accepting of the drinking or others. He gets "high" on acceptable occasions and still feels that he can control his drinking. Sometimes he may miss days of work, perform less well at work, experience the shakes, or lose his appetite.

Those who support a stage theory say a person may still control the time or occasion at which he wants to begin drinking, but once he starts, he cannot stop. It may become obvious to the drinker and to those around him that his drinking routine and behavior have changed. At this stage the person begins to rationalize his drinking, to think up excuses, and to blame everything but his drinking for the problems he is having. Relationships and job may suffer. Around this time he may begin to drink in the morning, drink alone, and require pick-me-ups throughout the day.

If the person continues to drink, his drinking may go out of control. He may stay drunk for weeks at a time, may be unable to go a day without drinking, and have severe withdrawal symptoms if he goes without drinking. Withdrawal symptoms usually begin six to twelve hours after heavy intake of alcohol has ceased. Symptoms generally reach their peak in one or two days and gradually subside after three to six days. Symptoms can be mild, such as lack of appetite, sweating, or nervousness, or they can be severe and potentially fatal such as severe tremors, convulsions, hallucinations, shock, and cardiac irregularity. When consumption stops or slows, dependency is signaled through the appearance of some of these symptoms. In these later stages there is often damage to the liver, nerves, heart, gastrointestinal tract, and other major organs. Relationships and work may continue to deteriorate.

A person may experience blackouts, periods of time of which he has no memory. One social work informant who is herself a recovering alcoholic described a therapy group she led for hospitalized alcoholics. When asking the men to describe the funniest thing that others had told them they had done during a blackout, she recounted the time she had directed traffic in the busy main street of her small town so that her friends could cross. One of the men countered with a memory of waking one morning in a large bed with a strange woman on either side of him. When she asked for painful memories of blackout behavior, one man said that he had slapped his elderly father in the face and another said that he had sexually assaulted his young daughter while he was drunk.

If the disease progresses, a person begins to think about how activities are interfering with his drinking, which becomes the focal point of his life. He becomes trapped in a life that revolves completely around alcohol: getting it, downing it, reacting to it, not getting it, reacting to that, and getting enough again. He may no longer take care of himself and may experience a great deal of remorse, resentment, defensiveness, debasement, and anxiety. Again, his social group may change to reflect the heavier, less socially acceptable, and sicker drinking pattern. With the late stages of the disease often come loss of job and family and physical deterioration.

With chronic use of alcohol, symptoms of acute intoxication include disorientation, an unsteady gait, and an abnormal cheerfulness or euphoria, as well as nystagmus, a rapid back-and-forth movement of the eyes. A chronically intoxicated person will have signs of nervous system abnormality in the form of confusion, incoherent speech, poor memory, intellectual impairment, and loss of dexterity. His attention span and ability to concentrate will be compromised. His psychological symptoms may include great self-absorption, impulsiveness, and ambivalence about almost anything. He may disregard dangerous situations, lack insight, and often be unable to distinguish fantasy from reality. At any time in the disease process some people continue to drink and others stop drinking. When an individual reaches the stage in which his organs are being damaged and persists in drinking, he will continue to deteriorate mentally, physically, and socially. Eventually he will die of the complications or consequences of alcoholism.

Etiology

Attempts to describe the causes of alcoholism and substance abuse focus on a range and mix of physiological, psychological, and social bases. Some see the use of drugs as an attempt at self-treatment for a condition causing distress to the abuser. Others says that abuse is evidence of an underlying character disorder that causes the person to seek immediate satisfaction despite long-term consequences. Some cite metabolic disturbances or a physiological susceptibility in which there is a biologically abnormal response to the substances. Some studies report that this response is familial. Some point to social causes, saying that abuse is an expression of rebelliousness against societal values, a reaction to socioeconomic pressures with no underlying psychopathology, evidence of delinquency, or the price of winning social acceptance. In many parts of our society there is incredible pressure to drink—with the boys, with the customers, with the boss, with the gang. Some people like the "high" feeling or behavior that the drug ingestion may allow them. Others may see alcohol as a tranquilizer, as a way to quell anxiety and to reduce the dangers felt in any situation. Some may want to avoid the "hangover" or sickness that accompanies withdrawal if they stop drinking.

Part of the difficulty in discussing the etiology of alcohol use in particular is in separating use from abuse. People say that they drink in order to relax and relate more easily to people. Some participate as a way to be part of their peer group or because peer pressure demands it. People also drink or take drugs to alter their mood, to avoid reality, or even, in some cases, to alter their identities, to have themselves be seen as jovial, outgoing individuals. It is often said that use becomes abuse when it interferes with a person's ability to perform his usual roles, his jobs and positions in society. For example, a teenager is expected to be a student and a family member; an adult is generally expected to work and to fulfill family obligations. Explanations of specific patterns of abuse are also debated. Some people drink heavily or take drugs at one point in their lives and then stop. Many people occasionally abuse alcohol, that is, get drunk and feel wretched the next day, but they would not be called abusers by anyone but a temperance society.

Definition and Classification of Alcohol Use

The attempt to define and classify alcoholism has a long, complicated history. In 1952, in a now classic article called "Phases of Alcohol Addiction," E. M. Jellinek approached the definition of alcoholism in terms of five observed patterns of drinking. Jellinek himself was concerned that his provisional attempts at description would be simplistically applied. However, his emphasis on differentiating between patterns of abuse, between the consequences of alcohol use and dependence on alcohol and sociocultural variation, laid the groundwork for research in the area.

The *Diagnostic and Statistical Manual of Mental Disorders,* third edition *(DSM III),* published in 1980, includes alcoholism within the separate category of substance abuse disorders. Based on the description of clinical features, *DSM III* presents five categories related to alcohol: alcohol intoxication, alcohol withdrawal, alcohol organic mental disorders, alcohol abuse, and alcohol dependency. Alcohol abuse is pathological use for at least one month that causes impairment in social or occupational functioning. Alcohol dependency subsumes abuse and also includes tolerance or withdrawal. This is a major revision from earlier versions of the *DSM,* which included alcoholism as a subcategory of personality disorder. It has been suggested that although *DSM III* provides reliable and valid identification of alcoholics in treatment situations, it may or may not be effective in identifying alcoholics in other situations.

The World Health Organization has attempted to develop a universal definition of alcoholism based on etiologic assumptions. The WHO typology presents two basic categories, which overlap yet define two distinct types of alcohol problems: alcohol dependence syndrome and alcohol-related disabilities. The dependence syndrome is an interrelated cluster of physiological, cognitive, and behavioral symptoms including the following elements: narrowing of the drinking repertoire to almost continuous daily consumption; salience of drink-seeking behavior where drinking is given highest priority; increased tolerance to alcohol; repeated withdrawal symptoms; relief drinking to relieve or avoid withdrawal, especially in the morning; compulsion to drink; and readdiction liability. On the other hand, alcohol-related disabilities consist of the physical, social, and psychological dysfunctions that result from excessive drinking and dependence. In this model both dependence and alcohol-related disabilities exist in degrees, as opposed to older binary, all-or-none classification schemes. The WHO definition is part of the international program on diagnosis and classification, which will recommend improvements in sections of the International Classification of Diseases (ICD) dealing with alcoholism, drug abuse, and mental health. The National Council on Alcoholism has approached the problem by providing a diagnostic instrument consisting of eighty-six criteria commonly associated with alcoholism, including such information as drinking patterns, information from family and friends, autopsy findings, and laboratory tests. The diagnostic tool allows an over-all review of the ways in which a person drinks and how his life is affected. Physical criteria are emphasized. There are many reliability and validity problems with the instrument, and it continues to be revised.

Some systems classify use, misuse, and abuse. "Use" generally means that the alcohol is taken in ways that are acceptable to the person's culture and do not harm him. Misuse refers to adverse consequences directly re-lated to drinking. For example, if a person gets drunk at parties or other social occasions and begins to abuse other people physically or behave in-appropriately in other ways, he is said to misuse alcohol. In abuse, chronic, recurrent drinking has both acute and chronic adverse effects. Others clas-sify dependency, heavy drinking, and alcohol-related problems. In this typology, those who drink irresponsibly and sometimes get into trouble but who are not dependent on alcohol would be classified as having al-cohol-related problems. The second type, heavy drinking, is measured by quantity-frequency indexes. Within heavy drinking there are two cate-gories: heavy binge drinking and steady heavy drinking. The third, al-cohol dependency, is characterized by blackouts, morning drinking, tremors, organ damage, loss of control, missing meals due to drinking, and continuous drinking for twelve hours or more.

In *Emerging Concepts of Alcohol Dependence,* Pattison, Sobell, and Sobell suggest that most of the classification systems just described are based on a unitary model of alcoholism that assumes a distinct entity in which alcoholics and prealcoholics are different from nonalcoholics; al-coholics experience an overwhelming physical or psychological craving to drink and a process of loss of control over initiation of drinking and/or an inability to stop drinking; and alcoholism is a permanent and irreversible condition, a progressive disease that follows an inexorable development through a series of fairly distinct phases. In varying degrees, there is evi-dence to contradict all of these assumptions. Therefore, Pattison and col-leagues propose a working multivariate model of the alcohol syndrome that links empirical evidence to corollary implications for treatment. The model lists eleven propositions, each of which includes several corollaries:

1. Alcoholism dependence subsumes a variety of syndromes defined by drink-ing patterns and the adverse consequences of drinking.
2. An individual's use of alcohol can be considered as a point on a continuum from nonuse, to nonproblem drinking, to various degrees of deleterious drinking.
3. The development of alcohol problems follows variable patterns over time.
4. Abstinence bears no necessary relation to rehabilitation.
5. Psychological dependence and physical dependence on alcohol are sepa-rate and not necessarily related phenomena.

6. Continued drinking of large doses of alcohol over an extended period of time is likely to initiate a process of physical dependence.
7. The population of individuals with alcohol problems is multivariate.
8. Alcohol problems are typically interrelated with other life problems, especially when alcohol dependence is long established.
9. Because of the documented strong relationship between drinking behavior and environmental influences, emphasis should be placed on treatment procedures that relate to the drinking environment of the person.
10. Treatment and rehabilitation should be designed to provide for continuity of care over an extended period, beginning with effective identification, triage, and referral, and extending through acute and chronic phases of treatment and follow-up.
11. Evaluative studies of treatment of alcohol dependence must take into account the initial degree of disability, the potential for change, and an inventory of individual dysfunction in diverse life areas, in addition to drinking behavior. Assessment of improvement should include both drinking behavior and behavior in other areas of life function, consistent with presenting problems. Degrees of improvement must also be recognized. Change in all areas of life function should be assessed on an individual basis. This necessitates using pretreatment and posttreatment comparison measures of treatment outcome.

Association with Other Diseases

Alcoholism increases the risk for many diseases. Cancers of the mouth, tongue, pharynx, esophagus, and pancreas are more common in alcoholics than in nonalcoholics. The heavy use of alcohol also effects the heart. Cardiac arrythmias (irregularities of the heart beat) can lead to heart failure. Cardiac myopathy, damage to the heart muscle, with symptoms ranging from shortness of breath and ankle swelling to heart failure, often occurs after ten or more years of heavy drinking. If a person already has heart disease, two ounces of whisky can suppress the pacemaking abilities of the heart. Excessive alcohol use also affects the liver with a range of syndromes from fatty liver to alcoholic hepatitis to cirrhosis.

Excessive drinking also causes blood abnormalities: enlarged red blood cells, anemia, and reduced white blood cell counts. It is thought that higher rates of infectious disease common in alcoholics are attributable to a diminished immune response. High alcohol intake also affects muscle tissue besides the heart. Many alcoholics experience muscle weakness and severe muscle pain as a result of cramping. Involuntary smooth muscle contractions are also affected.

In pregnancy, maternal alcohol misuse threatens the developing fetus. The most consistent result, lowered birth weight, is associated with greater risk for neonatal death, mental retardation, and neurological defects. Several studies have related maternal alcohol use to low IQ and motor development scores. Another possible result is fetal alcohol syndrome, characterized by prenatal and/or postnatal growth retardation, central nervous system involvement, and characteristic facial shaping such as unusually small head circumference and/or flattening of facial features. Alcoholism can also cause metabolic and physiological disturbances in the fetus. It is thought that 5 percent of total birth defects may be alcohol-related. Generally women who drink heavily are at greater risk for menstrual disorders, infertility, and repeated miscarriages. Men who drink heavily have a higher risk of decreased sex drive, impotence, testicular atrophy, and infertility related to reduced sperm counts, decreased sperm motility, and higher rates of sperm abnormalities.

Some disorders associated with alcoholism arise from malnutrition. One of them, pellegra, occurs as a result of niacin deficiency. The syndrome includes inflammation of the tongue, skin, and peripheral nerves of the extremities; spinal cord changes; anemia; and confusion. Hepatic encephalopathy is also associated with alcohol use; it consists of brain dysfunction resulting from severe liver disease, which allows high levels of ammonia to reach the brain causing organic brain syndrome. Many gastric abnormalities are also associated with alcoholism, but most of them are reversible after the intake of alcohol is discontinued.

In alcoholic dementia there are irreversible deficiencies of all mental faculties. In Wernicke-Korsakoff syndrome, which can follow delirium and toxic states, the person is disoriented as to time and place with grossly impaired recent memory, eye movement abnormalities, and ataxia (jerky movements and staggering). This syndrome occurs in alcoholics who have obtained almost all of their calories from alcohol for several months and have thus become vitamin B^1 (thiamine) deficient. Basically, if heavy drinking continues, alcoholism eventually damages every system of the body.

Diagnostic Procedures

Disagreement about definition and diagnostic criteria make the diagnosis of alcoholism difficult. The acceptance of a multivariate model of alcoholism in which multiple patterns of dysfunctional alcohol use result in multiple kinds of disability underscores the complexity of diagnosis. Many definitions, classification schemata, and tests have been developed to diagnose alcoholism. Those of the American Psychiatric Association (*DSM III*) and the World Health Organization have already been discussed.

With this conceptual work has come increased interest in the development of simple, accurate screening procedures that can identify alcohol dependence. Research on early identification has been in two areas: bio-chemical markers and and psychosocial assessment. Biochemical markers involve carrying out several laboratory tests that may be useful in the early detection of alcohol abuse. Serum gamma-glutamyl transpeptidase (GGTP) has been suggested as an indicator of heavy alcohol consumption. When it is interpreted with mean corpuscular volume (MCV) and other tests, its discriminatory ability is enhanced. Routine blood chemistries are also useful in conjunction with other tests for detecting alcohol abuse.

For many years personality tests were used in an attempt to differen-tiate an alcoholic personality type. Just as the definition of alcoholism has been enriched recently, the psychological testing has moved from seeking an alcoholic personality type to a more complex stance. The Minnesota Multiphasic Personality Inventory (MMPI) profile of diagnostic scales pro-vides information regarding the type, severity, and symptomatology of personality pathology. It is a very long test. The MacAndrews Alcoholism Scale is made up of forty-nine items from the MMPI and has been suc-cessfully employed in longitudinal studies. For example, it differentiated a group who were hospitalized for alcoholism later in life from a random sample of college students. The scale is unable to distinguish alcohol ad-diction from drug addiction.

The Michigan Alcoholism Screening Test (MAST) is a short screening test that asks direct questions about alcohol consumption. It is simple, gen-der-specific to men, and vulnerable to unconscious denial or deliberate falsification. The Munich Alcoholism Test combines clinical signs and symptoms as described by the physician with self-report material provided by the patient. Another self-report test, known as the Twenty Question Test or the Johns Hopkins Twenty Question Test, was developed by Dr. Robert B. Seliger. Questions include the following: (1) Do you lose time from work due to drinking? (2) Have you ever felt remorse after drinking? (3) Do you want a drink the next morning? (4) Do you drink alone? (5) Have you had memory losses because of your drinking? The Iowa Alco-holic Stages Index attempts to identify alcoholics and to measure their stage of alcoholism. To be classified as alcoholic in terms of this index, a person has to meet qualifying criteria on at least one of four subscales; trouble due to drinking, personal effects of drinking, preoccupied drinking, and uncontrolled drinking. A person's stage in the process can range from non-alcoholic (0) to advanced alcoholic (4).

Besides tests of this sort, a history and physical examination are im-portant. The history includes the history of a person's pattern of abuse including social, vocational, marital, medical, and psychiatric informa-tion. A person is asked about previous therapy and about his involvement with the law. Because alcohol is highly toxic, the physical examination is thorough, with a review of body systems, physical and mental status examinations, radiologic findings, and clinical pathology testing.

Treatments

Treatment for those who abuse alcohol has both self-help and professional components. Many times primary responsibility is carried by a counselor rather than a physician. Most treatment is nonresidential, but 10 to 15 percent takes place in rehabilitation facilities, hospitals, prisons, or day facilities.

Treatment comprises detoxification, correction of chronic health problems, and rehabilitation. Detoxification is the management of acute alcohol intoxication and the concomitant alcohol withdrawal syndrome. People often feel very sick at this juncture. Continuing to drink is not making them feel better, and drinking less is making them feel worse. If the need for detoxification was not sufficient to create a crisis in a person's life, the detoxification itself may do so. Specialized detoxification facilities were developed in the late 1960s and expanded rapidly after the Uniform Alcoholism and Intoxication Treatment Act decriminalized public intoxication. Some of these use "social setting" detoxification, in which the traditional use of drugs such as diazepam (Valium) and chloridiazepoxide (Librium) are avoided in favor of a supportive social climate meant to enhance further treatment. It is thought that "social setting" detoxification has expanded as a result of changing attitudes regarding the use of sedatives and tranquilizers in withdrawal management, the lower cost of such a setting, and evidence indicating that a significant percentage of people withdraw from alcohol without serious medical complications. The appropriate setting for detoxification depends on the person's physical condition, nutritional status, severity of alcohol dependency, and overall medical condition. As yet the different detoxification methods have not been adequately assessed and compared.

The second treatment goal is to correct chronic health problems and to teach the abuser how to care for his body. The third goal is to alter the person's long-term behavior patterns so that he is no longer drinking. Most research reports that the total social rehabilitation of a person who has abused alcohol depends on abstinence. Exceptions are studies that have determined that some alcoholics manage better with controlled amounts of tranquilizers, just as some studies about heroin addiction report that narcotics addicts live better on methadone maintenance. In both instances, the drug solutions to drug problems are meant to be temporary. Most self-help groups frown on what they consider to be drug substitution, but some professionals report that these temporary solutions expedite the rehabilitation process.

TREATMENT PROGRAM SPONSORSHIP

The largest treatment provider is the Veterans Administration, with one hundred Alcoholism Dependence Programs caring for about 50,000 people each year. In addition, thousands of job-based alcoholism programs sponsored by occupational groups, business management, and unions report great success in early intervention with stable, younger people with a real stake in retaining their jobs and families. In job-based programs, supervisors or managers confront employees whose drinking is interfering with their work with evidence of impaired performance and a simultaneous offer of support for rehabilitation. A specific written management policy that describes the principles on which interventions are based clarifies the program. These programs use the power of the subculture to pressure the person into confronting his drinking. By 1980 there were about 4,400 occupational programs reporting success of 75 to 85 percent. Directly descended from the alcoholism programs are the Employee-Assistance Programs (EAPs), which expand the strategies underlying the job-based alcohol programs to offer help with other kinds of personal problems that interfere with job performance.

While job-based programs are directed to employees whose job performance is deteriorating, drunk driving programs are directed toward those whose driving has been affected by alcohol. Alcohol is the single factor most often involved in fatal and serious traffic accidents. The risk of crash increases as the blood alcohol concentration (BAC) rises. Alcohol is present in about 16 percent of the drivers in crashes involving only property damage, but the proportion increases to 25 percent with about 11 percent above .10 percent BAC in personal injury crashes. For all drivers who are fatally injured, 40 to 55 percent have BACs of .10 percent or above, and 29 to 43 percent have BACs of .15 percent or above.

Most of the drunk driving programs are offered through Departments of Transportation. Referral is generally involuntary, resulting from arrests for driving under the influence of alcohol. Once individuals are part of these programs, they are encouraged to join voluntary community programs, which are ongoing and comprehensive. The results of the state alcohol safety schools are mixed. It is suggested that the person to benefit most from this approach is the social drinker. In 1970 the United States government implemented a demonstration project of thirty-five alcohol safety action programs, which coordinated five kinds of activities; enforcement, judicial and legislative, presentence investigation and probation, rehabilitation, and public information and education. The project was short-lived, but this kind of systems approach is thought to be useful.

The largest nonprofessional treatment sponsors are self-help groups. Even many of the previously described occupational and government programs require their clients to join self-help groups as part of their treatment. The largest and prototypical organization of this kind is Alcoholics Anonymous, which does not record its membership but is estimated to have about 1,250,000 members in 42,000 groups around the world. The only requirement for membership is a desire to stop drinking. AA has no dues or fees but relies on the contributions of members. Its primary aim is to help people to achieve sobriety and to stay sober.

Alcoholics Anonymous is as much a treatment modality or approach as it is a form of sponsorship. Basically it sees alcoholism as a sufficiently strong influence to rule a person's life. The fellowship's rules are firm and supportive. Anonymity allows a person to keep his identity a secret while he stabilizes his life. Through group meetings, which are available every day of the week, and a sponsor system that makes it possible for someone to have a combination partner-buddy-friend, it makes AA and its principles consistently available to the troubled person. In fellowship meetings, people first listen to others with similar problems. When new members are ready, they are encouraged to share their experiences.

The religious nature of much of the activity and the emphasis on a Power greater than the members is reassuring. Like a good parent, it demands and comforts at the same time, knowing that people will have a difficult time with sobriety but expecting that after a time the goal of the organization is achievable and necessary for the survival of its members. An informant described the experience as, "You have to surrender to win."

The philosophy and principles of Alcoholics Anonymous are embodied in the Twelve Steps, which suggest action to be taken as opposed to rules that must not be broken. Bill W., cofounder of AA, said that the Twelve Steps boil down to admission of alcoholism, personality analysis and catharsis, adjustment of personal relationships, the dependence on some Higher Power, and working with other alcoholics to help them develop the tools of sobriety. An informant calls it one drunk helping another. Alcoholics gather together and provide each other with the support necessary for sobriety and recovery. Most meetings, which can be found through the office of any chapter of AA, are open to visitors.

Al-Anon, separate but in many ways parallel to AA, describes itself as a fellowship for relatives and friends of alcoholics who share their experience, strength, and hope in order to solve their common problems and to help others. Throughout the world there are 20,000 Al-Anon groups, including 2,500 groups for teen membership called Alateen. They also help lone members who are in communities where no group exists. Just as AA does, they have established groups in hospitals, prisons, and other institutions. Al-Anon helps each member to deal with his alcoholic family member or friend, to help that person to get help for his problem and to live with sobriety. To do this it educates each member about alcoholism and helps him to support the alcoholic person while separating from his drinking. Some of Al-Anon's Rules of Thumb include remembering that you are emotionally involved and facing the reality that alcoholism is a progressive illness that gets increasingly worse as drinking continues.

TREATMENT MODALITIES

Alcoholism treatment methods include many forms of traditional and nontraditional psychotherapy, small group therapy, behavioral interventions, peer and educational group approaches, drug therapies, and family work. Multimodality approaches, which include various forms of therapy and self-help, are thought to be most useful. The overall focus remains the management of drinking, relationship abilities, self-concept, and stress.

Generally psychotherapeutic techniques are employed after a person has been detoxified. The therapist learns what aspects of the person's life he needs to rethink and reinterpret. Psychodynamically oriented psychotherapists suggest that the person's defense mechanisms, his inner means of protecting himself psychologically, should be redirected. Individual therapy can also be an occasion for someone to acknowledge his alcohol problems for the first time. Many alcoholics participate in group psychotherapy because the peer support, the development of interpersonal skills, and the sharing of experiences that occur in group therapy are thought to be important in managing alcoholism. Couples therapy is also thought to be useful for reopening communication that may have been lost and establishing an atmosphere of support and encouragement. In the same way family therapy has become important in the treatment of alcoholism since the alcoholism, as will be described later, can become a family problem. Psychodrama has also been used in the treatment of alcoholism. Using psychodrama, a group technique in which experiences are acted out in a theater-like atmosphere, allows people to explore unpleasant feelings and relationships that were previously managed through drinking and to have others react to their expression in a safe place.

Behavior therapy is sometimes used in the treatment of alcoholism. The oldest of the behavioral techniques are punishment of drinking behavior and the pairing of tastes, smells, and sights associated with drinking with aversive stimuli. In electrical aversive conditioning, painful shocks to the skin are paired with sips of alcohol. Chemical aversion involves nausea-inducing drugs administered intravenously; at the earliest sign of nausea the person is given drinks so that the person associates nausea and vomiting with drinking. None of these techniques has proved very popular. Behavioral therapists have also tried to teach alcoholics to drink moderately and to decrease their drinking by changing the atmosphere in which they drank.

Drug therapy is yet another approach. Disulfiram, known as Antabuse in the United States, is a deterrent drug rather than a treatment for alcoholism. Because drinking after taking Antabuse makes one violently ill, taking Antabuse is making a conscious choice not to drink that day. It is a means by which someone who has acknowledged his alcoholism can protect himself from drinking. There is considerable debate about Antabuse. Many members of self-help groups think it is an unnecessary crutch. For others it has proved highly effective.

Other modalities include cognitive restructuring, assertiveness and social skills training, and stress management. Except for the great success of Alcoholics Anonymous and job-based prevention and treatment programs which sponsors broad based rather than specific modalities, none of these approaches has been able to demonstrate great success by itself. Thus, treatment approaches are generally multidimensional and composed of myriad self-help and professional components.

Anticipated Course of the Treated Disease

If a person stops drinking before major organ damage has ensued and finds and uses psychological, social, and community support to maintain sobriety, he will have a reasonable chance of resuming his life. If he continues to drink, the disease will do greater damage to his body, relationships, abilities, and psyche. More than most other diseases, the anticipated course depends on determination of the ill person to stay sober.

Psychosocial Information

For some people the limited use of alcohol can be life-enhancing. For others who cannot control their use, alcohol and other drugs negatively affect their work, family relationships, friendships, and health. Getting the substance and maintaining its level in one's body becomes life's central theme. Eventually the nature of the abuse and the conditions under which it is maintained dictate every moment.

When someone is deeply involved with alcohol, he neglects himself. Thus one does not follow a nutritious diet; sleeps too much or not enough; does not follow a normal schedule; and does not exercise properly. Since avoidance of stress is such a clear impetus for people to take a drink, drinking becomes a relaxation technique. Thus, alcoholism interferes with all aspects of an individual's life-style.

One informant who is a highly placed executive in a large company and an alcoholic said that before he stopped drinking, his family life and his work revolved around his drinking. No matter how much he had drunk the day before or how terrible he felt each morning, he was always careful to wake himself at least a half an hour before his wife and family to belt down a few quick ones before he could go on to the rest of the day. He could get through breakfast and out to his car and be on the road before he needed another drink. With alcohol in his car, his office, and various places in his house, he could be blind drunk by evening, and no one would have seen him take one drink. Blackouts, during which there were great lapses in his memory, began to frighten him, and when he confided to his wife and a close friend that he was an alcoholic, no one believed him. Many alcoholics can maintain their life-styles for a long period, but the price is enormous.

Life-Style Interventions

In alcoholism the resumption of a normal life-style depends on restraint from the use of the substance as well as restraint from the activities that encourage one to drink. Although some professionals suggest that people who have been abusers can become users, they are in the minority. Most professionals and members of self-help groups insist that only abstinence can lead to full recovery.

Abstinence from drugs means a total restructuring of one's life-style. A nutritious diet helps to rebuild what is often a malnourished body. Because many of the drugs disrupt sleep patterns, one has to teach oneself all over to sleep and rest normally. Once drug use has stopped, one also has to teach himself to schedule his life around work, relationships, and other kinds of activities rather than around the next drink or dose.

Alcoholism and the Law

In 1962, in *Robinson* v. *California*, the Supreme Court of the United States eliminated the concept that one could be found guilty of being addicted to alcohol in itself. One could be found guilty only of antisocial behavior. In 1968, in *Powell* v. *Texas*, the Supreme Court ruled that chronic alcoholism was not by itself a defense. The mere fact that someone was intoxicated while doing something did not mean that he was not responsible for taking the first drink and committing the offense. Thus there is free will and choice in becoming intoxicated. In 1969, in *Jackie C. Packer* v. *State of Maryland*, the Maryland Court of Appeals ruled that one is able to decide freely whether to take the first drink, and that in his or her preexisting state, before drinking, was free of existing mental disease or defect.

Thus alcoholism is a disease characterized by loss of will to stop drinking and compulsivity to drink, so a person with such a disease cannot take a first drink. If he or she does take the first drink, all subsequent behavior resulting from compulsive aspects of the disease are the responsibility of the individual and not the disease or defense of alcohol.

LAW ENFORCEMENT

In 1980 law enforcement agencies made 9,686,940 arrests for crimes committed in 1980 or before. Of those, 1,303,933 were for driving when intoxicated, 427,829 were for commercial liquor violations, and 1,049,614 were for general drunkenness. Almost 10 percent of those under eighteen years old who were arrested were arrested for drug violations, and an additional 2.3 percent were arrested for drunk driving. The National Council on Alcoholism says that violent behavior attributed to alcohol use accounts for approximately 65 percent of murders, 60 percent of cases of child abuse, 55 percent of fights or assaults in the home, 40 percent of assaults, 35 percent of rapes, 30 percent of other sex crimes, and 30 percent of suicides. Public drunkenness remains a criminal offense in several populous states like Texas, California, and Pennsylvania. Often, even if public drunkenness has been decriminalized, an individual is still booked by the police on other related charges like disorderly conduct, vagrancy, or loitering. Those arrested are almost never legally represented, almost always found guilty and incarcerated. Recidivism is high. By 1981 thirty-four states, the District of Columbia, and the Virgin Islands had adopted a variation of the Uniform Act, the Uniform Alcoholism and Intoxication Treatment Act, which was adopted by the National Conference of Commissioners on Uniform State Laws in August 1971. The act says that alcoholics and intoxicated people should not be criminally prosecuted because of their alcohol consumption but rather should be given treatment to help them to live more productively. Still, when tossing a drunk person into the emergency room of a municipal hospital recently, a policeman said that it didn't make any difference to him whether he threw the old drunk into the emergency room or the lockup. It was the same difference to him, as long as he didn't have to smell him or touch him for long. Although the law has changed, much public opinion lags behind.

DRIVING

Driving under the influence of alcohol is illegal and a serious public health problem. Each year there are 50,000 traffic deaths and 2 million serious traffic-related injuries in the United States. The National Safety

Council and Department of Transportation's National Highway Safety Administration (NHSA) says that half the deaths and a significant percentage of the serious injuries are caused by drunk drivers. In the United States almost everyone drives, and 75 percent of the adults drink. Almost everyone has drunk and driven, so laws have tended to be very lenient and unenforced. However, the average person who is arrested for drunk driving has had at least fifteen drinks, according to the level of alcohol measured in the blood (BAC). This group is primarily middle-aged (25–44), but younger drivers are overrepresented because they have trouble driving at lower BAC levels. Combining alcohol with inexperience in driving greatly increases the risk of an automobile accident. There is also higher risk for unmarried people and for people who are recently divorced or recently released from prison.

In the last decade there has been a vigorous political action and public relations campaign against drunk driving organized by two groups: Mothers Against Drunk Driving (MADD) and Remove Intoxicated Drivers (RID). Both groups were founded by women who had lost children or husbands in accidents that involved drunk drivers. These groups have succeeded in persuading states to strengthen somewhat their drunk driving laws and to set standards of alcohol concentration in the blood (BAC), but the police and the courts have failed to enforce the stricter laws.

The threat of arrest has not acted as a deterrent, because drunk drivers are rarely stopped. It is estimated that people who are drunk make about two thousand trips while intoxicated before they are pulled over. Also, once they have been arrested, defendants use maneuvers like plea bargaining, repeated continuation of cases, and suspended sentences in order to avoid the maximum punishment, and the courts do not enforce the harsher laws because prisons are already crowded. Fines usually do not deter, and many people who have had their licenses suspended continue to drive. Thus, although there are laws on the books, they have not succeeded in controlling drunk driving.

Insurance

Alcoholics and their families have been found to use more medical services than average for a variety of problems related to excessive drinking. After the alcoholic enters treatment, total medical care costs for the family have shown a 40 percent median reduction in sick days and accident benefits. Thus insurance companies have impetus for supporting alcoholism treatment.

Insurance coverage is varied for people who are alcoholics. About 85 percent of the seventy Blue Cross plans nationwide recognize alcoholism as a covered condition. They offer benefits comparable to those offered for other conditions. Medicare classifies alcoholism and drug abuse within psychiatric or mental health services, with less coverage than is generally available for physical illnesses. Most Medicaid plans do not address the issue directly. NIAAA is working to expand benefits under Medicare and Medicaid.

The Federal government offers about fifty different health insurance plans, and most include alcoholism benefits. Aetna Life and Casualty and NIAAA are working on a project that will provide cost and utilization data for an expanded Aetna alcoholism benefit for 300,000 Federal employees. Under CHAMPUS, alcoholism benefits cover brief hospital care for detoxification, inpatient rehabilitation, and outpatient psychiatric care.

SOCIAL SECURITY DISABILITY

The 1982 *Social Security Handbook* reports that addiction to drugs or alcohol is not a basis for a finding of disability in itself. As with all other conditions, the disability determination is based on symptoms, signs, and laboratory findings. Once a person is determined to be disabled, he is referred to the appropriate state agency for treatment of his addiction. If he does not follow the course of treatment designated for him, it is likely that his eligibility will be suspended. Exceptions to this rule are made only when treatment facilities are unavailable or in some other rare circumstance. Payment cannot be made directly to the disabled person but instead must be made to a representative payee, because the beneficiary is considered incapable of managing the funds (205j and 1631a2 of the Social Security Act). The order of preference in selecting a payee for an adult is (1) the legal guardian or spouse or other relative who has actual custody or who demonstrates a strong concern for the welfare of the beneficiary, (2) a friend with custody or a similar personal concern, (3) a public or nonprofit institution having custody of the beneficiary, or (4) a properly licensed private institution having custody of the beneficiary. If the beneficiary regains his capabilities, evidence of his present abilities must be submitted. Once the beneficiary's abilities have been established, direct payments will be made to the beneficiary.

Relationships with Others

Substance abuse is as much a social problem as a medical one. Often people begin to use drugs and alcohol as a way to smooth social communication, to enhance social abilities, or to feel part of a group. In our society drinking, like driving, is a part of the passage to adulthood. Young adults proudly show identification to the waitress in the cocktail lounge to prove they are old enough to drink. Everyone laughs as he remembers getting

drunk on champagne punch or green beer or purple passions. The inter-
weaving of alcohol and social life continues as friends stop at a bar for
happy hour on the way home from work or pride themselves on knowing
which wine to serve with dinner. People are given a bottle of whisky at
Christmas as a bonus for a job well done, or as a sign of success in middle
age they join an exclusive club where only members can drink to their
hearts' content. Even the toasts people make before they drink depict alcohol as a positive, life-giving force. The French say, "A votre santé," to
your health; the Jews say, "L'chaim," to life; "Skoal," say the Scandina-
vians, pledging health in drinking.

Use turns to abuse when the substance makes life more difficult instead
of easier and when the desire for the substance is stronger than the desire
for the social parts of life. To justify the abuse, one turns from the very
activities that ingestion used to enhance. Other groups are sought that
value the drugs more than anything else.

FAMILY MEMBERS

Although people are able to find social groups that will condone their
behavior, their jobs and often their families will not be so tolerant. Families can either enter into the behavior, ingesting along with the individual, close ranks and push the person out, adapt, or seek help. The first
two solutions are clear. The third, adaptation, is a mode of family interaction that eventually becomes as much a syndrome as the addiction itself.
The syndrome has many names, among them co-dependency and enabling. In alcoholism, the syndrome is sometimes called co-alcoholism or
near-alcoholism. It begins as a way for the family to protect the abuser
because they fear his getting into trouble. Perhaps friends will desert or a
person will lose his job if people find out that he is drinking too much.
Part of the family's behavior is based on denial. Family members decide
that this is an occasional thing or that it will stop soon. Sometimes they
point to an area of responsibility that the person who is abusing substances
still maintains. Then, they say, how can she be an alcoholic if she takes
such good care of her kids, or how can he be an alcoholic if he goes to
work every day and his boss thinks so much of him? Spouses also use denial
to explain behavior to kids, saying, "Daddy didn't mean it. He was just
upset last night." Or "Mommy just doesn't feel well and that's why she
fell down and couldn't make dinner." Thus children don't know what is
true and what isn't. They are quickly taught to use the family myths and
to protect the abuser along with their nonabusing parent. They also become increasingly responsible for taking care of the house, themselves,
each other, and eventually the abusing parent. All this responsibility is
carried out without outside recognition, because it is part of the myth that

the parent is still doing what he is supposed to do. Families grieve chronically because the person does not die or even go away, in most cases. They have lost the parent or partner but not the person. Often accompanying the sense of loss is anger at the person who has done this to himself and guilt about having somehow been responsible.

One informant, the wife of an alcoholic who has been dry for twelve years, says that she looks back at that period of her life as a long nightmare. She was constantly exhausted from protecting the family, covering up for her husband with her children, being furious with him and furious with herself, mourning their former existence and her former life, and constantly being terrified that he would kill somebody else or himself when he was driving. Finally she moved the whole family out to the country, thinking that if there were no bars or liquor stores around, her husband would have no choice but to stop. At that point he chose to live by himself, near the bottle and away from the family. He also took the family car, so that she was marooned out in the country with three young children. When her husband blamed her for his drinking, she felt so guilty she was further immobilized. Then she was enraged and so depressed she became suicidal. At that point she got help for herself, and eventually her husband joined her.

Another response on the part of the family is to try to control the individual's intake. Family members hide or throw away the bottles. They water down the whisky, refuse to advance money, shame, accuse, and beg the person to stop. They ask for promises, then are incensed when the promises are broken. What begins out of caring only increases the anger of the abusing person. The individual, who has already lost control of his intake, feels manipulated and powerless. When he promises then breaks his promise, he feels remorse and guilt. In the meantime his spouse is caught in the spiral, one day so angry she could kill, the next day blaming herself for being cruel.

James Burgin, in the *Guidebook for the Family with Alcohol Problems*, says that these are all stages of the disease of the family. Thus far responses have been emotional and behavioral. By the next stage the family has progressed into the structural response, where the entire structure of the family has been reorganized to accommodate the dysfunctional substance-abusing member. The reorganization assumes that one member will be unpredictable and out of control. Just as the ingestion of the substance is the prime focus of the abuser, it now becomes the prime focus of the entire family. Children react to this solution by going to extremes in compliance or deviance. They are either the best-behaved children imaginable or absolute hellions. One informant described becoming the perfect child as her father's drinking increased and as her mother's accommodation became more extreme. She was always pleasant, always went along with the people in charge, got good grades, was a faithful church member, and never made any judgments on her own. By the time she grew up, she barely knew who she was.

The last stage in the family disease process is the crisis response. If the family has not split apart already, it moves toward some other crisis in which it is clear that something has to change. Sometimes it is a spouse who finally means it when she says if the person doesn't get some help and stop abusing, she is going to leave. The crisis can also come from outside the family. The most likely source is the job, where the employer says that the person will be suspended or lose his job if he doesn't involve himself in a treatment program. At other times it is physician pointing out the damage that the drugs have already done to someone's body and mind. If a person is involved in a religious institution, it can be his minister. The crisis has to be real, and the cost has to be very important to the abuser.

SEXUAL ACTIVITY

Alcohol is a depressant that affects sexual activity. Alcoholic men often experience decreased libido and/or impotence, testicular atrophy, and infertility. Among other responses to alcohol, the level of testosterone, a male hormone, is reduced within hours of having about seven drinks. In contrast, the level of estrogen, a female hormone, is raised. Alcoholic women often have severe gonadal failure, commonly manifested by reduced or absent menstruation, loss of secondary sex characteristics such as breast and pelvic fat accumulation, and infertility. Both alcoholic men and women show evidence of a defect in the control over sex hormone secretions by the brain. Although in women these hormones would be expected to increase in order to correct the gonad failure resulting from heavy alcohol intake, they remain will below expected levels. By the time people have moved from use to abuse, although they may be outwardly flirtatious, their interest in and capacity for sexual activity has waned. When people stop drinking, as their other activites return to normal, they are also able to resume normal sexual activity.

Ability to Work

Alcoholism can severely affect one's ability to work. Both alcohol-related absenteeism and impaired job performance cost the workplace billions of dollars, of which the bulk of the amount, an estimated $36.8 billion, represents the value of lost productivity. There is also a strong relationship between industrial accidents and alcoholism. Although there are not yet any national statistics, a 1982 Maryland study of workers who died in industrial accidents found that 11 percent had BACs over .08 percent. The workplace is also important in alcoholism treatment. The threat of job loss with its concomitant loss of income and prestige is a motivating factor for people to seek treatment for alcohol abuse.

Psychological Issues

Psychological issues relate to initial drinking motivation, to problems the person might have as a result of the drinking, and to the decision to abstain from drinking. Many issues related to the motivation to drink heavily have been discussed previously. The psychological problems that evolve as heavy drinking continues are also significant. Impairment of judgment and memory often begin early. For a while the person is able to cover up, but as the abuse progresses, the person is less able to make the distinction. As organ involvement proceeds, psychological symptomatology and impairment increase. The person uses massive denial in regard to not only his drinking but its effect. Alcoholism promotes psychological deterioration while promoting massive denial of its occurrence. It is as if you were drowning in a pond, and as you sank deeper and faster, your mind increasingly assured you that you were swimming just fine.

A relationship between alcoholism and depression has been demonstrated, but it is not yet known whether the affective disorder precipitates, predisposes to, aggravates, or is caused by the alcoholism. Continued abuse also brings a withdrawal from all close relationships. This isolation contributes to the loss of desire to be honest and to maintain one's contact with reality. Alcoholism and suicide are also related. The adult suicide rate in the United States is reported to be as high as 5 percent, but for people who abuse alcohol, studies report a suicide rate of up to 29 percent.

The decision to maintain sobriety is also ultimately psychological, although a person may feel great pressure from family or job. After all, drinking might feel like someone's only way of controlling his life. An informant said that at the bottom, a person feels as if he has four alternatives: He can become psychotic and require hospitalization, he can kill himself or someone else, he can drink himself into oblivion and eventual death, or he can stop.

Psychological difficulties extend to the early stages of an abuser's recovery. He feels that if he abstains, all will be well. Instead, for a period of at least six months to a year, things are harder than ever. Often a person both depends on and resents certain people who are close to him. He also experiences marked anxiety, which was suppressed for all the time he drank. With his natural coping abilities depleted, the anxiety is increased. New situations, changes, and crises are especially difficult.

A person who has stopped drinking experiences that strange phenomenon of being alone in a crowd. He has depended on alcohol to make him comfortable in social situations and to be able to communicate. Without the alcohol he feels alone. Denial also continues to be a particular problem. There is the feeling that abstinence will rectify everything, and the person denies that he has so deeply hurt some people that they might not forgive him or want anything to do with him even as he recovers.

Abuse of Substances Other Than Alcohol

Although alcohol is the most prevalent and prototypical form of substance abuse, it differs in many ways from the abuse of other substances. The percentage of polydrug abusers is not known, but many people use many combinations of drugs. Therefore, to describe substance abuse as fully as the other disease entities in this volume, it is necessary to fit alcoholism into its larger classification system. Medical and psychosocial aspects of each principal category will be presented.

Classification

Drugs of dependency are classified by the World Health Organization as (1) alcohol and barbiturate-type; (2) amphetamine-type; (3) cannabis-type; (4) cocaine; (5) hallucinogen-type; (6) khat; (7) opiate-type; and (8) volatile solvent-type. They can be classified further according to their mood-altering effects as depressants, stimulants, cannabis, hallucinogens, narcotics, and volatile substances.

DEPRESSANTS

Alcohol and barbiturate-type drugs are known as depressants because they depress the central nervous system. Included in this group are alcohol, barbiturates, nonbarbiturate sedatives like glutethimide (Doriden), meprobamate (Equanil), methaqualone (Quaalude), and ethchloroynol (Placity), as well as large amounts of minor tranquilizors like diazepam (Valium) and chlordiazepoxide (Librium). Unlike narcotics, these drugs are not analgesics, they do not diminish pain. Within this category, barbiturates are classified according to length of action: Phenobarbital is long-acting, butibarbital is intermediate, secobarbital is short-acting, and pentobarbital is ultra-short-acting. Side effects include skin rashes, nausea, and vomiting. These drugs are often used in suicide.

Regular use of high doses of these drugs produces physical dependency. The length of time required for such dependency varies. One example is Valium, for which a physical dependency can develop with regular use of high doses in six weeks. If the drug is abruptly terminated without properly monitored detoxification, a life-threatening syndrome like delirium tremens can occur. This syndrome can produce myriad symptoms, including restlessness, hallucinations, delusions, excitement, sweating, anxiety, gastrointestinal problems, and violence.

HALLUCINOGENS

Hallucinogens, also known as psychedelics, are so named because they cause hallucinations. They fall into two broad chemical categories. The first group is called indoles because they contain a molecular structure known as the indole ring. The indole group is related to hormones made in the brain by the pineal gland and elsewere. Using these drugs makes people feel high very rapidly; the drugs reach their peak in an hour or two. Indole hallucinogens are LSD (lysergic diethylamide), morning glory seeds, mushrooms (psilocybe cubensis and other species), ibogaine, DMT (dimethyltryptamine), and Yage. LSD, which is semisynthetic, is the most notorious of all the psychedelics. It received a great deal of attention in the 1960s when some people reported fabulous mind-expanding, long-lasting experiences with the drug, and others reported very negative experiences.

The second group of hallucinogens comprises drugs that do not contain the indole ring. They resemble molecules of the amphetamines and adrenaline. The onset of their reaction is more gradual, and they do not reach their peak for several hours. Included in this group are peyote and mescaline, STP (DOM), MDA (methylenedioxyamphetamine), and related drugs.

The greatest danger in using hallucinogens is an adverse psychological reaction, often referred to as a bad trip, which takes the form of overwhelming anxiety, intense fear, or even immobilization. Bad trips can be related to the quantity of the drug taken, something else mixed with the drug about which the person is ignorant, or even unsupportive settings in which the drug is taken. People who are unstable, paranoid, or depressed before taking the drugs are more likely to have bad trips than those who are stable. Because there are no legal sources for these kinds of drugs, people do not know exactly what they are buying. Often they do not know the source of the drugs or anything about the seller.

Hallucinogens may be found in plants or synthesized. They are usually ingested orally. Soon after ingestion, there is an increase in heart rate, enlargement of pupils, a dry mouth, nervousness, and overactivity. In the next phase colors appear brighter, sounds become more distinct, and there is an increased awareness of body sensations. One next experiences visual distortions. After that there is a distortion of thought processes. People report ecstatic or horrifying insights into the workings of the universe. The duration can be short or as long as twenty-four hours, depending on the

drug and the dose. Some people also report flashbacks in which hallucinations occur without their having ingested the drug again.

The life-style of those who are frequent users of these drugs can cause
them to neglect themselves. There are rarely drug-related deaths, and these
deaths occur only from very high doses. Regular users tend to be unstable
in relationships, in work and in school. They are shown on psychological
tests to be impulsive, pleasure-seeking, and rebellious, like heavy marijuana users. Frequent hallucinogen users generally have high rates of unemployment and are poor achievers. The drugs are ineffective if used daily.
Effects are less on the second day and almost absent on the third. There
must be at least four to six days in between in order to feel the full effect
of the drug. Effects of the drug are unpredictable each time it is used.
Even with that lack of predictability, the trip becomes ordinary after a
while, so people tend to terminate use after a few years unless they are
polydrug users who continue to mix hallucinogens with other drugs.

The National Survey on Drug Abuse reports that the highest lifetime
prevalence statistics for hallucinogens is for young adults. About one-fourth
of young adults have used hallucinogens at one time, but one-fourth to
one-third of them have only tried a drug of this category once or twice.
Only 4 percent report having used them in the past year.

PCP

PCP (phencyclidine), often called angel dust, is popular among young
adolescents. It is thought that the drug is more prevalent than it is reported
to be and that the number of deaths associated with it are also considerably higher than the reported numbers. In 1979 more than three hundred
deaths were reported as associated with PCP intake. Approximately 8 million Americans are thought to have used the drug, about 5,500,000 of
them betwen the ages of twelve and twenty-five. By 1980 surveys reported
that almost 2 million of the 124 million Americans over twenty-five had
used PCP. Many users of PCP use other drugs as well. Patterns of use
studies have reported that 81 percent are white, 65 percent are men, and
88 percent were between ten and twenty-nine years of age. PCP can act
as a depressant, a stimulant, or a hallucinogen, so its classification is mixed.
CODAP reported 8,000 PCP admissions in 1979.

NARCOTICS

Narcotics are central nervous system depressants that include morphine, heroin, methadone, and meperidine (Demerol). These drugs have
positive uses in that they reduce one's awareness of pain and calm the
emotional responses that generally accompany severe pain. Some research
has suggested a relationship between narcotic abuse and the role of en-

dorphin, which is secreted in the brain and attaches itself to the surface of the cells responsible for the awareness of pain in order to limit pain. These sites are the same for heroin and morphine as they are for endorphin. Side effects include the depression of the depth and frequency of respiration, itching, constipation, and pupillary contraction. Withdrawal symptoms associated with dependence on this group of drugs include enlarged pupils, perspiration, runny nose, eye-tearing, yawning, gooseflesh, irritability, restlessness, muscle twitching, loss of appetite, rapid breathing, and diarrhea. Users look for ways in which to avoid the withdrawal symptoms as well as to gain any other effects from the drugs. Withdrawal begins around four hours after the administration of heroin, six hours after morphine, and twelve hours after methadone.

Fatalities can occur in several ways. An intentional or unintentional overdose can lead to the gradual slowing of respiration and finally to complete failure of breathing. This condition can be treated with narcotic antagonist drugs if the person receives treatment in time. Death can occur also through pulmonary edema as the lungs fill with fluid and asphyxiate the abuser.

Some complications arise not from the drugs but from the vehicle used to administer them. Injection can cause blood-borne infections (septicemia), infected clots, pulmonary emboli, and endocarditis or abscesses at the site or at a distance. A user can contract hepatitis through the sharing of needles and syringes with infected fellow abusers. The injection of insoluble material may cut off the blood supply to limbs or vital organs, causing gangrene. Sniffing the drugs can cause the nasal septum to perforate. Finally, users are more susceptible to infection, hepatitis, pneumonia, and tuberculosis.

In terms of personal neglect the reduction in the awareness of pain leads to higher rates of tooth decay and infection and to cigarette burns on hands and arms. Most physical effects can be reversed once someone has stopped taking the drugs. Psychological impairment is harder to address because of the membership of hard drug users in antisocial subcultures that support their drug use and condone the kinds of illegal activites (primarily stealing and prostitution) that support the high cost of a drug habit. Thus, mistrust, unreliability, and lying become part of a narcotics user's routine.

The number of Americans who have used heroin is smaller than the number who have used the other drugs included in this chapter. The extent of its use is not known, because the activity surrounding it takes place in the underworld. Most statistics are based on indicators like the size of the population of methadone maintenance programs and other treatment facilities. It has been suggested that about 500,000 people in the United States are addicted to heroin. Of those, 100,000 are estimated to be located in the area of New York City. About 95,000 heroin abusers were admitted to CODAP clinics in 1979. The majority of heroin addicts are reported to be under thirty years old.

VOLATILE SOLVENTS

Users of volatile solvents are generally boys between the ages of eleven and eighteen. The most common users are Hispanic boys, and it has also been a problem with native American boys. To get high, people put some gasoline, cleaning fluid, airplane glue, or aerosol spray into a plastic bag and inhale the fumes. Symptoms include a brief period of drunk behavior with slurred speech, a lack of coordination, stumbling gait, and falling. Complications include blood disturbances like anemia, the malproduction of white blood cells, brain damage, liver and kidney damage, inflammation of the pancreas, upper respiratory lesions, and pneumonia. The most common cause of death is asphyxiation, as the user inhales fumes, then loses consciousness, then stops breathing.

Federal drug authorities estimate that one out of ten people under seventeen and a total of 7 million people have experimented with inhalants. A 1980 national survey on drug abuse reported that the lifetime prevalence of inhalants was 9.8 percent among 12–17 year-olds, 16.5 percent among 18–25-year-olds, and 3.9 percent among those over twenty -five. Men have used inhalants ten to one over women; American Indians and Hispanics are overrepresented and blacks are underrepresented in the use of inhalants.

STIMULANTS

Amphetamines, cocaine, methylphenidate (Ritalin), and caffeine (contained in tea, coffee, and chocolate) are central nervous system stimulants that speed mental processes and allow the brain to take in more from the environment. They can be taken by mouth, injected, or, in the case of cocaine, sniffed. Symptoms from these drugs include restlessness, nervousness, and inability to sleep. People are overactive, hyperalert, talkative, and sometimes quite aggressive. Their physical symptoms include weight loss, rapid heartbeat, elevated blood pressure, dilated pupils, and dry mouth.

People who abruptly cease taking drugs from this group also experience withdrawal symptoms. Depression, apathy, and feeling of exhaustion can last for two to four months after drug use has stopped. People sometimes sleep excessively and develop paranoid psychoses, obsessive compulsive reactions, or catatonic schizophrenia. Sometimes they remain hypomanic for months, talkative, cheery, and overactive. Many physical complications can occur as a result of abuse of stimulants, including death from stroke, acute heart failure, high fever, and complications from injections in a vein. Psychosocial symptoms include deterioration of personality, a blunted moral sense, and antisocial behavior.

About 13 million Americans have used amphetamines without medical supervision. Approximately 20 percent of young adults report using amphetamines in this way. It is thought that this report may be higher than the accurate number, because often people buy over-the-counter stimulants that resemble amphetamines or have similar names, and then report having taken amphetamines. CODAP reported 15,000 amphetamine admissions in 1979.

By 1980 approximately 27.5 percent of the 32 million Americans between the ages of eighteen and twenty-five had used cocaine. About 10 million Americans have tried the drug, and it is second only to marijuana in popularity. Of adult users, one-quarter have used the drug once or twice; one-third, three or four times; and one-third, eleven to ninety-nine times. Use is highest in the Western part of the United States and in large cities. CODAP reported about 8,000 admissions in 1979.

CANNABIS

Marijuana and hashish are both products of the hemp plant, the species *Cannabis sativa*. A sticky resin exuded from the flowering tops of the plants houses the intoxicating properties. When the resin is made into patties or lumps, it is called hashish. Marijuana can be smoked or eaten. When eaten, it can stay in the body for a long time, because it is stored in the fat. The effects of small doses of marijuana resemble those of mild alcohol intoxication. The first few times one uses marijuana, he may feel no reaction at all. When he does respond to the drug, he generally feels relaxed and less inhibited. Time seems to slow down, and perceptions of shapes and colors are distorted. Sometimes one experiences organized hallucinations. Often there is extraordinary hunger, and people appreciate the tastes and textures of food in a new way. Sometimes people experience acute panic states in which they are highly anxious; they feel detached from themselves and their situation, and memory may be impaired. Fatigue and sleepiness signal the end of the drug effect. The effects of the drug usually diminish in about an hour and disappear in two or three. Hashish is sometimes associated with psychotic behavior.

Complications include a rapid heart rate, tremor, conjunctivitis (inflammation of the inner surface of the eyelid), some dryness of the mouth, and urinary frequency. Occasional uses and doses available in the United States do not usually result in physical disability. By itself, marijuana use does not produce symptoms of obvious toxicity. Overdose just causes people to feel disoriented, hung over, and stuporous. Problems begin when people use marijuana with other drugs or use marijuana daily. Age is a significant factor. Adolescents who use the drug daily have many more social and psychological problems than do adolescents who use the drug minimally or not at all. The primary symptoms that may be experienced with daily use are apathy and laziness. Regular and long-term use can cause dry coughs like those of heavy cigarette smokers through irritation of the respiratory tract.

Marijuana ingestion interferes with some brain activities, including short-term memory, coordination, the ability to learn, and the ability to make judgments. These effects are thought to be temporary. It is also thought that smoking marijuana over a long period of time may increase one's risk of lung cancer and other respiratory difficulties. Since marijuana causes a temporary increase in heart rate, it is thought to be dangerous for people with heart conditions, high blood pressure, or other circulatory problems.

Habitual marijuana use causes problems of the reproductive system for both men and women. For example, habitual use causes a decrease in sperm number and movement. It is not yet clear whether it has an effect on overall male fertility. For women, some research has demonstrated links between frequent marijuana use and abnormal menstrual cycles. It has also been demonstrated that THC, the main ingredient in marijuana contributing to the high feeling, passes through the placenta in pregnancy to the fetus. It has also been found in breast milk of mothers who smoke marijuana. Of all the drugs discussed, this is the one many users are convinced is not dangerous.

More than 50 million people have used marijuana. They represent all socioeconomic classes, all age groups, and all areas of the country. In 1981 about one-third (34 percent) of high school seniors reported having used marijuana before entering high school. The age of first use has declined over the past fifteen years, with many children starting to use it as early as the sixth grade. As of 1980, surveys reported that in the 18–25 age group, 21 million people (68 percent) had tried marijuana and about 10 percent of this group has used it more than one hundred times. Reports of the association of marijuana with other drug use are contradictory. Some studies report that marijuana use is associated with other drug use, some suggest that people begin with marijuana and move on to other drugs and some report no association. CODAP reported more than 38,000 people admitted to affiliated clinics with marijuana as their primary drug problem in 1979.

POLYDRUG USE

Many substance abusers use more than one kind of drug. Some people who are primarily alcoholics also abuse other kinds of drugs, and some people who are primarily abusers of drugs also abuse alcohol. Polydrug use often produces additive and synergistic effects, and such combined use is increasing. Problems occur because the drugs can sometimes cause conflicting responses in the body. For example, amphetamines cause a neurophysiological response that is opposite to that produced by the ingestion of alcohol.

The mix of drugs is quite variable according to age, ethnosocial variables, and availability. The use of alcohol by heroin users is increasing, and the combination can be deadly, because heroin and alcohol have an additive effect. This can be a serious problem in methadone maintenance programs, especially for those who stay in treatment for several years but do not change their life-styles.

The most common combination for youth is alcohol and marijuana. Neither is necessarily a stepping stone to the use of hard drugs, but both drugs are commonly found in society and are used and abused more frequently by those who eventually do use hard drugs. Women who mix drugs tend to use tranquilizers and sedatives along with alcohol. It has been reported that more than 80 percent of women alcoholics have used other drugs and alcohol, and about half of the other drugs were sedatives and/or tranquilizers.

The prognosis for polydrug users is poorer than it is for single drug users because they have more psychological problems and a higher anxiety level. Polydrug users also have to be very carefully detoxified, because sometimes they are being withdrawn from one substance when they are addicted to or reacting to an entirely different substance.

Drugs and the Law

Unlicensed production, possession, use, sale, and transportation of these substances are illegal. By making drug activity illegal, society basically decides that all users and addicts are criminals. The United States government has tried three ways of dealing with the problem of drugs in the United States. It has tried to control the supplies of the drugs, to punish suppliers and users through criminal penalties, and to treat the users with medical regimens and self-help techniques. Since 1914 these methods have been used with little success. At that time the Harrison Act was passed, which taxed opium and coca products and mandated those who handled them to register and keep records of all transactions. In 1937 the Marijuana Tax Act placed marijuana in the controlled category. The Boggs Act of 1951 and the Narcotic Control Act of 1956 increased the penalties and introduced mandatory sentences. The Drug Control Amendments, also called the Harris-Dodd Act, classified amphetamines, barbiturates, and hallucinogens as dangerous drugs and brought them under federal control. These amendments are meant to crack down on those trafficking in the drugs, but penalties are considerably more lenient than those of the Narcotic Drug Control Act of 1956. Under the Harris-Dodd Act, no one can possess any of the proscribed drugs, exept for personal or veterinary purposes; records are required by authorized persons; and prescriptions are limited to five refills with none refilled after six months.

In 1966 the Narcotic Addict Rehabilitation Act (NARA) was passed. It considered drug addiction a medical problem but committed addicts to programs for treatment.

The first important federal drug legislation since the Harrison Act was the Comprehensive Drug Abuse Prevention and Control Act of 1970. This repealed and replaced all old statutes. Generally possession penalties were reduced, trafficking penalties were extended, and new controls were imposed on previously unregulated narcotic and nonnarcotic drugs. Title II of this act is the Controlled Substances Act, which requires registration of and detailed record-keeping by every person involved in drug distribution. The prevalence of abuse has increased, as have the laws and the bodies that police the laws.

In 1972 the Drug Abuse Office and Treatment Act reorganized the effort by changing the roles of state and local governments in planning and funding, allocating more money, and deciding that each state had to have one organization to coordinate all its programs.

By 1973 there was a change in direction. President Nixon made a victory statement about the war on drugs and then disengaged from the war when the election was over. After all, the numbers of addicted Vietnam veterans had been greatly exaggerated and the interest of the public lessened. In 1973 the National Institute on Drug Abuse (NIDA) was formed within the Department of Health, Education, and Welfare. Now policies remain basically the same. There is faith in the power of criminal sanctions to deter illicit drug use, based on two assumptions: that there are certain drugs that no one should use and that the government can prevent their use.

Treatment Programs for Drug Abuse

Goals for the treatment of drug and alcohol abuse are similar: detoxification, treatment of chronic health problems, and rehabilitation. In the same way the programs are a mix of self-help and professional interventions. Approximately 3,600 drug-abuse treatment units throughout the United States, serving about 235,000 people each year, are coordinated by CODAAP, the Coordinating Office for Drug and Alcohol Abuse Programs. About 80 percent of their facilities are outpatient clinics. Two-thirds of the clients are treated in drug-free modalities and one-third are treated with drug maintenance in order to achieve physical and social stabilization. Those people in maintenance programs are to be slowly withdrawn until they are drug-free.

Almost half of the participants in CODAAP programs are abusers of heroin (95,000 people) or other opiates, and about 16 percent report marijuana as their primary drug. Only 7 percent of CODAAP participants report their primary drug to be alcohol. Another 7 percent (15,000 people) are treated for amphetamine abuse, and 3 percent (7,000 people) are treated for abuse of tranquilizers.

Treatment for heroin abusers is primarily through methadone maintenance programs and less often through therapeutic communities. Methadone maintenance is used to extinguish drug-seeking behavior of heroin addicts and to reinforce a drug-free state. Methadone diminishes the high the person would feel if he shot heroin and allows him to feel well enough and to have sufficient energy to lead a responsible life. At this time there are more than 100,000 people enrolled in methadone maintenance programs in this country. Thus, 13 to 20 percent of people who are addicted to narcotics are involved in methadone maintenance at any one time. At the beginning of treatment the centers require daily attendance. As the addicted person demonstrates that he is free of other drugs and is working or looking for work, he is given several days' worth of methadone to maintain him until his next visit to the center. However, this right is hard to earn and easy to forfeit through noncompliant behavior. The program requirements of full participation and almost daily attendance are stringent. Methadone ingestion has several unpleasant side-effects, including increased sweating (experienced by almost half the people who take methadone), constipation (20 percent), decreased libido (about 20 percent), and orgasmic difficulty (about 15 percent). In many clinics a person has to have a note signed from his counselor saying that he had completed that day's psychotherapy in order to receive methadone.

When someone chooses a program of this nature, his alternatives are generally less desirable. Some people are given a choice of a maintenance program or a prison sentence by the courts. Others need a respite from the street. Some try to beat the system by dealing methadone in much the same way as they deal any other drug. Since the presence of these drugs can be detected in urine, centers use urinalysis to see if someone is clean of other drugs. This method is fraught with problems, since abusers become highly adept at substituting the urine of nonaddicted people for their own. Counselors say they expect to be conned in this way and others. Confronting abusers with the negative effects of relating in this way is all part of treatment.

The therapeutic community, a highly structured social organization that exerts a twenty-four-hour-a-day influence on an individual in order to change his life-style completely, is also a treatment modality for substance abusers. Examples of therapeutic communities established primarily for the treatment of drug abusers are Synanon, Daytop, and Odyssey House. The groups insist on voluntary entry and put new members through a powerful indoctrination period. Intensive group psychotherapy and extraordinary peer pressure are used to eliminate criminal behavior and to teach positive values and attitudes. Real work experiences, vocational counseling, and training develop the work skills of the members. Although the communities were at first only concerned with the rehabilitation of the abuser, they now offer family counseling and often make family involvement a condition for entering the community.

Besides methadone, antagonist drugs have been developed that will block the action of narcotics. When taken daily, they render the abuser immune to the effects of the narcotics. The use of these drugs is not yet widespread.

Following the pattern established by Alcoholics Anonymous, other self-help groups have been formed for abusers of cocaine, narcotics, marijuana, and other drugs. Cocaine abuse also has recently become a concern to traditional family and mental health agencies, because its use has spread from the very rich to the middle class. A self-help network called Recovery, which was formed to help former mental patients, has been useful for some substance abusers.

How to Be Helpful in Cases of Substance Abuse

Support and confrontation are most important to someone who is or has been abusing drugs. Support means offering the person a safe atmosphere in which he is respected. Confrontation means a willingness to deal directly with the person's problem in respect to its effect on the person and, when it is appropriate, on you. To offer a safe haven without confrontation is to lose the person to the substance. To confront without support is to lose the person, for he may well leave the situation. It is as if you and the abuser are together fighting the part of the person that wants to use the drugs. For a long time after he has stopped using drugs, the person is both attracted to and repelled by the drug. Some say the attraction lasts a lifetime.

Abusers are effective in involving people in their drug-taking. They are able to convince people that they need the drugs, they will be sick without them, and others should help them pay for drugs or even obtain the drugs for them. They blame, enrage, and chastise those around them in order to maintain the involvement. To be helpful one should remain outside this process. The person will have to manage that part of his behavior himself.

Since through years of drug-taking the abuser has lost the ability to judge his capacities correctly or express his feelings, he must learn again how to sort out capabilities and responsibilities, how to acknowledge anxiety and anger, and when to take action on his own behalf. When the person has stopped abusing and expects his life to turn around instantly, it is up to the people around him to remember that his expectations may be unrealistic. That is the most important time of all to be supportive but firm. It may take a year for the person to resume a healthy, fulfilling life.

11

Conclusions

CHRONIC ILLNESS IS usually perceived unidimensionally. The physician or nurse sees the disease and its effect on the body; the social worker sees the effects on family, work, and social life; the speech therapist is most concerned with the person's ability to communicate; the physical therapist, with ambulation and self-care; the occupational therapist, with work in all of its guises; the personnel director, with the ability to manage a particular job; the minister, with a person's spiritual comfort. Specific tasks, time limitations, and exigencies of place often prevent a comprehensive point of view. Gerontology and other like specialties solve this problem, to some degree, with a focus that demands a multidimensional approach. In the same way *Understanding Chronic Illness* presents a multidimensional picture spanning physical, social, legal, and psychological aspects of illness. It allows the reader to realize the process through which the ill individual and those around her learn about, react to, and adapt to chronic disease.

The medical process is explored through discussion of the classification and natural history of a particular disease followed by a description of means for diagnosis and treatment. This section attends to the physical aspects of an illness—how the disease presents itself, progresses, and affects and limits the body. Information about prevalence, incidence, and populations at risk describes the groups of people who are most likely to have a disease and those who may develop it in the future. Association with other diseases indicates the frequency with which people have more than one disease and underscores the complexity of treating illnesses of this sort.

Knowledge of ways in which a disease affects the body and of the medical and technological means used in diagnosis and treatment diminishes some of the magic and fear with which these subjects are often approached. In the same way use of this framework demystifies the systems of health care so that acute hospitalization, rehabilitation facilities, nursing home care, and home care can be seen as separate steps in the process. In the past decade health maintenance organizations and hospice programs have become part of health care delivery. Such systems seem to rely heavily on nurses and general practitioners to be gatekeepers to physician and other specialists. As the government becomes more involved in containing the escalating costs of health care, more alternatives to the traditional systems will surely develop. The consumer will have to become more of an authority about all aspects of health care.

Modifications in life-style such as diet, exercise, and daily schedule act as a bridge from the medical to the psychosocial aspects of disease, because they are considered part of treatment and are methods people commonly use to keep themselves healthy. Ways of modifying life to adapt to illness may mean restriction from certain activities, such as specific kinds of work or recreation. Sometimes, too, laws may restrict the activity of people with certain illnesses. In addition, laws also spell out rights and entitlements that can affect some or all chronically ill people. In some illnesses the primary legal concern is guardianship. In others it may be the right to retraining, special education, or disability payments. Again, one aspect of the framework relates to another, for entitlements are often related to complicated and variable public systems of insurance.

Next, the framework turns to social life—relationships with family members and strangers, and the effect on work and recreation. Age of onset, previous family functioning, and the severity of the disease are important factors in understanding the impact of the disease. Roles and obligations are often exchanged when an illness is acute. Times when an illness is in remission require renegotiation. Families who remain open and flexible seem to do best. Relationships with strangers, work, and recreation are affected both by the limitations a disease imposes and by its visibility. Chronic illness can affect strength, stamina, memory, and self-expression.

A discussion of social life and work leads to the psychological aspects of chronic illness, particularly self-concept, emotional response, and patterns related to the illness itself. Altered mood and affect can ensue also from medication or the depression felt as a result of being ill. A person can become less sexually responsive because of illness, fatigue, or a change in how she feels about herself. Thus, by including medical, legal, social, and psychological aspects, the framework allows for a rich understanding of chronic disease. The framework can be used to inform oneself about any specific illness.

Common Themes in Chronic Illness

Despite differences among the diseases, there are certain common themes that suggest ways to think about chronic illness. First, they all do some unalterable physical damage that must be dealt with, or the results will be increasingly disabling even when the disease process is in remission. Second, most of the illnesses share continuous cycles of recurrence, followed by remission, followed by recurrence, which remain unpredictable as to timing, duration, and extent of severity. The nature of the dread event differs, so that a stroke has different meaning from a newly aching joint or a new tumor, but there is almost always a dread event—the alarming physical signal of attack. All the illnesses involve fatigue, unseen by others but an added drain on the ill person. The degree to which symptoms are visible also differs according to the kind and severity of disease. Nonetheless, visibility is a common theme.

In diagnosis and treatment there are also commonalities. Along with the labeling process of diagnosis comes prognosis, with its concomitant fears and panic reactions. "You have cancer" or "You have rheumatoid arthritis" or "You have emphysema" or "You have epilepsy" is almost always met with denial or a terrible foreboding of the worst someone has ever seen or read or heard about the illness. If one wants to understand what is happening, one has to be able to take herself through the medical process—diagnosis, treatment, and follow-up. Part of the understanding is sharing the tedium, the detail of trying to leave nothing to chance in managing the disease.

Common, too, in most of these diseases is the place of the regimen in the life of the ill person and family, whether it be medicine or diet, radiation or exercise. Once the diagnosis is made and treatment is prescribed, self-management becomes most important, and anticipating, observing, preventing, and treating become themes in the life of anyone who is chronically ill. Closely aligned with this theme is the notion that one can make the best of resources and minimize limitations through good self-management, but the illness may progress despite the best adherence to regimen.

In treatment there is also the common theme of risk tradeoffs in decision-making. Here the physician and the ill person play the odds, gamble with percentages. "If you do this, there is a 50 percent chance of that." "A large percentage of people who try this get these side effects." "If we don't do this test, you will probably die. If we do the test, there is a 10 percent chance you will die as a result of the test." Sometimes the person has to decide if the discomfort of the treatment or the side effects are worth the possible gain. Many of these diseases cause various kinds of death. Stroke and heart attack kill tissue. Through cancer and diabetes, people can lose limbs and other body parts. Severe dementia causes intellectual and social death.

Because many of these illnesses offer little or no chance of cure, ill people and their families sometimes become desperate. When conventional and sometimes experimental treatments do not work, some people resort to unfounded promises of cure, wearing objects that promise to rectify the situation, following diets, or even taking medicines that have to be obtained illegally, at great expense, or out of the country.

There are several common social and psychological themes in chronic illness that depend largely on prognosis and the degree of permanent disability. The most significant and universal is a feeling of loss of control, which the ill individual and his loved ones share. It often begins at the time of diagnosis, when there is a pervasive feeling of powerlessness. From that point one can no longer take her body for granted or even trust it any more. And she knows that, even with long remissions, she can never again be free of the specter of illness or disability. This also precludes the closure that one can usually hope for in other difficult situations in life. One can say, "I can leave this job," "the term will end," "the war will be over," but one can never again be completely free of the knowledge that one's body has betrayed her and may again. Some say that one's body can be sufficiently altered by the disease process for her to feel it as alien. The knowledge of the presence of disease can alter one's aspirations and even her fantasy life. There is a lack of predictability. One cannot pretend to know, negatively or positively, what lies ahead.

Chronic illness can be accompanied by increased dependence on others to do not only what one has previously been able to do for herself but what society expects. Families and friends often contribute to the increasing confinement and isolation. A wife, for example, may turn down invitations from family and friends because "I never know how he will be." When this becomes a pattern, the couple will be invited less often, and the well spouse will become increasingly isolated as well. Thus everyone involved with the ill person must work to counteract the isolation and inactivity. All these themes increase one's sense of vulnerability.

Stress is another common theme in chronic illness. There has been much speculation about the role of stress in the etiology of illness. Knowledge of the progression of the disease is thought to add to the stress levels of the ill person. It has also been posited that the recurrence of some diseases is stress-related. With varying rates of success, researchers have tried to identify the relationship of stress to heart disease, cancer, substance abuse, arthritis, and diabetes, for example.

There are also many common themes in the social aspects of chronic illness. For example, at some point in the disease process almost all of those dealing with chronic illness are confronted with the redefinition of roles, especially in terms of work, family responsibilities, and self-care. To a great extent people must suit their work to their physical capacities. In this society great value is placed on being self-supporting; but the issues around work are much more than financial. Self-esteem, sense of purpose, and status come from one's work.

Family roles are often affected by chronic illness. It is common for spouse to take care of spouse and even child to take care of parent. At times, when an illness is active, well family members must assume responsibility for their dependent relatives. When an acute phase has passed, some families redefine roles and some do not. Thus role definition is complicated by the kind and degree of disease, as well as the degree of family flexibility and dependency. It is always an issue.

Each illness is accorded some part in the identity of the ill individual. Some people make the illness one part of themselves. Some deny that they are ill. If the signs of the illness are not visible, some people try to pass, that is, pretend that they are not ill. Passing adds stress to an already stressful existence. Others have their lives revolve around their illness and, in fact, almost become the illness. In these circumstances, a person sees herself as a cardiac, an arthritic, or a diabetic rather than a person with a disease.

The use of denial and other defenses is also common in chronic disease. To some degree these defenses are useful, helping the person cope with the illness. However, there are points at which the disease must be acknowledged so that the person's health will not be endangered. There is a difference, too, between denying the presence of the disease and denying the limitations the disease suggests. Denial of the disease can be destructive; denial of some limitations may be helpful. The psychological response usually evolves over time. There is usually depression at the time of diagnosis and prognosis, hope and sometimes euphoria at the first remission, great despair at the first recurrence, then somewhat of a flattening of the highs and lows as the cycles continue.

People commonly experience feelings of isolation. Part of the isolation is paradoxical. The ill person says, "No one knows how I feel and, if people knew how I felt, they wouldn't want to be around me." For many, the isolation increases as the illness progresses. If the illness becomes severely disabling or terminal, one's isolation is compounded with fear of abandonment.

Another theme, related to several already mentioned, is loss—of health, control, certain kinds of ability, a positive body image, self-esteem, of attractiveness, aspects of sexuality, and many adult roles. These losses can range from mild to severe, but for people to adjust to their illness there must be an acknowledgment of loss and appropriate grieving.

Finally, there is the stigma of the disease. Again, the degree of stigma is related to the ways in which society judges each illness. For example, it is less stigmatizing to have heart disease than cancer. With a chronic illness, society sees you as a less-than-perfect person. Sometimes the stigmata are unattractive, like deformed joints or a dragging limb. More often the stigmata are internal, in what the person feels about herself as someone who has such a disease.

Many of the psychological and social themes in the response of family members to the illness echo the themes of the ill individual. Because physical demands require that the family be deeply involved with its management, the illness almost but never quite becomes theirs. The family must grieve about the losses the illness has created for them as well as their ill relative. Spouses, especially, lose many of the aspects of partnership. At times their spouse's body becomes unpredictable. When the illness is in crisis, work and social responsibilities are curtailed. The presence of the illness also makes the future less certain.

The burden of the care falls to family members, and the burden is not just physical and social, but financial as well. If the ill person lives with her family, the burden is constant. If the person is severely disabled, family members can become completely responsible, as they would for an infant with an adult's body, in some cases, or an adult with the physical ability of an infant, in others. If the ill person lives alone, the family constantly wonders whether she is all right.

Many family members feel that in some way they have caused the illness or that they should have been the ones who got sick. Sometimes family members develop their own devastating cycle of guilt, then overwork, and a period of refusing to look after themselves, followed by anger and resentment that this has happened to them, followed again by guilt for having such nasty thoughts. Another cycle that sometimes befalls family members is an alternation of overprotection and rejection, holding the ill member so close that she is stifled, then pushing her away, then pulling her breathlessly close again.

Since these illnesses are of such long duration, there is rarely a sense of completion. Generally neither cure nor death is imminent. When the illness is in remission, one waits for a crisis. When the illness is in crisis, one looks for signs of remission.

When cure is possible, some families have difficulty redistributing responsibility and authority. They have become comfortable in their adjustment to life with a precariously sick member. When death becomes inevitable, families have difficulty adjusting to its finality. Some have not resolved their guilt or allowed themselves to grieve. Others have difficulty, after trying so hard to keep a loved one alive, in letting her go.

Life outside the family also makes things difficult for family members. Many chronic illnesses are stigmatizing to the families as well. People shun whole families, are afraid that illnesses are contagious or that they won't know how to behave or what to say. The longer friends and colleagues stay away, the easier it is to stay away. Thus families are abandoned along with their ill relative.

It is ironic that in polite society we are taught not to point out that someone's slip is showing, or someone has a spot on his tie. One looks away and says nothing. Never point out that someone or something is different. You also are expected to know what the other person is capable of and how he feels. But none of these conventions will work in relating to someone who is chronically ill. You have to assume that you don't know what illnesses feel like or understand the kinds of limitations they impose. One cannot assume symptoms or performance, because many symptoms are not visible and are variable from instance to instance and person to person.

What one can probably assume is that the illness is a significant part of the person's life, undeniable and undesirable and inexorable, but a part, not the whole. Pretending that the illness does not exist is not helpful. Lending false hope that everything will be all right places extra stress on the individual to act well. This can be physically damaging to the person and damage your relationship. It is also important not to be so overly protective and do so much for the person that she feels devalued because she is unable to reciprocate. This problem is compounded when one's relationship to the ill individual is not well defined. How much does one do for a colleague, a supervisee, a friend of short duration? That issue is more easily defined when one asks, how much does one do for a patient, a client, or a spouse? To understand requires intimacy. When intimacy does not exist, one can ask about symptoms, limitations, and the degree of help a person wants or needs. To be effective and enduring, this asking must be matched by an openness and a willingness to share on the part of the other person in the relationship. When an ill person does not respond to overtures, allow her to refuse just as you would in any other kind of relationship. But do not confuse refusal with rejection and become angry as a result.

The kinds of formalized help available constitute another point in common among the chronic diseases. In addition to the health teams made up of physicians, nurses, social workers, psychologists, and specialty therapists, every group of ill people stresses the need for clear information about the disease process and for lists of available community resources and support networks. Such information and support are provided, to a great extent, by the self-help organizations generally available in each disease category. In areas where self-help groups are not available, national organizations will provide systematic help for beginning one.

Self-help groups nonjudgmentally act as mirrors of understanding, reflecting back shared experiences and advice. They assume that problems arise not because of personality issues but because of the impact a particular illness has on a situation. In these ways self-help groups become an important social outlet for people who are isolated and in crisis.

The following chapter-keyed appendix provides the names and addresses of self-help organizations and government agencies devoted to a particular chronic disease, condition or group of conditions. Self-help organizations are generally eager to have interested people participate in support groups, public education, advocacy activities. They are pleased when someone wants to know more about the illness and will help someone to educate herself. The federal government funds many research and education projects in chronic disease. Some government agencies, like the National Cancer Institute and the National Institute of Drug Abuse, publish materials at every level of sophistication. These agencies are interested in prevention as well as treatment. Often there are parallel state and local programs as well. In educating oneself, consulting laymen's sources is also useful. Books on particular diseases in the public library ranging from "Everything You've Always Wanted to Know About . . ." to "My Life as a . . ." supplement the more scholarly publications. Often one book may present a slanted view, so it is important to read several. Once one has read enough to familiarize oneself with professional vocabulary (one of the reasons why glossaries were included in this book), one can read a good deal of professional literature with some degree of comfort.

How to Be Helpful to People Who Are Chronically Ill

Be willing to learn about the illness. Remember that the ill person is the treatment manager and is generally very knowledgeable about the disease. Ask her about capabilities and limitations rather than assuming them. Help the person to take care of herself by, in part, not letting her get lost in the disease. Encourage the person to involve herself in self-help organizations, because they provide support, education, and means for advocacy and are usually aware of the newest and best in research and treatment. Self-help organizations often arm themselves with interpretations of laws affecting those with their particular disease. Many such organizations are working to change or expunge unfair laws. Support the families of ill people in helping their ill relative and in continuing to live for themselves. Basically, to be helpful is to understand the disease. Such understanding requires education, involvement, and empathy. It allows one to say, "I have some knowledge of what life is like for a person with this illness."

Appendix

Resources for Those
Who Are Chronically Ill

Chapter 1: Introduction

Accent on Information
P.O. Box 700
Bloomington, Ill. 61701
  (309)–378–2961

Computerized retrieval service for health devices.

Bureau of Education for the Handicapped
U.S. Office of Education
Washington, D.C. 20202

Clothing Research and Development Foundation
P.O. Box 347
Milford, N.J. 08848

Types and sources of clothing for the disabled.

Directory of Living Aids for the Disabled
Superintendent of Documents
Government Printing Office
Washington, D.C. 20402

Hospice Action
P.O. Box 32331
Washington, D.C. 20003

Mainstream, Inc.
1200 15th Street, N.W.
Washington, D.C. 20005
  (800)–424–8089

Medic Alert Foundation International
P.O. Box 1009
Turlock, Calif. 95380

Comprehensive emergency medical identification system for individuals.

National Amputation Foundation
12–45 150th Street
Whitestone, N.Y. 113357
  (212)–767–0596

National Association of Area Agencies
  on Aging
Room 400
1828 L Street, N.W.
Washington, D.C. 20036
  (202)–223–5010

National Association of the Physically
Handicapped
2 Meetinghouse Road
Merrimack, N.H. 03054

National Center for Law and the
Handicapped
P.O. Box 477
University of Notre Dame
Notre Dame, Ind. 46556
(219)–283–4536

Works for equal protection under the law
for all handicapped individuals through
education, research, assistance, and referral.

National Council for Homemaker-
Home Health Aide Services
67 Irving Place
New York, N.Y. 10003
(212)–674–4990

National Health Information Clearinghouse
1550 Wilson Boulevard
Suite 600
Rosslyn, Va. 22209
(703)–522–2590

National Hospice Organization
1901 North Fort Myer Drive
Suite 402
Arlington, Va. 22209

National Information Center for the
Handicapped
P.O. Box 1492
Washington, D.C. 20013

National Library of Medicine
National Institutes of Health
8600 Rockville, Md. 20209
(301)–496–6095

National Library Service for the Blind
and Physically Handicapped
Washington, D.C. 20542

National Rehabilitation Information
Center
4407 Eighth Street, N.E.
The Catholic University of America
Washington, D.C. 20017
(202)–635–5822

National Wheelchair Athletic Association
40–24 62d Street
Woodside, N.Y. 11377

Office of Technology Transfer
(Veterans Administration)
252 Seventh Avenue
New York, N.Y. 10001
(212)–620–6659

Information on new devices and techniques
developed by the V.A.

People-to-People Committee for the
Handicapped
1028 Connecticut Avenue, N.W.
Washington, D.C. 20036

Physicians for Automotive Safety
50 Union Avenue
Irvington, N.J. 07111

Rehabilitation Services Administration
Office of Human Development Services, HEW
Switzer Building
Washington, D.C. 20201
(202)–245–0322

Self-Help Reporter
c/o National Self-Help Clearinghouse
Graduate School and University Cen-
ter/CUNY
33 West 42d Street/1206S
New York, N.Y. 10036

Social Security Administration
6401 Security Boulevard
Baltimore, Md. 21235
(301)–594–7700

Society for the Advancement of Travel
for the Handicapped
26 Court Street
Brooklyn, N.Y. 11242

Talking Book Topics
United States Library of Congress
Division for the Blind and Physically
Handicapped
Washington, D.C. 20542

Therapeutic Recreation Information
Center
Department of Physical Education
and Recreation
University of Colorado
Box 354
Boulder, Colo. 80309
(303)–492–7333

Travel Information Center
Moss Rehabilitation Hospital
12th Street and Tabor Road
Philadelphia, Pa. 19141

Veterans Administration
810 Vermont Avenue, N.W.
Washington, D.C. 20420
(202)–393–4120

Chapter 2:   Arthritis

Architectural and Transportation
Barriers Compliance Board
330 C Street, S.W.
Washington, D.C. 20201

Arthritis Foundation
3400 Peachtree Road, N.E.
Atlanta, Ga. 30326

Arthritis Information Clearing House
P.O. Box 34427
Bethesda, Md. 20034

Independent Living for the Disabled
Office

HUD
7th and D Streets, S.W.
Washington, D.C. 20410

International Rehabilitation Film Review Library
20 West 40th Street
New York, N.Y. 10018

The Lupus Erythematosis Foundation
120 Tremont Street
Boston, Mass. 02108

Moss Rehabilitation Hospital
Travel Information Center
12th Street and Tabor Road
Philadelphia, Pa. 19141

National Center for a Barrier-Free
Environment
Seventh and Florida, N.E.
Washington, D.C. 20002

National Institute of Arthritis, Diabetes, Digestive, and Kidney Diseases
9000 Rockville Pike
Bethesda, Md. 20205

Rehabilitation International
20 West 40th Street
New York, N.Y 10018

Publications and films.

Rehabilitation Services Administra-
tion
Department of Health, Education and
Welfare
Washington, D.C. 20201

Sister Kenny Institute
A/V Publication Department #266
27th at Chicago Avenue
Minneapolis, Minn. 55407

Stanford Arthritis Center
Health, Research and Policy Building

Room 109C
Stanford, Calif. 94305

United Scleroderma Foundation
P.O. Box 724
Watsonville, Calif. 95076

Chapter 3: Cancer

American Cancer Society
777 Third Avenue
New York, N.Y. 10017

Can Surmount: Trained volunteers, also cancer patients, meet with patient and family in hospital or home for support and education.

I Can Cope: Eight-session, hospital-based course that educates patients and families about cancer and methods for dealing with psychological problems.

Reach to Recovery: Volunteers help women who have had mastectomies toward physical and natural recovery.

Cancer Information Service
National Cancer Institute
   (800)–638–6694

Candle Lighters
123 C Street, S.E.
Washington, D.C. 20003

Support groups for childhood cancer patients.

ENCORE (postmastectomy groups)
National Board, YWCA
600 Lexington Avenue
New York, N.Y. 10022

Hospice Action
P.O. Box 32331
Washington, D.C. 20003

National Hospice Organization
765 Prospect Street
New Haven, Conn. 06511

International Association of Laryngectomees
American Cancer Society
777 Third Avenue
New York, N.Y. 10017

Leukemia Society of America
800 Second Avenue
New York, N.Y. 10017

Make Today Count
514 Tama Building
Box 303
Burlington, Iowa 52611

Mastectomy Counseling to Men
American Cancer Society
Santa Clara County Unit
1537 Parkmoor Plaza
P.O. Box 26007
San Jose, Calif. 95126

National Cancer Institute
Office of Cancer Communication
National Institutes of Health
Building 31, Room 10A18
Bethesda, Md. 20205

National Hospice Organization
301 Tower Suite 506
301 Maple Avenue West
Vienna, Va. 22180

Ronald McDonald Houses
c/o Golin Communications
500 North Michigan Avenue
Chicago, Ill. 60611

Located in several large cities; accommodation for families of seriously ill children while the children are being treated.

United Ostomy Association
2001 W. Beverly Blvd.
Los Angeles, Calif. 90057

United Cancer Council
1803 N. Meridian Street
Indianapolis, Ind. 46202

Federation of voluntary cancer agencies, providing service, education and research.

Chapter 4: The Dementias

Alzheimer's Disease and Related
  Disorders Association
2501 West 84th Street
Bloomington, Minn. 55431
  (612)–888–7653

Alzheimer's Disease Society
1435 Tenth Street
Fort Lee, N.J. 07024

Alzheimer Society
2 Surrey Place
Toronto, Ontario, Canada M5S2C2

Alzheimer's Disease Center
Albert Einstein College of Medicine
1300 Morris Park Avenue
Bronx, N.Y. 10461

ASIST (Alzheimer Support Information Service Team)
1197 112th Street, N.E.
Bellevue, Wash. 98004

National Institute on Aging
Bldg. 31, Rm. 5C–36
National Institutes of Health
Bethesda, Md. 20205

National Institute of Neurological and
  Communicative Disorders and
  Stroke
Office of Scientific and Health Re-
  ports
Bldg. 31, Room 8A–06
National Institutes of Health
Bethesda, Md. 20205

Chapter 5: Diabetes

American Association of Diabetes Ed-
  ucators

Box 56
North Woodbury Road
Pitman, N.J. 08071
  (609)–589–4831

American Diabetes Association
Two Park Avenue
New York, N.Y. 10016
  (212)–683–7444

American Foundation for the Blind,
  Inc.
15 West 16th Street
New York, N.Y. 10011
  (212)–924–0420

American Printing House for the Blind
P.O. Box 6085
Louisville, Ky. 40206
  (502)–895–2405

Diabetes Education Center
4959 Excelsior Boulevard
Minneapolis, Minn. 55416
  (612)-920–6742

Diabetes Group Insurance Trust
Jon W. Hall and Associates, Inc.
P.O. Box 14868
Shawnee Mission, Kans. 66215

Diabetic Self-Care Newsletter
344 East 63d Street
New York, N.Y. 10021

Garfield G. Duncan Research Foundation, Inc.
Diabetes Information Center
829 Spruce Street, Suite 302
Philadelphia, Pa. 19107

Good Control (monthly newsletter)
Stephanie M. Ryder, RN
Box 2112
Scottsdale, Ariz. 85252

Health-O-Gram, Sugar Free Center
  for Diabetics

Mantiliza Avenue
P.O. Box 114
Van Nuys, Calif. 91408

The Infuser: Newsletter
  for people on insulin pump
c/o Terry Miller
P.O. Box 273
Running Springs, Calif. 92382

International Diabetes Federation
3–6 Alfred Place
London WC1 E7EE, England

Joslin Diabetes Foundation, Inc.
One Joslin Place
Boston, Mass. 02215
  (617)–732–2400

Juvenile Diabetes Foundation
23 East 26th Street
New York, N.Y. 10010
  (212)–889–7575

Library of Congress
Division for the Blind and Physically
  Handicapped
1291 Taylor Street, N.W.
Washington, D.C. 20542
  (202)–882–5500

National Association for the Visually
  Handicapped
305 East 24th Street
New York, N.Y. 10010
  (212)–889–3141

National Diabetes Information Clearinghouse
7910 Woodmont Avenue, Suite 1811
Bethesda, Md. 10014
  (301)–654–0897

Chapter 6: The Epilepsies

Epilepsy Foundation of America
1828 L Street N.W., Suite 406
Washington, D.C. 20036

National Institute of Neurological
  and Communicative Disorders and
  Stroke
National Institutes of Health
Building 31, Room 8A–06
Bethesda, Md. 20205
  (301)–496–5751

Progressive Epilepsy Network
1315 Walnut Street, Suite 624
Philadelphia, Pa. 19107
  (215)–545–7000

Chapter 7: Heart Disease

American Heart Association
44 East 23d Street
New York, N.Y. 10010

Zipper Club (for those who have had open
heart surgery).

High Blood Pressure Information
  Center
National High Blood Pressure
  Education Program
120/80 National Institutes of Health
Bethesda, Md. 20205
  (301)–652–7700

International Association of Pacemaker Patients (now Heartlife)
P.O. Box 54305
Atlanta, Ga. 30308
  (404)–524–0826

Mended Hearts
7320 Greenville Avenue
Dallas, Tex. 75231

National Heart, Lung and Blood
  Institute
National Institutes of Health
Building 31, Room 4A21
Bethesda, Md. 20205
  (301)–496–4236

Sharing and Caring Groups
  (contacted through local hospitals).

Chapter 8:   Respiratory Disease

American Lung Association
1740 Broadway
New York, N.Y. 10019

Asthma and Allergy Related
    Foundation of America
19 West 44th Street
New York, N.Y. 10036

Cystic Fibrosis Foundation
6000 Executive Boulevard, Suite 309
Rockville, Md. 20852

National Asthma Center
875 Avenue of the Americas
New York, N.Y. 10010

National Clearinghouse for Smoking
    and Health
Parklawn Building 1–16
5600 Fishers Lane
Rockville, Md. 20857
    (301)–443–1690

National Heart, Lung and Blood
    Institute
National Institutes of Health
Building 31, Room 4A21
Bethesda, Md. 20205
    (301)–496–4236

National Institute of Allergy
    and Infectious Disease
National Institutes of Health
Building 31, Room 7A32
Bethesda, Md. 20205

National Institute of Arthritis,
    Metabolism and Digestive Diseases
National Institutes of Health
Building 31, Room 9A04
Bethesda, Md. 20205

National Jewish Hospital/
    National Asthma Center

3800 Colfax Avenue
Denver, Colo. 80206

Office on Smoking and Health
Technical Information Center
Parklawn Building, Room 1–16
5600 Fishers Lane
Rockville, Md. 20857

Chapter 9:   Stroke

American Heart Association
7320 Greenville Avenue
Dallas, Tex. 75231
    (214)–750–5414

American Physical Therapy
    Association
1156 15th Street, N.W.
Washington, D.C. 20005

American Speech-Language-Hearing
    Association
10801 Rockville Road
Bethesda, Md. 20852

Congress of Organizations
    of the Physically Handicapped
7611 Oakland Avenue
Minneapolis, Minn. 55423

Consumer Product Information
    Service
Public Documents Distribution
    Center
Pueblo, Colo. 81009

Friederich's Ataxia Group in America
    Newsletter
Box 1116
Oakland, Calif. 94611

Green Pages: A Directory of Products
    and Services for the Handicapped
641 West Fairbanks
Winter Park, Fla. 32789

High Blood Pressure Information
  Center
National High Blood Pressure
  Education Program
120/80 National Institutes of Health
Bethesda, Md. 20205
  (301)–652–7700

National Center for a Barrier Free
  Environment
8401 Connecticut Avenue, N.W.
Washington, D.C. 20015

National Center for Law and the
  Handicapped, Inc.
1235 North Eddy Street
South Bend, Ind. 46617

National Easter Seal Society
2023 West Ogdin Avenue
Chicago, Ill. 60612
  (312)–243–8400

National Heart, Lung and Blood
  Institute
National Institutes of Health
Building 31, Room 4A21
Bethesda, Md. 20205
  (301)–496–4236

National Institute of Neurological
  and Communicative Disorders
  and Stroke
National Institutes of Health 31,
  8A–06
Bethesda, Maryland 20205

Sister Kenny Institute
Division of Abbot-Northwestern Hos-
  pital
Chicago Avenue at 27th Street
Minneapolis, Minn. 55407
  (612)–874–4149

Society for the Advancement
  of Travel for the Handicapped
26 Court Street
Brooklyn, N.Y. 11242

Stroke Clubs of America
805 12th Street
Galveston, Tex. 77550

Talking Books Topics
United States Library of Congress
Division for the Blind and Physically
  Handicapped
Washington, D.C. 20542

Chapter 10: Substance Abuse

American Council on Marijuana
  and Other Psychoactive Drugs
6193 Executive Blvd.
Rockville, Md. 20852
  (301)–984–5700

Al-Anon Family Group World Service
  Office (includes Alateen and Ala-
  tot)
P.O. Box 182
Madison Square Station
New York, N.Y. 10010

Alcoholics Anonymous
Box 459
Grand Central Station
New York, N.Y. 10017

Center for Alcohol Studies at Rutgers
  University
P.O. Box 969
Piscataway, N.J. 08854
  (201)–932–2190

Cocaine Anonymous
Cocaine Hot Line
  (800)–Cocaine

Hazelden Educational Materials (for
  alcoholism)
Box 176
Center City, MO 55012

Mothers Against Drunk Driving
  (MADD)

5330 Primrose
Suite 146
Fair Oaks, Calif. 95628
   (916)-966-MADD

Narcotics Anonymous World Services
   Office
P.O. Box 622
Sun Valley, Calif. 91352

National Association of Gay Alcoholism Professionals
204 W. 20th Street
New York, N.Y. 10011

National Clearinghouse for Alcohol
   Information
P.O. Box 2345
Rockville, Md. 20852
   (301)-468-2600

Part of the National Institute on Alcohol
Abuse and Alcoholism

National Clearinghouse for Drug
   Abuse Information
National Institute for Drug Abuse
Alcohol, Drug Abuse and Mental
   Health Administration, HEW
5600 Fishers Lane, Room 10-A53
Rockville, Md. 20857
   (301)-443-6500

National Council on Alcoholism
733 Third Avenue
New York, N.Y. 10017
   (212)-986-4433

Components include:

American Medical Society on Alcoholism
Research Society on Alcoholism
National Nurses' Society on Alcoholism

National Institute on Alcohol Abuse
   and Alcoholism
5600 Fishers Lane
Rockville, Md. 20857

National Institutes on Drug Abuse
5600 Fishers Lane
Rockville, Md. 20857

Pyramid Project—a resource network
   for drug abuse prevention
Western office: Pacific Institute
   for Research and Evaluation
3746 Mt. Diablo Blvd.
Suite 200
Lafayette, Calif. 94549
   (800)-227-0438

Eastern office: 7101 Wisconsin
   Avenue
Suite 1006
Bethesda, Md. 20014
   (301)-654-1194

Remove Intoxicated Drivers (RID)
P.O. Box 520
Schenectedy, N.Y. 12301
   (314)-768-0692

Glossary

Abduction. Moving a limb away from the center of the body.

Acetabulum. Cup-shaped cavity into which the large bone of the thigh (femur) fits.

Adduction. Moving a limb toward the center of the body.

Adrenocorticotropic Hormone (ACTH). A hormone produced by the pituitary gland that stimulates the action of the adrenal gland.

Alignment. Proper positioning of the body parts.

Allopurinol. The generic name for a drug used to control the production of uric acid in the body. Used in the treatment of gout, its brand name is Zyloprin.

Analgesic. Pain-relieving.

Arthritis. Inflammation of joints.
  Ankylosing: now generally called *atrophic* or *rheumatoid arthritis*, a type of arthritis in which the joint stiffens and becomes fixed or will not move as it should.
  Atrophic: a form of arthritis recognized as a chronic inflammatory disease that will eventually destroy the affected joint and lead to crippling and deformity; also called *rheumatoid arthritis*.
  Degenerative: a chronic and progressive form of arthritis that generally in-

293

volves several joints and is characterized by the destruction of the cartilage; also called *hypertrophic arthritis* or *osteoarthritis*.

Gouty: arthritis that occurs as a result of gout; the joint or joints are irritated by deposits of uric acid crystals, which collect as a result of the body's inability to use properly and eliminate this acid.

Hypertrophic: another name for *degenerative arthritis*.

Infectious: arthritis that occurs as a result of an infection in the body, which settles in one or two joints; generally disappears after the infection is treated and cured.

Juvenile: a form similar to, but in many ways different from, rheumatoid arthritis in adults, but found in children generally between the ages of six weeks and sixteen years.

Proliferative: similar to *ankylosing arthritis*; refers to the rapid growth of the synovia, which then causes immobility of the joint.

Rheumatoid: the most serious form of arthritis, which eventually results in crippling and destruction of the joint or joints involved; generally affects the entire body.

Traumatic: a type of arthritis generally the result of a severe shock or prolonged stress.

Arthrodesis.   The fusion or freezing of a joint in a fixed position. A surgical procedure used to provide stability to a joint severely deformed by rheumatoid arthritis.

Arthroplasty.   A surgical procedure to rebuild a joint by using the joint's own material, by inserting metal supports, or by replacing the joint with an artifical one.

Articular cartilage.   A protective coating of connective tissue on the front surface of the bones of movable joints that allows the bones to move against each other with a minimum of friction.

Atrophy.   Wasting away of a body part or tissue.

Autosuggestion.   Technique for influencing one's own attitudes, behavior, or physical condition by mental processes other than conscious thought.

Biofeedback.   Technique for making one conscious of involuntary body processes in order to manipulate them through mental control; control is learned through awareness.

Bursa.   A small sac filled with fluid, located between a tendon and a bone.

Bursitis.   Inflammation of the bursa.

Corticosteroid.   Compound produced naturally by a properly functioning adrenal gland.

Diathermy.   Generation of heat in tissues by electrical currents.

Extension.   Moving into a straight position.

Fibrocartilage.   Type of connective tissue containing many fibers, which serve to stabilize and prevent movement.

Fibrositis.   Inflammation of fibrous tissue of the body resulting in pain and stiffness.

Flexure contraction.   Inability to straighten joint, caused by shortening of muscle.

Ibuprofen.   Generic name for a nonsteroidal anti-inflammatory drug effective in the treatment of osteoarthritis and rheumatoid arthritis (Motrin).

Indomethacin.   Nonsteroidal anti-inflammatory drug (Indocin).

Isometric exercise.   Exercise involving great amount of muscle contraction but no joint motion, in which opposing muscles are contracted with little shortening but great increase in tone of muscle fibers involved.

Joint.   Generally movable place of connection between two or more bones.

Ligament.   Fibrous band of tissue connecting bones or supporting organs in place.

Metacarpophalangeal.   Pertaining to the five bones that form the part of the hand between the wrist and fingers (metacarpus) and the small bones of the fingers (phalanges).

Muscle spasm.   Strong, painful contraction or tightening of a skeletal muscle.

Myositis.   Inflammation of a voluntary muscle.

Naproxen.   Drug for reduction of swelling and stiffness and pain in rheumatoid arthritis (Naprosyn).

NSAID.   Nonsteroidal anti-inflammatory drugs.

Osteoarthritis.   A degenerative disease of joints which involves the progressive deterioration of the joint cartilage. Associated with aging and daily wear and tear of the joints. The most common type of arthritis.

Osteomyelitis.   Inflammation of bone.

Osteonecrosis.   Death of bone.

Osteophytes.   Bony outgrowths caused by disease.

Osteoporosis.   Thinning of the bones, making them very brittle.

Osteotomy.   Surgical cutting of bone to improve alignment and to alter the joint's weight-bearing surfaces to reduce pain and excess wear.

Oxyphenbutazone.   Potent anti-inflammatory drug (Oxalid, Tandearil).

Phenylbutazone.   Nonsteroidal anti-inflammatory drug (Azolid, Butazolidin, Sterazolidin).

Probenecid.   A uricosuric agent that aids in the increase of urinary excretion of uric acid. Used in treatment of gout and gouty arthritis (Benemid, Colbenemid, Polycillin, PRB).

Rheumatic fever.   An inflammatory disease exhibiting high fever, swelling of joints, and inflammation of the heart muscles and valves.

Rheumatism.   A general term for conditions involving soreness, swelling, or stiffness of the muscles or joints.

Rheumatoid factor.   An agent found in the blood of a large number of people with rheumatoid arthritis; frequently tested for as an aid to diagnosis.

Rheumatologist.   A physician who specializes in the diagnosis and treatment of rheumatic and arthritic diseases.

Sacroiliac.   Joint connecting the hip bones and the lower vertebra of the spine.

Salicylates.   Drugs used to relieve the pain and/or inflammation of rheumatic and arthritic muscles and joints. Aspirin is the most commonly used salicylate in the treatment of arthritis.

Scleroderma.   Disease, in which swelling of the skin is followed by hardening, atrophy, deformity, and ulceration. Can become generalized, resulting in immobility of the face, contraction of the fingers, and excessive fibrous tissue in the heart muscle, kidneys, digestive tract, and lungs.

Sclerosis.   A hardening of the underlying bone of a joint destroyed by arthritis; caused by new bone formation as a result of repeated efforts to use the joint.

Subluxation.   Incomplete dislocation of a joint, which can be corrected manually.

Synovectomy.   Removal of the lining of the capsule of a joint.

Synovial fluid.   Transparent lubricating fluid secreted by synovial membrane; resembles white of an egg.

Synovial membrane.   Membrane that secretes synovial fluid; found in *bursae*, joint cavities, and tendon sheaths.

Systemic lupus erythematosus.   Generally serious disease characterized by arthritic symptoms and changes in the blood system. Usually identified by a "butterfly" rash appearing across the bridge of the nose.

Tolmetin sodium.   Generic name for an anti-inflammatory drug (Tolectin).

Tophi.   Chalky lumps of solidified uric acid crystals found on the elbows, earlobes, and joints of the hands and feet, which are generally a sign of gouty arthritis.

Ulnar deviation.   Displacement of the hand in the direction of the little finger.

Ultrasound.   Vibrations with the same physical nature as sound but with frequencies above the range of human hearing; sometimes used to treat musculoskeletal disorders.

Uric acid.   Acid formed by urine; excess is a symptom of gout.

Valgus deformity.   A type of deformity in which the body part is bent outward from the center of the body.

Chapter 3: Cancer

Adjuvant treatment. Drugs or x-rays administered before or after surgery as a precautionary measure when uncertain if a cancer has spread beyond the site of the original tumor.

Ames test. Test to identify chemicals that alter the genetic structure of cells. Chemicals that do so are usually cancer-causing.

Anaplastic. Lacking in differentiated structure; reversion (of cells) to a more primitive type.

Antibody. Protein produced by the body's immune system in response to an intruder; serves to render intruders harmless.

Anticarcinogen. Agent that offers protection against a carcinogen.

Antigen. Protein that serves to identify intruders that have invaded the body. Antigens provoke immune systems to form antibodies.

Ascites. Accumulation of fluid in the abdominal cavity.

Atrophic. Wasted or shrunken; describes tumors where the scarring is so intense that the surrounding tissues are contracted.

BCG. Bacillus-Calmette-Guérin, a vaccine for immunization against tuberculosis.

Benign tumors. Abnormal growths, almost always enclosed in a fibrous capsule, that do not spread to other parts of the body.

Biopsy. Removal and microscopic examination of tissue from the body for the pupose of diagnosis.

Blood count. Count of the number of white and red blood cells and platelets in a sample of blood; abnormalities in the blood count may indicate infection, anemia, or hemorrhaging.

Bronchus. Main air passages leading from the trachea (windpipe) to the lungs.

Cachexia. Malnutrition and wasting of the body.

Cancer. General term for the disease characterized by uncontrolled cell growth.

Carcinogen. Cancer-producing substance or condition.

Carcinoma. Cancer of the epithelial cells, which make up the skin and line the surfaces of body organs.

Chemotherapy. Drug treatment to destroy cancerous cells.

Colostomy. Opening for feces constructed in the abdominal wall when the rectum has been removed.

Cyst. Small sac filled with fluid or diseased matter.

Cytostasis. Slowing of the proliferative rate of cells.

Cytotoxic. Able to destroy cells.

Differentiated cells. Mature cells that perform a specific function in the body, for example, blood cells, skin cells, or bone cells.

Dysplasia. Faulty or abnormal development or growth.

Edema. Presence of swelling caused by large amounts of fluid in the intercellular spaces of the body.

Electron microscopy. Technique for visualizing material through the microscope that uses beams of electrons instead of light beams, thereby permitting clearer magnification than is possible with the ordinary microscope.

Electron therapy. Direct cancer therapy by electrons.

Epidemiology. Scientific study of factors determining the frequency and distribution of disease.

Epithelium. Outer layer of cells covering the skin and other surfaces.

Estrogen. Female sex hormone.

Gene. Segment of a chromosome that contains a unit of genetic information.

Gonadectomy. Excision of an ovary or testis.

Hodgkin's disease. Cancer of the lymphatic system.

Hormone. A chemical produced by a gland. Each type stimulates its target organ to specific action.

Immune system. Body's line of defense against disease. Body forms antibodies against bacteria and viruses that cause disease.

Immunosuppression. Suppression of the body's immune responses. Certain chemicals initiate immunosuppression.

Immunotherapy. Treatment of cancer by increasing the response of the body's immune system so that it destroys cancer cells.

Initiation. The silent beginning of the cancer process.

In situ. Confined to a small site of origin.

Interferon. Special proteins made by cells to fight virus infection.

Interphase. "Resting" period of cell, when it is not dividing.

Ionizing radiation. Radiation that separates molecules into charged particles (ions), such as X-rays.

Jaundice. Yellowish staining of the skin and other tissues by bile pigments.

Laryngectomy. Surgical removal of the vocal cords or voice box.

Leukemia. Cancer of the blood-forming organs such as bone marrow, with marked increase in the number of white blood cells (leukocytes).

Linear accelator. A machine producing high-energy radiations.

Lymph. The fluid that flows in the lymphatic system and eventually empties into the venous circulation, almost colorless, composed of tissue fluids, proteins, and some blood cells.

Lymphatic system. A drainage system that cleanses the fluid between cells and deposits the wastes from that fluid into the body's blood system.

Lymph node (lymph gland). A discrete collection of lymphocytes situated at the junction of lymphatic vessels; fluids in vessels pass through lymph nodes to be cleansed.

Lymphocytes. White blood corpuscles arising in lymph glands and nodes, instrumental in the immunological processes of the body.

Lymphoma. Cancer of the lymph tissue, which is part of the body's immune system.

Macrophase. A large cell with the ability to destroy bacteria and dead or abnormal cells.

Malignant. Life-threatening.

Malignant tumor. A tumor showing invasive properties.

Mammography. X-ray examination of the breast. A mammogram can detect breast tumors while they are still too small to be felt.

Mastectomy. Surgical removal of the breast.

Melanoma. A serious skin tumor usually containing dark pigment.

Metastasis. Secondary tumor centers at a distance from the original tumor, resulting from the transportation of tumor cells by blood or lymph streams.

Metastatic pathway. The path traveled by cancerous cells when they spread from a tumor to distant parts of the body.

Mucous membranes. Secretion producing lining tissue of such organs as the mouth and the intestine.

Mutation. A change in the structure of a gene.

Neoplasm. Any abnormal new growth or tumor, either benign or malignant.

Oncology. The branch of medicine that studies tumors.

Oncologist. A physician specializing in the treatment of cancer.

Oxygen effect. Enhancement of radiosensitivity of cells because of the presence of oxygen.

Palliative.   Anything that serves to eliminate the symptoms of, but cannot cure, a disease.

Palpation.   Application of the fingers to the body for the purpose of diagnosis.

Pap smear.   Microscopic examination of cells taken simply and painlessly from the cervix to detect cancer of the cervix before a tumor can be seen or felt.

Platelet.   Irregularly shaped disc in the circulating blood essential for blood clotting.

Polyp.   A mass of swollen tissue projecting into a body cavity, usually benign, often occurring in the mouth, bladder, or intestine.

Precancer.   Lesion that has a significant probability of developing into cancer in the course of time.

Primary tumor.   Original, or the first, cancerous tumor to have developed in a patient's body.

Prosthetic device.   Artificial device used to replace a part of the body.

Rad.   A measure of the amount of ionizing radiation absorbed by tissues.

Radiation sickness.   Illness sometimes caused by radiation therapy; characterized by nausea, lack of appetite, vomiting, and diarrhea.

Radiation therapy.   Use of x-rays, electrons, neutrons, gamma rays, etc., to destroy malignant tumors.

Radical mastectomy.   Removal of the breast, tumor, pectoral muscles and lymph nodes of the axilla.

Radiotherapy.   See *Radiation therapy*.

Remission.   Temporary lessening in the severity of a disease.

Resectable.   Amenable to surgical removal.

Resection.   Surgical removal of an organ or part of an organ or tissue.

Reticulo-endothelial system.   System of lymphocytes and other macrophages capable of destroying foreign cells, present in the network of the spleen, lymph nodes, and other organs.

Reticulosis.   Malignant disease of some part of the reticulo-endothelial system.

Sarcoma.   Cancer of the supporting structures of the body like bone, cartilage, and muscle.

Secondary tumor.   A tumor that develops in a person who already has cancer.

Staging operation.   Series of biopsies on various organs and lymph nodes throughout the body to determine how far a cancer has spread.

Telecobalt unit.   Machine producing high-energy radiations.

Tissue. Collection of different cells organized to perfrom a specific function.

Tumor. Abnormal growth of tissue, benign or malignant, that serves no useful purpose in the body.

Tylectomy. Operation restricted to the local removal of a tumor.

Undifferentiated cells. Immature cells incapable of performing their proper function in the body.

Urostomy. Opening for urine constructed in the abdominal wall of a patient whose bladder has been removed.

White blood cells. Produced in the bone marrow and the lymph nodes, help fight infection.

Wilms' tumor. An embryonal tumor of the kidney.

Xerography. X-ray examination of the breast; uses more radiation and produces clearer pictures than a mammogram.

Chapter 4: The Dementias

Abstract thinking. Ability to put together concepts in new forms and combine ideas; ability to do things like arithmetic and reading.

Acetylcholine. Chemical substance used by neurons to communicate with each other.

Activities of daily living. Specific activities encountered during the normal daily routine—bed, eating, hygiene, dressing, utilities, communication, locomotion, toileting.

Activity level. Refers to how frequently a person engages in various activities, such as walking or sleeping.

ADL. See *Activities of daily living*.

Agitation. State of extreme restlessness and apprehension.

Agonist. A muscle in a state of contraction, opposing the action of another muscle, called the antagonist, which relaxes at the same time.

Aluminum. Metallic element sometimes found in abnormal amounts in the brains of people who have Alzheimer's disease.

Alzheimer's disease. Disorder that affects the cells of the brain, resulting in a type of dementia that progressively worsens and cannot be cured.

Apathy. Lacking feeling or emotion; indifference.

Ataxia. Lack of muscular coordination; inability to control movement.

CT scan (Computerized Tomography).   Type of x-ray that gives an accurate picture of the brain, revealing type and extent of damage.

Catastrophic reaction.   See Panic Reaction.

Catabolism.   The breakdown of chemical compounds by the body into smaller particles, which results in the production of energy and the accumulation of waste products.

Cerebral cortex.   Also called "gray matter" of the brain, outer part of the cerebrum where most of the cells are located.

Chemical imbalances.   Abnormal concentrations of various substances in the blood; can be caused by malnutrition.

Chromosomes.   A group of threadlike structures, composed of genes; humans have twenty-three pairs of chromosomes.

Clot.   A semisolidified mass of blood cells.

Conservatorship.   Also known as *guardianship of property*; the appointment by the court of a legal guardian to act for another person in financial matters when a person has been declared incompetent.

Controlled environment.   An environment set up by an occupational therapist to test a person's ability to manage ADLs.

Creutzfeldt-Jakob disease.   A type of encephalopathy characterized by dementia that progresses quickly, resulting in total helplessness or death within a year; believed to be caused by a virus.

Cryptococcal infections.   Fungus infections that affect the central nervous system.

Custodial care.   A level of care designated by nursing homes, meaning that the person requires no acute or skilled (requiring an R.N. or M.D.) care but needs supervision and continuous assisitance with ADLs.

Day care.   A program which the person attends during the day, the focus of which is therapeutic recreation and socialization for the person and respite for his family.

Death.   The cessation of life.

Degeneration.   Deterioration of tissues, resulting in function loss.

Dementia.   Deprived of mind.

Dementia pugilistica.   Abuse of the brain, generally occurring in boxing, which can cause swelling, bleeding, and eventual damage.

Depression.   Emotional state characterized by loss of interest in one's surroundings and lack of energy; great sadness.

Dehydration.   Loss of water from the body.

Diuretics.   Drugs that increase the discharge of water through urination.

Disorientation.   Mental confusion as to person, place, or time.

Drug reactions.   Chemical process by which one drug reacts adversely with another, resulting in side effects or decreased effectiveness of the drugs.

Electrocardiogram (ECG, EKG).   A graphic record of the electric currents produced by the contraction of the heart muscle.

Electroencephalogram (EEG).   A graphic record of the electric current activity of the brain. The test is done by applying electrodes to the surface of the scalp.

Face–hand test.   Determines whether a disorder is due to a functional or organic cause; the person closes his eyes and places his hands on his knees, while the physician strokes his cheek and the back of his hand and asks the person which side is being stroked.

Fibers.   Thin threadlike structures

Flattening of affect.   The absence of appropriate emotional responses.

Focal signs.   Neurological signs, such as limb weakness, that help to diagnose Alzheimer's

Gait.   Manner of walking.

Gait ataxia.   Inability to coordinate movements when walking.

Genetic.   Hereditary; the passing of traits through successive generations.

Grasp reflex.   The immediate grasping of an object placed in the hand; occurs normally in infants.

Guardian of Property.   See *Conservatorship*.

Guardian of person.   Legal guardian appointed by the court to decide issues about the person's care, such as nursing home placement.

Guardianship of property procedure.   A petition is filed with the court asking for determination of the person's competency to manage his affairs. If subject is found incompetent by a judge, a legal guardian will be appointed to act for the person in financial matters.

Hardening of the arteries.   *Arteriosclerosis*: Mineral and fatty deposits on the wall of the artery make it narrow and stiff, resulting in high blood pressure; the most serious form involves the blood vessels of the heart and brain.

Huntington's disease.   A hereditary, progressive, degenerative disease that results in mental deterioration, characterized by involuntary jerky movements of the trunk and limbs (chorea).

Hypoglycemia.   Too little glucose in the blood.

Immunological defects.   Occur when the body produces substances that destroy normal tissue.

Immune system.   System of protection against disease and infection.

Incontinence.   Inability to voluntarily control the discharge of feces and/or urine.

Infarct.   Death of tissue.

Infectious agents.   Bacteria that cause disease.

Impairment.   A physiological or mental loss resulting from a disease or accident.

Involuntary function.   Those bodily functions automatically performed without thought, such as breathing.

Learning.   Ability to acquire, understand, and use new information.

Lumbar puncture.   Insertion of hollow needle between the third and fourth vertebrae to remove a sample of spinal fluid for examination.

Malnutrition.   Inadequate amount or the wrong proportion of nutrients.

Manganese.   Metallic element which, when accumulated in the brain, is thought possibly to cause Alzheimer's.

Manic-depressive illness.   Mental disorder characterized by states of elation, talkativeness, flight of ideas, followed by state of emotional withdrawal, irritability, and anger.

Memory.   Process of recalling, reproducing, and recognizing that which was learned in the past.

Memory loss.   The inability to recall, reproduce, or recognize things previously learned.

Meningitis.   Inflammation of the membranes covering the brain and spinal cord, caused by infection of the cerebrospinal fluid. Symptoms include sore throat, dullness, fever, chills, rapid pulse, rash, body aches, vomiting, and severe pain; effective treatment is available, resulting in recovery.

Mental impairment.   Loss of intellectual ability of sufficient severity to interfere with memory, judgment, and personality functioning.

Mental status examination.   A series of eight questions that indicate a person's orientation to time and place, his recent and remote memory, and his alertness. The eight questions all concern level of ability to independently control bladder and bowel functions, transfer from bed to chair, do personal care such as combing one's hair and teeth brushing, dress, cook, bathe, shop, do housekeeping, and travel.
>   Severely impaired.   Unable to do any of these things
>   Moderately impaired.   Able to wash, dress and undress
>   Mild to moderately impaired.   Able to cook, bathe, and shop
>   Mild to unimpaired.   Able to travel alone safely

Metabolic.   Process of consumption of oxygen and nutrients for energy production and maintenance of healthy tissue.

Multi-infarct dementia.   Type of dementia caused by a series of strokes. Accounts for 10 to 20 percent of people with dementia.

Multiple sclerosis. Nervous system disorder marked by degeneration and scarring of the nervous tissue over a period of years; movement of the limbs becomes spastic and jerky, eventually resulting in paralysis; speech becomes slurred and difficult; eventually affects basic systems such as digestion, resulting in total functional loss. Onset before forty; cause unknown.

Muscle spasm. Sudden involuntary contraction of a muscle, causing pain.

Myoclonus. See *Muscle spasm*

Myoclonic. Muscle spasm characterized by alternating contraction and relaxation of the muscle.

Neurosis. An emotional disorder not accompanied by severe personality change; the feeling of unconscious anxiety in certain situations.

Neurofilaments. Small, tubular structures inside nerve cells, which become twisted and tangled in Alzheimer's disease.

Nucleus basalis. An area of the brain located below the cortex; sends information to the cortex.

Over-the-counter drugs. Drugs that can be bought without a prescription.

Palmomentel reflex (palm-chin). When the palm of the hand is scratched, the muscles of the chin, on the same side of the body, twitch.

Panic reaction. Extreme fear or anxiety.

Parkinson's disease. A progressive disorder characterized by stiffness and slowness of voluntary movement, stooped posture, shuffling gait (festinating), rigidity of facial expressions, and shaking of limbs. Onset between fifty and sixty-five; cause unknown.

Pernicious anemia. Blood disorder caused by inability to absorb Vitamin B_{12}.

Petition. Process of appealing to the court for guardianship.

Pick's disease. Progressive dementia characterized by atrophy of the *cerebral cortex* of the brain.

Physostigmine (salicylate). Drug that improves the tone and action of skeletal muscle.

Plaques. Areas of degeneration in the brain.

Proteins. Compounds built up of amino acids and essential for growth and repair of the body.

Pseudo-dementia. A condition of apathy that results in dementia, but without any real loss of intelligence; usually caused by or related to depression or other psychiatric syndrome.

Reactive depression. Depression resulting from a specific incident, such as death of a spouse; distinguished from dementia by its rapid onset and response to treatment.

Reflexes.   Involuntary reaction to a stimulus.

Sedimentation rate.   Rate at which red cells settle out of blood that has been prevented from clotting.

Senile dementia.   Mental deterioration associated with increasing age.

Severely impaired.   See *Mental status examination.*

Snout reflex.   Primitive reflex present in normal newborns and adults with diffuse brain disease.

Tangles.   Pathologically twisted neurofilaments.

Testamentary capacity.   Ability to make a will under one's own discretion when legally considered mentally competent.

Thyroid hormone, thyroxin.   Insufficient amount leads to stunted growth and mental deficiency; excessive production leads to restlessness and rapid heartbeat.

Toxin.   Poison.

Transmitter.   Chemical that is put out by one cell to communicate a message to an adjacent cell that is translated into an electrical impulse or unit.

Tuberculosis.   Infectious disease spread through the body by the lymph and blood vessels; infection may or may not be localized in one area of the body; symptoms include fever, emaciation, and night sweats.

Virus.   Minute infectious agent capable of living and reproducing only in living cells.

Chapter 5: Diabetes

Alpha cells.   Cells of the pancreas that produce *glucagon.*

Beta cells.   Cells of the pancreas that produce insulin.

Blood glucose testing.   Testing for glucose levels in the blood.

Blood sugar levels.   The concentration of glucose in the blood.

Blood sugar dynamics.   Pattern of changes in blood sugar levels that emerges for each individual when assessing food intake, medication, exercise, stress, and other variables.

Brittle.   A form of diabetes particularly sensitive to changes in blood sugar and insulin levels, also called labile, unstable, insulin-sensitive.

Carbohydrate.   Fuel for the body easily changed into simple sugars, mainly glucose.

Coma.   Loss of consciousness, which may occur as a result of severe acidosis or blood sugar levels that are too high or too low. Unconsciousness due to low blood sugar is generally called an *insulin reaction.*

Control. Keeping blood sugars as close to the normal range as possible, usually between 60 and 120 mg/dl.

Dead space. The space between the needle and the hub of an insulin syringe, which can retain between 4 and 8 units of insulin and thus cause an improper dose to be administered when mixing insulins.

Diabetes mellitus. Inability of the cells of the body to use carbohydrates properly due to a lack of insulin, also called *diabetes.*

Diabetologist. A physician who specializes in the treatment of patients with diabetes mellitus.

Dietetic foods. Foods for special diets, *not necessarily* intended for diabetic diets.

Exchange lists. Lists of foods used in the exchange system of meal planning.

Exchange system. Technique for allocating foods of similar value into groups so that substitution can be made in a basic meal pattern.

Exercise plan. Pattern of daily exercise, based on blood sugar dynamics and food intake, that helps maintain normal blood sugar levels.

Fasting blood sugar (FBS). Blood glucose test on people who have had no food for eight to twelve hours.

Fat. Fuel available for the body to use, processed less rapidly than carbohydrates and proteins. Fat that is not used immediately is stored in fat cells until it is needed.

Gangrene. Death of tissue, usually due to loss of the blood supply, usually seen in the feet.

Glucagon. A protein hormone secreted by the alpha cells of the pancreas, which raises blood sugar levels and helps mobilize stored sugar and counteracts hypoglycemic reactions.

Glucose. The chief source of energy in humans, also known as dextrose or blood sugar.

Glucose tolerance test. A test for detecting diabetes.

Glycogen. Stored form of sugar in the liver.

Home blood glucose testing. A drop of blood from a finger prick deposited on a test strip, with color development measured by the eye or a meter indicating the amount of glucose present.

Hyperglycemia. A condition in which the blood sugar is higher than normal.

Hypoglycemia. A condition in which the blood sugar is lower than normal.

Impotence. Inability to have and sustain an erection.

Insulin. A protein hormone, secreted by the beta cells of the pancreas, which regulates the glucose going from the blood into body cells.

Insulin-dependent diabetes. Formerly *juvenile diabetes.* Usually occurs early in childhood or adolescence and indicates that person requires insulin therapy.

Insulin-independent diabetes.   Also called *maturity-onset diabetes.*

Ketoacidosis.   A condition in which the amount of ketone bodies in the blood increases when a diabetic has too little insulin and there is a rapid breakdown of fat.

Ketone bodies.   Substances formed during digestion of fat which may indicate infection.

Ketonuria.   The presence of ketones in the urine.

Maturity-onset diabetes.   Diabetes that can be managed by meal planning alone or a combination of meal planning and oral hypoglycemic agents. Also called *insulin-independent diabetes.*

Meal Plan.   Eating plan used to distribute calories, carbohydrate, protein, and fat throughout the day.

Nephropathy.   A degenerative kidney disease.

Neuropathy.   A disorder of the nerves from many causes. In diabetes, affected nerves to the feet and legs can produce changes in sensation and reflexes when severe; bowel and bladder function may also be affected.

Ophthalmologist.   A medical doctor who specializes in diseases of the eye and their treatment.

Oral hypoglycemic agent.   A medication that lowers blood glucose levels and is taken by mouth.

Pancreas.   A gland located behind the lower stomach that contains the cells that produce insulin and glucagon.

Periodontal disease.   Disease of the gums and other tissues that support and maintain the teeth in the jaws.

Photocoagulation.   A process that uses laser beams to repair damaged retinas.

Podiatrist.   A health professional with intensive training in the care of the lower extremities.

Polydipsia.   Excessive thirst.

Polyphagia.   Excessive hunger.

Polyuria.   Excessive urination.

Postprandial.   After a meal.

Postprandial blood sugar test.   Test for blood glucose performed on patients after a meal or after drinking a glucose solution of 100 grams of carbohydrate.

Protein.   A fuel for the body that is used more slowly than glucose.

Pruritis.   Genital itching, which may develop in women with persistently elevated blood sugar levels; sometimes a clue to uncontrolled diabetes.

Reagent strip.   A chemically treated strip of paper that reacts to blood or urine in a testing procedure.

Retina.   A multilayered portion of the eye that receives light and transforms it into energy, which is transmitted to the brain through the optic nerve.

Retinopathy.   Disease or injury of the retina.

Sulfonylureas.   A group of drugs used for oral treatment of diabetes.

Syringes.   Tool used to measure and inject insulin.

Urine testing.   Testing of urine to detect blood sugar levels.

Vitreous (corpus).   A clear, jellylike substance that supports the inside of the eye between the lens and retina.

Chapter 6: The Epilepsies

Absence.   A form of seizure characterized by momentary lapse of consciousness or attention (also called *petit mal*).

"Active" epilepsy.   Seizures not yet under control for five years with medicine.

Akinetic seizure.   A form of generalized seizure lasting from about a half a minute to several minutes, observed especially in children, characterized by loss of mobility and falling, even though muscle tone is preserved, and by loss of consciousness or clouding.

Angiogram.   An X-ray film series demonstrating the arterial system after injection of a radio-opaque material into an artery.

Anticonvulsant.   Medication that prevents or arrests seizures.

Ataxia.   Loss of muscle coordination.

Aura.   A premonition, a peculiar sensation or warning immediately preceding an epileptic attack, which the patient recognizes as the beginning of a seizure; may be noises in the ears, flashes of light, vertigo, etc.

Biofeedback.   A training technique used to enable an individual to gain some voluntary control over automatic body functions.

Blood level monitoring.   Laboratory tests to determine the level of medication in the bloodstream in order to measure the therapeutic effectiveness.

Carbamazepine.   An *anticonvulsant* as well as an analgesic drug used for neuritic pain (Tegretol).

Cerebellum.   The posterior brain mass, lying beneath the posterior portion of the cerebrum, above the pons and medulla; chief functions are the coordination of fine voluntary movements and posture.

Cerebral palsy.   A defect of motor function and coordination related to damage of the brain.

Cerebrum. The largest and uppermost portion of the brain, including the cerebral hemispheres, basal ganglia, and rhinencephalon.

Complex partial seizures. Partial seizures characterized by subjective symptoms like feelings of strangeness or familiarity, by visions or illusions, or by involuntary and apparently purposeful activities followed by amnesia for these events; the old term for these seizures is "psychomotor seizures"; commonly arise in the temporal lobe.

Computerized tomography, CT Scanning. A diagnostic technique that provides cross-sectional X-ray pictures of the brain; has proven useful in the diagnosis of the causes of certain types of epilepsy.

Congenital malformation. A defect existing at birth, due to either heredity or some influence during gestation.

Cortical excision. Surgical removal of a portion of the cortex of the brain.

Convulsion. Involuntary contractions of the body musculature, usually discontinuous and repetitive.

Dilantin. See *phenytoin*.

Electroencephalogram (EEG). A graphic recording of the electrical activity of the brain.

Electrode. An electrical terminal designed to make contact with a structure for stimulating or recording.

Epilepsy. A chronic brain disorder of various causes characterized by recurrent seizures due to excessive discharge of cerebral neurons.

Epileptic personality. A term suggesting erroneously that epileptics exhibit certain behavioral characteristics specific for epilepsy; instead, a variety of behavioral and affective disorders of diverse origins may occur in individuals who suffer from epileptic seizures.

Epileptic psychosis. Hallucinatory paranoid psychosis occurring in subjects with epilepsy, particularly temporal lobe epilepsy; tends to occur in subjects whose seizures are tapering off either spontaneously or in response to treatment.

Febrile seizures. Convulsions that accompany a high fever, typically occurring in childhood.

Grand mal. Severe, generalized seizures involving loss of consciousness and muscular contractions.

Ictal. Referring to the seizure event.

Idiopathic. Denoting a disease of unknown cause.

Infantile spasms. A form of epilepsy occurring usually in the first year of life and characterized by frequent tonic epileptic seizures of brief duration.

Meningitis. Inflammation of the membranes of the brain or spinal cord; common causes are bacterial or viral.

Metabolic disorders.   Disturbances of the complex of physical and chemical processes involved in the maintenance of life.

Myoclonic seizure.   A generalized convulsive epileptic seizure of particularly brief duration, commonly manifesting itself as a sudden massive jerk of the entire body, which may throw the subject to the ground.

Neurological impairment.   A impairment of the structure or function of part or all of the nervous system; may occur in many disorders including epilepsy, cerebral palsy, and mental retardation.

Neuropathy.   Any disease of the peripheral nervous system.

Partial seizures (focal or local).   Seizures originating locally in some part of the brain as opposed to those which affect the brain generally from the onset of the seizure. Partial seizures with elementary symptomatology may begin with sensation or movement of some part of the body, or with visual or auditory sensations; partial seizures with complex symptomatology (psychomotor seizures) begin with changes in thought or feeling and involve coordinated movement (see *complex partial seizures*); nature of the onset of the seizure depends upon the part of the brain in which the focus is located.

Petit mal epilepsy.   A form of primary generalized epilepsy characterized by attacks of brief impairment of consciousness often associated with flickering of the eyelids and mild twitching of the mouth (also called *absence*).

Phenobarbital.   A commonly used anticonvulsant also having a sedative and hypnotic action.

Phenytoin.   An anticonvulsant drug commonly used for generalized tonic-clonic and partial seizures (diphenylhydantoin, Dilantin).

Pneumoencephalogram.   The X-ray picture of the skull and its contents taken after introducing air or gas into the subarachnoid space, rarely done since the advent of *CT scanning*.

Postictal.   Referring to the time period following a seizure.

Primary generalized seizure.   Seizure have onset characterized by sudden loss of consciousness, appearing to affect the brain as a whole from the onset; most common forms are tonic-clonic (*grand mal*) and absence (*petit mal*); also included are *myoclonic seizures, akinetic seizures,* and *infantile spasms.*

Primidone.   An anticonvulsant drug used in the treatment of grand mal and psychomotor epilepsy (Mysoline).

Psychomotor epilepsy.   See *complex partial seizures.*

Seizure.   Attack of cerebral origin affecting a person in apparent good health or causing a sudden aggravation of a chronic pathological state; such attacks consist of sudden and transitory abnormal phenomena of a motor, sensory, autonomic, or psychic nature resulting from transient dysfunction of part or all of the brain.

Sodium valproate.   A newer anticonvulsant medication with actions against absence and generalized motor seizures (Depakene).

Status epilepticus.   A condition in which one major attack of epilepsy succeeds another with little or no intermission.

Subarachnoid space.   The space beneath the arachnoid membrane, between it and the pia mater; contains cerebrospinal fluid.

Tonic seizures.   A state of continuous muscular contraction, as opposed to intermittent contraction.

Chapter 7:   Heart Disease

Acidosis.   Metabolic condition in which the acid content of the blood or body tissues is too great; may result from failure of the lungs to remove carbon dioxide or from an overproduction of acid substances in the body's tissues.

Adrenal glands.   Pair of endocrine (hormone) secreting glands; the adrenal medulla, the inner portion of each, secretes epinephrine, a heart stimulant, and norepinephrine, a blood vessel constrictor. The outer portion, the adrenal cortex, secretes steroid hormones that influence the body's handling of salt water, carbohydrates, and other aspects of metabolism.

Adrenalin.   Same as *epinephrine*, a hormone which stimulates the rate and contractile force of heart.

Adrenergic blocking agents.   Used to decrease heart rate and vigor of heart contraction and to suppress constriction of blood vessels; block the normal response of an organ or tissue to nerve impulses transmitted to the adrenergic portion of the autonomic nervous system.

Aneurysm.   Ballooning out of the wall of a vein, artery, or the heart due to the weakening of the wall.

Angina pectoris.   Commonly referred to as angina, episode of chest pain usually caused by decreased blood flow to the heart.

Angiography.   The study of blood vessels, either arteries or veins, made by the injection of a radio-opaque substance, permitting visualization by x-ray.

Anoxia.   Absence of oxygen; condition most frequently occurs when blood supply to a certain part of the body is cut off.

Antiarrhythmic drugs.   Used to correct heart rate and rhythm; examples are lidocaine, procaine amide, *quinidine, digitalis.*

Anticoagulants.   Delay coagulation, clotting of the blood; examples are *heparin* and *coumarin* derivatives.

Antihypertensive drugs.   Used to control high blood pressure. *Diuretics* promote elimination of excess fluids. Some others, like *hydralazine*, dilate the arteries. Others, like *reserpine*, dampen the nerves that signal the arteries to constrict.

Aorta.   Main artery carrying blood from the heart to the rest of the body.

Arrhythmia.   Any variation from the normal rhythm of the heartbeat.

Arteriogram. X-ray picture of the channel of an artery made by injecting a radio-opaque substance into the blood.

Arterioles. Small muscular vessels formed from the small branches of arteries, which branch to form the capillaries.

Arteriosclerosis. Disease of arteries, often referred to as hardening of the arteries; includes and is often used synonymously with *atherosclerosis*. While the latter term refers primarily to disease of intima, arteriosclerosis may also include disease of the arterial media.

Arteritis. Inflammation of arteries.

Artery. Vessel carrying blood from the heart to body tissues.

Asymmetric septal hypertrophy (ASH). Disease of the heart muscle in which there is an enlargement of the interior walls of the left ventricle.

Atheroma. Also called *plaque*: deposit of fat and cholesterol in the inner lining of the artery wall.

Atherosclerosis. Form of *arteriosclerosis* that causes most strokes and heart attacks.

Atropine. Drug for treatment of slow heart rate, among other things.

Bacterial endocarditis. Bacterial inflammation of the inner lining of the heart affecting the heart valves.

Ball valve principle. A ball that fits in a cage over a cup-shaped opening in the seat. As the ball rises, fluid or air escapes through the opening in the seat.

Blood pressure. Force the flowing blood exerts against the artery walls. Expressed by two numbers, one over the other. Systolic (upper) pressure occurs every time the heart contracts. Diastolic (lower) pressure occurs when heart relaxes.

Bypass operation. A surgical procedure in which a graft is attached to an artery above and below the site of obstruction for the purpose of providing a normal blood flow distal to the diseased vessel.

Cannula. A tube used for insertion into a blood vessel or the heart.

Cardiac. Pertaining to the heart; sometimes refers to a person who has heart disease.

Cardiac arrest. Heartbeat ceases, blood pressure drops abruptly, and circulation of the blood ceases.

Cardiac reserve. Difference between the cardiac output at rest and at the maximum physical effort.

Cardiomyopathy. Diagnostic term for diseases involving the heart muscle.

Carditis. Inflammation of the heart.

Carotid arteries. The principal arteries that supply blood to the brain.

Catheter. Thin, flexible tube that can be guided into body organs.

Cerebrovascular accident. See under "Chapter 9: Stroke."

Coagulation. Formation of a clot; thickening of a liquid.

Coarctation of the aorta. Narrowing of the aorta.

Congestive heart failure. With the heart unable to pump required amount of blood, body tissues become congested with fluid accumulating in abdomen, legs, and/or lungs.

Coronary bypass surgery. Improves blood supply to heart muscle by constructing detours through which blood can bypass narrowed portions of coronary arteries.

Coronary heart disease. Also called *coronary artery disease* and *ischemic heart disease:* decreased blood supply to heart caused by narrowing of coronary arteries.

Coronary occlusion. Obstruction in a branch of one of the coronary arteries, which hinders the flow of blood to some part of the heart muscle.

Collateral circulation. Other blood vessels begin to supply that area of the heart muscle supplied formerly by the damaged artery.

Coumarin. *Anticoagulant.*

Cyanosis. Blueness of skin caused by insufficient oxygen in the blood.

Defibrillation. Treatment, usually with electric shock, to stop fibrillation.

Diastole. See *Blood pressure.*

Digitalis. Drug from leaves of the foxglove plant that stimulates pumping of the heart.

Diuretic. Drug that promotes excretion of urine.

Dyspnea. Shortness of breath.

Echocardiography. A diagnostic tool in which pulses of sound (ultrasound) are transmitted into the body and the echoes returning from the surfaces of the heart and other structures are electronically plotted and recorded.

Edema. Swelling due to abnormally large amounts of fluid in the tissues of the body.

Electrocardiogram. Also referred to as *ECG* or *EKG*; graphic record of electrical currents generated by the heart.

Embolism. Defined under "Chapter 9: Stroke," below.

Endarterectomy. Surgical removal of the innermost lining of an artery when it is thickened by fatty deposits and blood clots.

Endocarditis. Inflammation of the inner lining of the heart, usually associated with acute rheumatic fever or some infectious agent.

Endocardium. Thin, smooth membrane forming the inner surface of the heart.

Epicardium. Outer layer of the heart wall. Also called the *visceral pericardium.*

Epinephrine. See *adrenaline*.

Femoral artery. Main blood vessel supplying blood to the leg.

Fibrillation. Kind of cardiac arrhythmia. Individual muscle fibers take up independent irregular contractions. *Atrial fibrillation* involves very rapid, irregular contractions of the atria, followed irregularly by contractions of the ventricles. *Ventricular fibrillation* involves contractions of the ventricles that are irregular, haphazard, and ineffective.

Fluoroscope. X-rays are passed through the body onto a fluorescent screen, where the shadows of the beating heart and other organs can be seen.

Gallop rhythm. An extra heart sound that, when the heart rate is rapid enough, resembles a horse's gallop.

Heart attack. Death of a portion of heart muscle as a result of an obstruction preventing an adequate supply of oxygen to the heart. Sometimes referred to in terms of the obstruction (*coronary occlusion, coronary thrombosis,* or *coronary*) and sometimes in terms of muscle damage (*myocardial infarction, infarct,* or *MI*).

Heart block. Electrical impulse that triggers heartbeat as slowed or blocked.

Heart failure. A condition in which the heart is unable to pump the amount of blood required to maintain normal circulation.

Heart–lung machine. A machine through which the bloodstream is diverted for pumping and oxygenation, for example, during heart surgery.

Heart massage. Also called *cardiac massage*; an emergency technique using compression of the heart to keep the blood pumping through the body in the event the heart stops pumping effectively.

Hemoglobin. The oxygen-carrying red pigment of the red blood cells.

Heparin. An *Anticoagulant*.

High blood pressure. Also called *hypertension*; blood pressure elevated above normal.

Hydralazine. Used to control high blood pressure.

Hypertension. See *high blood pressure*.

Hypertrophy. Enlargement or overgrowth of an organ or body part.

Hypotension. Low blood pressure.

Hypothermia. Use of low body temperature to reduce cardiac output, pulse rate, blood pressure, and oxygen consumption, since cells survive longer when chilled.

Intima. The internal coating of the blood vessel.

Ischemic. The state in which a cell or tissue has an insufficient supply of oxygen.

Lumen. The space inside a tubular structure.

Malignant hypertension. Severe high blood pressure that may cause damage to the blood vessel walls in the kidney, eye, and other organs.

Mitral insufficiency. Incomplete closing of the mitral valve between the upper and lower chamber in the left side of the heart, which permits a backflow of blood in the wrong direction.

Mitral stenosis. A narrowing of the mitral valve.

Mitral valvulotomy. A surgical operation to widen the opening of the mitral valve.

Murmur. An extra heart sound, sounding like fluid passing an obstruction, heard between the normal heart sounds.

Myocardial infarction. Death of an area of heart muscle.

Myocarditis. Inflammation of the heart muscle.

Myocardium. Muscular tissue of the heart.

Nitroglycerine. Drug that provides rapid relief of chest pain within one to three minutes in an attack of *angina pectoris*.

Pacemaker. The *sinoatrial node*; a small bundle of muscle fibers and nerves within the right atrium, which sends out electrical impulses at regular intervals to cause contraction of the heart.

Pacemaker, artificial. A mechanical device that can be used to control the heart rate and take the place of the patient's own natural pacemaker.

Pericarditis. Inflammation of the pericardial sac.

Pericardium. The saclike covering of the heart.

Peripheral vascular disease. Refers to diseases of any of the blood vessels outside of the heart and to diseases of the lymph vessels.

Plaque. See *atheroma*.

Platelets. Elements of the blood that are involved in the clotting mechanism.

Primary hypertension. Also called *essential hypertension*; high blood pressure of unknown origin.

Pulmonary artery. Vessel transporting blood from the right ventricle to the lungs.

Pulmonary edema. Failure of left ventricle to pump adequately, causing fluid to accumulate within the lungs.

Pulmonary embolus. Blood clot breaks loose and becomes lodged in one of the arteries of the lung.

Pulmonary hypertension. High blood pressure in the blood vessels of the lungs.

Quinidine. Drug to treat abnormal heartbeat.

Radioisotope scanning. Diagnostic technique in which radioisotopes injected into the bloodstream label tissues and organs for scanning.

Rales.   Crackling noises in the chest, indicative of accumulated fluid.

Rauwolfia.   Family of antihypertensive drugs from powdered whole root of Indian snake root plant.

Red blood cells.   Blood elements that carry oxygen by means of hemoglobin.

Reserpine.   Antihypertensive drug, one of the substances in the Indian snake root plant (see *Rauwolfia*).

Rheumatic fever.   An inflammatory disease that usually follows an infection by a Group A beta-streptococcal organism.

Rheumatic heart disease.   The damage done to the heart, particularly the heart valves, by one or more attacks of rheumatic fever.

Sinoatrial node.   See *Pacemaker*.

Sphygmomanometer.   An instrument for measuring blood pressure in the arteries.

Stasis.   Stopping or slowing of blood or fluid flow in body.

Stenosis.   Narrowing of an opening.

Stress test.   Diagnostic tool to determine body's response to physical exertion. As person exercises, measurements are taken in relation to heart activity.

Stroke.   See under "Chapter 9: Stroke."

Syncope.   Fainting.

Systolic.   See *Blood pressure*.

Tachycardia.   Abnormally fast heart rate.

Thrombosis.   Clot in blood vessel or heart cavity.

Ultrasound.   High-frequency sound vibrations used in diagnosis.

Vasoconstrictors.   Agents that raise blood pressure by narrowing the lumen of arterioles.

Vasodilators.   Agents that lower blood pressure by causing lumen of arterioles to widen.

Vasoinhibitors.   Agents that inhibit the action of vasomotor nerves, preventing the normal response of blood vessels to stimuli.

Vasomotor.   Any agent that affects the caliber of the vessel.

Vascular.   Pertaining to blood vessels.

Ventricle.   One of two main pumping chambers of the heart.

Venule.   Small vein.

White blood cells.   Defensive elements in blood; destroy foreign bodies.

Chapter 8:   Respiratory Diseases

Anoxia.   Deficiency of oxygen in the tissues.

Antibiotic.   Drug that can kill or inhibit the growth of bacteria (not viruses).

Autonomic nerves.   Nerves that control involuntary functions such as breathing.

Antidepressant.   Drug used to relieve symptoms of depression (Elavil and Haldol are examples).

Bacteria.   Organisms that cause infection.

Basal state.   Lowest possible level of metabolism in which the least amounts of oxygen are required.

Black lung disease.   Form of *pneumonoconiosis* arising from exposure to coal dust; industrial disease of coal miners.

Black pigment.   Black, sooty material found in the lungs when affected by emphysema and chronic bronchitis.

Blebs.   Large blisters that can be found in the lung, can contain fluid, and may reduce lung functioning.

Blood gas.   Measurement of oxygen and carbon monoxide levels in the blood that has passed through the lungs.

Breath sounds.   Sounds of air going through the lungs.

Breathalyzer.   Instrument used to analyze the contents of exhaled air.

Bronchial hygiene.   Method of cleansing the lungs of irritants and excess mucus, which involves use of bronchodilator, inhalation of moisture, and coughing to expel secretions.

Bronchial crisis.   Fits of coughing that can cause weakness in the limbs.

Bronchodilators.   Drugs that help clear the airways.

Bronchospasm.   Muscle spasm of the bronchi that causes contraction in the airways.

Bronchi.   Two tubes into which *trachea* divides at its lower end; singular is bronchus.

Bronchial tubes.   Divisions of the bronchi after they enter the lungs.

Bullae.   Large watery blisters that can occur in lungs.

Capillaries.   Network of the smallest blood vessels connecting terminal arteries with veins. Thin walls of capillaries allow for exchange of nutrients and waste products between tissues and blood.

Catarrh.   Inflammation of mucous membrane associated with chronic cough.

Chronic obstructive pulmonary disease (COPD).   Category of diseases characterized by persistently blocked bronchial air flow.

Cilia. Hairlike structures that extend from the surface of the airways and beat rhythmically to move mucus, dust particles, and other irritants from the lungs.

Cortisone drugs. Used to reduce inflammation, made to resemble cortisone, a principal hormone of the adrenal gland.

Decongestion. Reduction of nasal passage swelling.

Dust disease. See *pneumonoconiosis*.

Dyspnea. Shortness of breath.

Edema. Condition in which body tissues retain excess fluid, causing swelling.

Effluent. Streaming outward like a mist.

Expectorant. Drug that thins mucus, making it easier to expel secretions.

Humidification. Addition of moisture to the air.

Inspiration. Taking air into the lungs.

Lymph glands. Glands that help fight infection.

Macrophage. Scavenger cell of the lung that has ability to ingest inhaled irritants and remove them.

Mucolytic agent. Drug used to thin secretions.

Mucous glands. In the normal lung, glands that provide mucus for cleansing.

Nebulizer. Apparatus for spraying fine mist from liquid.

Particle size. Relates to size of water particles produced by nebulizer.

Pleura. Membrane enfolding lungs and lining thorax and diaphragm walls.

Pneumonoconiosis. *Dust disease*; formation of excessive fibrous tissue in the lungs caused by long inhalation of dust in industrial occupations. Examples are *black lung disease, silicosis,* and *asbestosis*.

Pneumonectomy. Removal of a lung.

Pneumonia. Inflammation of the lungs.

Pneumonitis. Inflammation of the lung tissue.

Postural drainage. Positioning of the body to cause expectoration or elimination of mucus and thus drain secretions from the lung.

Respirable-size particles. Small particles that can be deeply inhaled into the lung.

Respiration. Processes of moving air into (*inspiration*) and out of (expiration) the lungs; breathing.

Respiratory center. Region of the brain that regulates the movements of *respiration*.

Respiratory distress syndrome. *Dyspnea* in the newborn, especially found in premature infants. Symptoms include severe retraction of chest wall, cyanosis (in which skin turns blue from lack of oxygen), increased respiratory rate, and expiratory grunt.

Respiratory failure. Inability of the lungs to provide normal oxygenation and carbon dioxide removal.

Somnolence. Excessive sleepiness; may occur during periods of respiratory distress when oxygenation and the removal of carbon dioxide are impaired.

Spirometer. Apparatus that measures gases exhaled.

Tenacious. Refers to thick secretions difficult to remove.

Thorax. Bony part of chest.

Trachea. Tube connecting larynx with bronchial tubes.

Tracheostomy. Surgical opening in the trachea.

Tracheostomy tube. Tube inserted in the airway to ease breathing, avoiding dead space and airway obstruction.

Chapter 9: Stroke

Ageusia. Impairment of taste sense.

Agnosia. Inability to recognize an object.

Agrammatism. Reduction in grammatic flexibility and use.

Agraphia. Inability to express oneself in writing.
  Acoustic: from hearing to writing.
  Literal: inability to write letters of the alphabet.

Akinetic mutism. Unresponsiveness to the environment, except possibly with eye movement.

Alexia. Word blindness.
  Motor: patient understands but cannot read aloud.
  Musical: loss of ability to read music.
  Optical: sensory aphasia.

Amaurosis fugax. Transient monocular blindness.

Amusia. Loss of musical appreciation or expression, for example, singing.

Anarthria. Inability to articulate words properly.

Anomia. Loss of ability to name familiar objects.

Anosmia. Loss of ability of identify odors.

Anosognosia. Denial of a defect or illness not due to loss of memory; may include confabulation and evasion.

Anton's syndrome. Visual denial.

Aphasia.   Loss or partial loss of ability to understand speech or to speak.
   Amnesic: nominal.
   Anomic: loss of ability to name familiar objects.
   Auditory: word deafness.
   Broca's: expressive.
   Central: syntactical.
   Expressive-receptive: global.
   Global: all communications functions.
   Graphomotor: writing loss.
   Lichtheim's: loss of spontaneous speech but not ability to repeat words.
   Nominal: loss of ability to name objects.
   Receptive: sensory.
   Semantic: inability to recognize the significance of words.
   Sensory: inability to understand meaning of words.
   Syntactical: inability to speak sequentially.
   Tactile: inability to name objects touched.
   Transcortical: inability to repeat words.
   Verbal: expressive.

Apraxia.   Disorder of motor activity without paralysis. Errors in purposeful activity, especially as noted in dressing.
   Constructional: unable to copy simple designs.
   Ideational: inability to carry out a complex act.
   Ideomotor: knowledge of how to do it but not correctly; usually unilateral.
   Kinetic: instinctive grasping.

Astereognosis.   Loss of ability to recognize objects by handling with eyes closed.

Asymbolia.   Difficulty with visual imagery.

Asynergia.   Lack of voluntary coordination of muscles.

Ataxia.   Loss of voluntary motion.

Atopagnosia.   Loss of ability to locate a sensation.

Berry aneurysm.   Small saclike aneurysm attached to a cerebral artery through a narrow opening.

Brain scan.   A two-dimensional map of the gamma rays emitted by a radioisotope through the skull.

Cerebral embolism.   Sudden plugging of a cerebral vessel by a clot.

Cerebal hemorrhage.   Bleeding into the brain.

Cerebral infarction.   Death of part of the brain caused by obstruction of blood flow in arteries that supply the brain.

Cerebral thrombosis.   Formation or presence of a cerebral artery thrombosis.

Cerebrovascular accident (CVA).   Sudden diminution of blood supply to the brain; stroke.

Cerebrovascular disease (CVD).   Changes in the brain and in functioning due to impaired blood circulation to the brain.

Cerebrovascular event.   Same as stroke; cerebrovascular accident.

Circle of Willis.   Continuum of arteries at base of brain.

Completed stroke.   A stroke in which signs and symptoms have become stable.

Computerized tomography (CT scanning).   A diagnostic technique that provides cross-sectional x-ray pictures of the brain which illustrate the area of the brain damaged by stroke.

Diplopia.   Perception of two images of an object; double vision.

Disability score factors.   Examples include changes in posture, gait, speech, reflexes, visual fields, voluntary motions, limb strength, clonus, tremor, touch sense, and apraxia, among others.

Doppler ultrasound blood velocity detector.   A machine that sends out ultrasounds that pick up velocity of blood flow through the vein and are transmitted as sounds.

Dysarthria.   Defect in movement or coordination of organs of articulation, slurring of consonants, variations in stress and speed of speech.

Dysgraphia.   Inability to write properly.

Dyslexia.   Failure to read comprehendingly.

Dysphasia.   Loss of ability to speak or understand words in proper sequence.

Dyspraxia.   Partial loss of ability to perform motions meaningfully.

Epidural hematoma.   Collection of blood between dura mater and skull.

Hemianopia.   Defective vision of half of the visual field.
  Homonymous: both right halves or both left halves of field affected.
  Quadrantic: one-fourth of field in each eye affected.

Hemiparesis.   Muscular weakness of one side of the body.

Hemiplegia.   Paralysis of one side of the body.

Hemiplegia alterna.   Lesion in basis pedunculi.

Hemiplegia, lacunar.   Syndrome related to lacunae around cerebral vessels.

Hemiplegic posture.   Patient carries weight on good side and leans in that direction.

Ingravescent stroke.   Stroke-in-evolution; stroke in which symptoms are progressing.

Lacunae.   Softening around cerebral vessels found at autopsy in many hemiplegics.

Limbic system.   Part of brain that regulates behavior patterns; includes olfactory bulb, mamillary body, fornix, and hippocampus; related to memory.

Metamorphopia.   Distortion of size and shape of object.

Monoplegia.   Paralysis of a single limb.

Neurologic index of mental impairment (NIMI).   A standard objective examination of mental status.

Palilalia.   Reiteration of ongoing speech.

Pallhypesthesia.   Diminished vibration sense.

Paragraphia.   Mistakes in spelling or use of wrong words in writing.

Paralexia.   Transposition of words or syllables inappropriately in reading.

Parosmia.   Interference with smell.

Perseveration.   Continuation of an activity after its stimulus has been removed.

Proprioceptive neuromuscular facilitation.   Therapeutic method that relies on positioning and abnormal reflexes.

Profile, stroke prone.   Outline of major signs and symptoms that often precede stroke, like TIA, obesity, hypertension, congestive heart failure, arteriosclerosis, elevated blood lipids, diabetes, high red cell count, or blood uric acid.

Progressive stroke.   Stage of stroke before it becomes stabilized.

Prosopagnosia.   Inability to recognizes faces.

Reflex.   An involuntary action or movement.

Spasticity.   Increased muscle tone with exaggerated tendon reflexes and increased response to passive stretch.

Steal.   Shift of blood supply to an area other than where it normally would go.

Stroke.   See *Cardiovascular accident*.

Subarachnoid hemorrhage.   Bleeding into subarachnoid space.

Subdural hematoma.   Accumulation of blood between dura mater and arachnoid membrane.

Synkinesis.   Usually symmetrical unintentional movement of one limb when motion is willed in another.

Transient ischemic attack (TIA).   Reversible short-lasting symptoms resulting from interference with cerebral blood supply.

Chapter 10: Substance Abuse

Abusers.   People who use substances in ways that threaten their health or functioning.

Abstinence.   Refraining completely from using any drugs or alcohol.

Addiction. A pattern of consumption marked by compulsive taking of a substance, the need for increasing doses over time to maintain the same effect (*tolerance*), and the appearance of symptoms when it is stopped that disappear when it is reinstated (*withdrawal*).

Alcohol. A colorless, volatile, slightly aromatic, flammable liquid, one of the products of vinous fermentation, which is the intoxicating ingredient in wines and spirits. Also called *ethyl alcohol* and *ethanol*.

Alcoholism. Any form of drinking which in its extent goes beyond the traditional and customary dietary use or the ordinary compliances with the social drinking customs of the whole community concerned, irrespective of the etiological factors leading to such behavior and irrespective also of the extent to which such etiological factors are dependent upon hereditary, constitutional or acquired physiopathological and metabolic influences.—World Health Organization

> Alcoholism is a disease which is characterized by a compulsive drinking of alcohol in some form. It is an addiciton to alcohol. The drinking of alcohol produces continuing or repeated problems in the patient's life.—American Medical Association

Amphetamines. Stimulant drugs which increase the activity of the central nervous system (Methedrine, Benzedrine, Dexedrine, etc.).

Analeptics. Drugs that act as stimulants or restoratives to the central nervous system, like caffeine or amphetamine.

Barbiturates. *Depressant* drugs that decrease the activity of the central nervous system, include sleeping pills and most tranquilizers.

Blackout. Amnesia for the events of any part of a drinking episode, without loss of consciousness.

Cannabis. Drugs derived from the hemp plant: marijuana, hashish, etc.

Central nervous system (CNS). The brain and spinal cord.

CNS depressant. Any agent that will depress the functions of the central nervous system; also, a drug which may produce a calming effect or relief of emotional tension or anxiety; or drowsiness, sedation, sleep, stupor, coma or general anesthesia; or increase the pain threshold; or produce depression or apathy; or disorientation, confusion, or loss of mental acuity.

CNS stimulant. Any agent that temporarily increases the activity of the central nervous system; also, a drug which may produce extended wakefulness; elation, exhilaration, or euphoria; or alleviation of fatigue; or insomnia, irritability, or agitation; or apprehension or anxiety; or flight of ideas, loquacity, hypomania, or transient deliria.

Cocaine. A short-acting but powerful stimulant refined from the coca plant that is pharmacologically similar to the amphetamines; effects include euphoria, restlessness, and excitement.

Cocaine free base. Elaborate, hazardous do-it-yourself chemical process for converting street cocaine into a much stronger substance that is rapidly absorbed by the lungs and carried to the brain in a few seconds. Posthigh is so uncomfortable that to maintain the high, smokers often continue smoking until they are exhausted or have run out of cocaine.

Controlled substances. Plants and chemicals listed in the Federal Controlled Substances Act, the law regulating disapproved psychoactive drugs and those approved only for medical use.

Delirium. State of mental confusion marked by disorientation and hallucination; fever and certain drugs are common causes.

Delirium tremens (DTs). The most severe form of withdrawal from alcohol, marked by agitation, hallucinations, and other mental and physical imbalances.

Dependence, physical. Adaptive state that manifests itself by intense physical disturbances (*withdrawal syndrome*) when the drug is suspended from use.

Dependence, psychological. Feeling that periodic, continued administration of the drug is necessary to find pleasure, in order to avoid discomfort.

Depressant. Any agent that will decrease a body function or nerve activity.

Detoxification. Supervised withdrawal from drugs and/or alcohol in ways that prevent *withdrawal syndrome* while ridding the body of toxins.

Endorphins. Substances produced by the body that resemble the opiates in their abilities to minimize pain and produce a sense of wellbeing.

Flashback. Recurrence of symptoms associated with *LSD* or other *hallucinogens* some time after the actual drug experience.

Freebase. A smokable form of cocaine; to smoke cocaine in this form.

Fetal alcohol syndrome. Association of maternal alcoholism with congenital malformations and delayed psychomotor development; major clinical features are cerebral dysfunction, growth deficiency, and distinctive facial appearance.

Habituation. Desire but not a compulsion to take a drug with little tendency to increase the dose, some psychological but no physical dependence, and little detrimental effect on the individual.

Habit-forming drugs. May produce compulsive use; euphoria; personality changes; transient psychoses, twilight state, hallucinoses, or deliria; increased tolerance or need or desire to increase the dosage.

Hallucination. The perception of something being there that is not there.

Hallucinogens. Drugs that stimulate the nervous system and produce varied changes in perception and mood, also known as *psychedelics*; can alter orientation to time and place, consciousness, sensory pleasure, motor coordination, mood and affect, ideation, and/or personality.

Hangover. After effects of drinking; headache, oversensitivity to light and sound, etc.

Hashish. Resin from cannabis sativa plant; considerably more potent thant marijuana; high content of *THC*.

Heroin.   Narcotic and opiate derived from the poppy plant, sometimes referred to as smack, H, or horse).

Hypnotic.   Drug that induces sleep.

Intoxication.   Being under the influence of a drug, with effects ranging from stimulation and exhilaration to stupefaction and loss of consciousness.

Intramuscular.   Within a muscle, like the injection of a drug into the muscle of an arm or leg.

LSD-25.   Lysergic acid diethylamide, the principal hallucinogen used in the United States.

Marijuana.   Flowering tops of the cannabis plant.

Mescaline.   A hallucinogenic alkaloid produced synthetically or derived from peyote.

Methadone.   An opioid used in detoxification and maintenance treatment of heroin addiction; prevents heroin withdrawal symptoms, blocks the effects of heroin, has lasting effects for twenty-four hours a dose, is administered orally, and can be dispensed at a treatment center.

Methadone maintenance.   Ambulatory treatment program for maintaining heroin addicts on Methadone.

MIAO inhibitors.   Used as mood elevators, related chemically to amphetamines, potentiate alcohol, amphetamines, depressants, antihistamines, sedatives, esthetic drugs, and insulin.

Narcotic.   Class of drugs which induce sleep and stupor and relieve pain; includes opiates, anesthetics, and others.

Narcotic antagonist.   Drug that blocks or contracts the effects of opiate narcotics.

Opiates.   Narcotic drugs derived from opium: morphine, cocaine, heroin.

Opioids.   Synthetic drugs manufactured to act like opiates.

Paranoia.   Delusions of persecution.

PCP.   Phencyclidine; a synthetic depressant.

Peyote.   Anhalonium williamsii, cactus.

Polydrug use.   Use of more than one drug at a time.

Potency.   In pharmacology, the measure of relative strength of similar drugs; if a lower dose of drug A produces the same effect as a higher dose of drug B, A is said to be more potent than B.

Potentiation.   The effect of two drugs, usually sedative, which is greater than the sum of the effects of each drug taken alone. One drug intensifies the effects of the other.

Psychedelic.   Consciousness-expanding.

Psychoactive drugs.   Drugs that affect the mind, especially mood, thought, or perception.

Psychosis.   Loss of ability to distinguish reality as perceived by others from one's own private mental productions, often marked by hallucinations, delusions, and disturbances of mood.

Recreational drugs.   Any drugs used nonmedically for enjoyment or entertainment.

Rush.   Sudden change in consciousness and body sensation resulting from inhaling or injecting certain psychoactive drugs.

Skin popping.   Injecting drugs under the skin rather than in a vein or muscle.

Solvents.   Volatile liquids that can dissolve other substances, which when inhaled produce a brief euphoria followed by a long dreamlike state; some components like lead are quite toxic.

Sniff.   To inhale the fumes of organic solvents.

Snort.   To inhale a powdered drug.

Stimulants.   Drugs that increase the activity of the nervous system, causing wakefulness; caffeine, cocaine, and amphetamines.

STP.   Longest-lasting psychedelic (lasts up to three days).

Synergism.   In pharmacology, the interaction of two drugs to produce a combined effect greater than the simple sum of their individual effects.

Synthetic drugs.   Manufactured drugs that are man-made.

THC (tetrahydrocannabinol).   Active agent in marijuana and hashish.

Tolerance.   The need for increasing doses of a drug overtime to maintain the same effect.

Toxic.   Poisonous, harmful, or even deadly.

Withdrawal.   The process of stopping the use of a drug that has been taken regularly.

Withdrawal syndrome (or symptoms).   Physiological reactions following abrupt withdrawal of a drug after a period of prolonged and/or excessive use.

A Limited Glossary of Drug Slang

Acid.   LSD.

Angel dust.   Slang term for PCP (phencyclidine).

Back track.   To allow blood to come back into the syringe during injection.

Bale.   A pound of marijuana.

Bang.   To inject.

Bennies.   Amphetamines.

Big c.   Cocaine.

Blasted.   To be intoxicated.

Blow one's mind.   To break with reality.

Blow a stick.   To smoke a marijuana cigarette.

Blue heavens.   Amytal.

Blue velvet.   Combination of paregoric and antihistamine for intravenous use.

Bombita.   Amphetamine for injection.

Boo.   Marijuana.

Boost.   To shoplift.

Bummer.   An unpleasant drug experience.

Burn.   To cheat in a drug transaction.

Busted.   Arrested.

Can.   Ounce of marijuana.

Candy.   Cocaine.

Cap.   Packet of heroin.

Cartwheels.   Amphetamines.

Charlie.   Cocaine.

Chipping.   The practice of using narcotics such as heroin on an occasional basis.

Coke.   cocaine.

Cold turkey.   Abrupt withdrawal from narcotics without medication.

Come down.   End of a drug experience.

Cooker.   Receptacle in which drugs are heated before injection.

Cop.   Acquire a drug.

Crash.   To fall asleep after drug experience.

Crystals.   A crystalline form of methamphetamine (Methedrine).

Cut.   To dilute with a variety of materials including milk sugar.

Dealer.   Drug seller.

Deck.   Packet of heroin.

Dexies.   Dexedrine.

Dime bag. $10 worth of drugs.

Dolly. Methadone (Dolophine).

Downers. Depressant drugs.

Drop. Take pills by mouth.

Fix. Injection of narcotics, a dose.

Flip out. To lose mental and/or emotional control following use of drugs, especially powerful hallucinogens; to become psychotic.

Freak out. Same as above.

Floating. Intoxicated.

Footballs. Combination of dextroamphetamine and amphetamine.

Fuzz. Federal agents or police.

Gin. Cocaine.

Give wings. To inject somebody with heroin by vein or to teach him to inject himself.

Goofballs. Barbiturates.

Grass. Marijuana.

H. Heroin.

Hash. Hashish.

Hay. Marijuana.

Head (pothead, acid head). Someone who is constantly high on LSD, marijuana, or hashish.

High. Under the influence of drugs.

Hit. A single dose.

Holding. Possessing illegal drugs.

Hooked. To be dependent on drugs, usually meaning addiction to heroin.

Horse. Heroin.

Hung up. Enmeshed in personal problems.

Hustle. Be a prostitute.

Joint. Marijuana cigarette.

Joy pop. Intermittent use of heroin.

Junkie. Addict.

Key (or kilo). 2.2 pounds of marijuana.

Lid. Approximately one ounce of marijuana.

Lit up. Under the influence of drugs.

Mainline.   To take drugs intravenously.

Maryjane.   Marijuana.

Meth.   Methedrine or methamphetamine.

Narc.   Narcotics officer.

Nickel bag. $5 supply of drugs.

Nod.   Be lethargic and sleepy when under the influence of narcotic drugs.

OD.   Overdose of narcotics, often lethal.

Pot.   Marijuana.

Purple hearts.   Phenobarbital (luminal).

Push.   To sell drugs.

Rainbows.   Tuinal (amobarbital and secobarbital).

Red birds, red devils, reds.   Seconal.

Reefer.   Marijuana cigarette.

Roach.   Marijuana cigarette butt.

Score.   Obtain drugs.

Shoot.   Take drugs by needle.

Shooting gallery.   A place where people gather to inject drugs.

Skin pop.   To inject drugs under the skin.

Smack.   Heroin.

Snipe.   Marijuana cigarette butt.

Snort.   To take drugs by sniffing through the nose.

Snow.   Cocaine.

Spacy.   Detached from reality.

Speed.   Stimulants, especially amphetamines.

Speed ball.   Heroin mixed with cocaine or amphetamine.

Speed freak.   Someone constantly high on amphetamines.

Spike.   A needle used for injecting drugs.

Spoon.   A measure of drug to be injected.

Stash.   To hide illegal drugs.

Stick.   Marijuana cigarette.

Stoned.   High on drugs.

Trip.   Session with hallucinogenic drugs.

Uppers.   Stimulant drugs.

Twenty-five.   LSD.

Weed.   Marijuana.

Wired.   To be addicted or habituated.

Yellow jackets.   Nembutal (pentobarbital).

Bibliography

Chapter 1: Introduction

ANDERSEN, S. V., AND E. BAUWENS. *Chronic Health Problems: Concepts and Applications.* St. Louis: C. V. Mosby, 1981.

AUTHIER, J.; G. STARR; AND K. AUTHIER. "Impact of Illness on the Family." In R. E. Rakel, (ed.), *Family Practice.* 3d ed. Philadelphia: W. B. Saunders, 1984, pp. 102–17.

BRACHT, N. F. "The Social Nature of Chronic Disease and Disability," *Social Work in Health Care,* no. 5, 12 (1979): 129–44.

BUTRYM, Z., AND J. HORDER. *Health, Doctors and Social Workers.* London: Routledge & Kegan Paul, 1983.

CAMPION, E. W.; A. BANG; AND M. I. MAY. "Why Acute-Care Hospitals Must Undertake Long-Term Care." *The New England Journal of Medicine,* 308, no. 2 (January 13, 1983): 71–74.

CASSEL, E. J. "The Nature of Suffering and the Goals of Medicine." *New England Journal of Medicine* 306, no. 11 (March 18, 1982): 639–45.

CASSILETH, B. R., et al. "Psychosocial Status in Chronic Illness: A Comparative Analysis of Six Diagnostic Groups," *New England Journal of Medicine,* 311, no. 2 (August 23, 1984): 506–11.

CRANSHAW, R. "In Praise of Chronic." *Journal of Chronic Disease* 35 (1982): 79–80.

Directory of National Information Sources on Handicapping Conditions and Related Services. U.S. Department of Health, Education, and Welfare, 1980.

FELLER, B. A. "Americans Needing Help to Function at Home." *Advancedata,* 92 (September 14, 1983): 1–12.

"Financing Medicare: Exploration in Controlling Costs and Raising Revenues." *Milbank Memorial Fund Quarterly: Health and Society*, vol. 62, no. 2, 1984, special issue.

FRIES, J. F., AND G. E. EHRLICH. *Prognosis: Contemporary Outcomes of Disease.* Menlo Park, Calif.: Addison-Wesley, 1981.

FUCHS, V. R. "Though Much Is Taken: Reflections on Aging, Health and Medical Care," *Milbank Memorial Fund Quarterly: Health and Society*, 62, no. 2 (1984): 143–66.

GILLICK, M. R. "Is the Care of the Chronically Ill a Medical Prerogative?" *New England Journal of Medicine*, 310, no. 3 (January 19, 1984): 190–93.

Green Pages: A Directory of Products and Services for the Handicapped. 641 West Fairbanks, Winter Park, Fla. 32789.

LANSDOWN, R. *More than Sympathy: The Everyday Needs of Sick and Handicapped Children and Their Families.* London: Tavistock, 1980.

MCCOLLUM, A. T. *The Chronically Ill Child: A Guide for Parents and Professionals.* New Haven: Yale University Press, 1981.

MILLER, J. F., ed. *Coping with Chronic Illness.* Philadelphia: F. A. Davis, 1983.

ROSENBERG, M. L. *Patients: The Experience of Illness.* Philadelphia: W. B. Saunders, 1980.

SMITH, M. S., ed. *Chronic Disorders in Adolescence.* Littleton, Mass.: PSG Incorporated, 1983.

Social Security Handbook. 7th ed. Social Security Administration, 1982.

STOLOV, W. C., AND M. R. CLOWERS. *Handbook of Severe Disability.* Washington, D.C.: U.S. Department of Education, 1981.

STRAUSS, A. L. *Chronic Illness and the Quality of Life.* St. Louis: C. V. Mosby, 1975.

TRAVIS, G. *Chronic Illness and Disability.* Stanford, Calif.: Stanford University Press, 1976.

"Vocational and Educational Opportunities for the Disabled." Insurance Company of North America, Human Resources Center, Willets Road, Albertson, N.Y. 11507.

WERNER-BELAND, J. A., ed. *Grief Responses to Long-Term Illness and Disability.* Reston, Va.: Reston Publishing Company, 1980.

ZOLA, I. K. *Missing Pieces: A Chronicle of Living with a Disability.* Philadelphia: Temple University Press, 1982.

———, ed. *Ordinary Lives: Voices of Disability and Disease.* Cambridge, Mass.: Apple-Wood Books, 1982.

Chapter 2: Arthritis

"Arthritis: The Basic Facts." Atlanta: Arthritis Foundation, 1981.

Arthritis Health Professions Section. *Self-Help Manual for Patients with Arthritis.* Atlanta: Arthritis Foundation, 1980.

Boss, G. R., AND J. E. SEEGMILLER. "Hyperuricemia and Gout: Classification, Complications and Management," *New England Journal of Medicine*, 300 (1979): 1459–68.

BREWER, E. J. *Juvenile Rheumatoid Arthritis*. Philadelphia: W. B. Saunders, 1982.

EDEN, D. *Arthritis and Rheumatism: The Facts*. New York: Oxford University Press, 1981.

EHRLICH, G. *Rehabilitation Management of Rheumatic Conditions*. Baltimore: Williams & Wilkins, 1980.

FRIES, J. F. *Arthritis: A Comprehensive Guide*. Reading, Mass.: Addison-Wesley, 1979.

FRIES, J., AND G. EHRLICH. "Arthritis and Connective Tissue Disease." In J. Fries and G. Ehrlich, eds., *Prognosis: Contemporary Outcomes of Disease*. Menlo Park, Calif.: Addison-Wesley, 1981, pp. 341–97.

GARDINER, B. M. "Psychological Aspects of Rheumatoid Arthritis," *Psychological Medicine*, 10 (1980): 159–63.

HART, F. D. *Overcoming Arthritis*. New York: Arco Publishing, 1981.

HEALEY, L. A.; K. R. WILSKE; AND B. H. HANSEN. *Beyond the Copper Bracelet: What You Should Know About Arthritis*. 2d ed. Bowie, Md.: Charles Press, 1977.

HOCHBERG, M. C. "Adult and Juvenile Rheumatoid Arthritis: Current Epidemiologic Concepts," *Epidemiologic Reviews*, 3 (1981): 27–44.

HORNER, J. *That Time of Year: A Chronicle of Life in a Nursing Home*. Amherst: University of Massachusetts Press, 1982.

KATZ, W. A. *Rheumatic Diseases: Diagnosis and Management*. Philadelphia: J. B. Lippincott, 1977.

KELLEY, W. N., et al. *Textbook of Rheumatology*. Philadelphia: W. B. Saunders, 1981.

KREWER, S. *The Arthritis Exercise Book*. New York: Simon & Schuster, 1981.

McCARTY, D. J., ed. *Arthritis and Allied Conditions*. Philadelphia: Lea & Febiger, 1979.

MELVIN, J. *Rheumatic Disease: Occupational Therapy and Rehabilitation*. Philadelphia: F. A. Davis, 1982.

"The Mismanagement of Arthritis," *Consumer Reports*, vol. 44, June/July 1979 (reprint).

NICHOLAS, J. J. "Rheumatic Diseases." In W. C. Stolov and M. R. Clowers, eds., *Handbook of Severe Disability*. Washington, D.C.: U.S. Dept. of Education, 1981, pp. 189–204.

RESNICK, D., AND G. NIWAYAMA. *Diagnosis of Bone and Joint Disorders*. Philadelphia: W. B. Saunders, 1981.

RODMAN, G. P., et al. *Primer on the Rheumatic Diseases*. Atlanta: Arthritis Foundation, n.d.

ROGERS, M.; M. H. LLANZ; AND A. J. PARTRIDGE. "Psychological Care of Adults with Rheumatoid Arthritis," *Annals of Internal Medicine*, 96 (1982): 344–48.

ROSENBERG, A. M. *Living with Your Arthritis*. New York: Arco Publishing, 1979.

SCHWARTZ, L. M.; R. MARCUS; AND R. CONDON. "Multidisciplinary Group Therapy for Rheumatoid Arthritis," *Psychosomatics*, 19, no. 5 (May 1978): 289–93.

SMITH, J. L. "Psychological Aspects of Arthritis," *The Arthritis Reporter*, New York, n.d. (reprint).

SPENGEL, P.; G. E. Ehrlich; and G. Glass. "The Rheumatoid Arthritic Personality: A Psychodiagnostic Myth," *Psychosomatics* 19, no. 2 (1978): 79–86.

SPIEGEL, T. M. *Practical Rheumatology*. New York: Wiley, 1983.

WEST, A. "Understanding Endorphins: Our Natural Pain Relief System," *Nursing*, 1 (February 1981): 50–53.

WEINER, C. L. "The Burden of Rheumatoid Arthritis: Tolerating the Uncertainty," *Social Science and Medicine*, 9 (1975): 97–104.

WILSON, R. W., AND B. J. UMASSIAN. "Endorphins," *Ameican Journal of Nursing*, April 1981, pp. 722–25.

ZEITLIN, D. "Psychological Issues in the Management of Rheumatoid Arthritis," *Psychosomatics*, 18, no. 8 (August 1977): 7–14.

ZIEBELL, B. *Wellness: An Arthritis Reality*. Dubuque, Iowa: Kendall/Hunt Publishing Company, 1981.

Chapter 3: Cancer

ABRAMS, R. D. *Not Alone with Cancer: A Guide for Those Who Care—What to Expect, What to Do*. Springfield, Ill.: Charles Thomas, 1976.

BARSTOW, L. F. "Working with Cancer Patients in Radiation Therapy," *Health and Social Work*, 7, no. 1 (February, 1982): 35–40.

BLUMBERG, B.; M. FLAHERTY; AND J. LEWIS, eds. *Coping with Cancer*. Bethesda, Md.: National Cancer Institute, NIH Publication #80-20801, 1980.

Breast Cancer Digest. *A Guide to Medical Care, Emotional Support and Educational Programs*. Bethesda, Md.: National Cancer Institute, 1979.

"Cancer Care: The Relative's View," *The Lancet*, November 17, 1983, pp. 1188–89.

Cancergram. Abstracts of selected cancer-related articles dealing with specific subjects recently published in 3,000 journals, National Cancer Institute.

CASSILETH, B. R., ed. *The Cancer Patient: Social and Medical Aspects*. Philadelphia: Lea & Febiger, 1979.

CASSILETH, B. R., AND J. A. DONOVAN. "Hospice: History and Implications of the New Legislation," *Journal of Psychosocial Oncology*, 1, no. 1 (Spring 1983): 59–69.

Division of Cancer Treatment. *Summary Report VII*, October 1, 1981–September 30, 1982, National Cancer Institute.

FRIEDENSBERG, I., et al. *Psychosocial Aspects of Cancer: Annotated Bibliography*. Washington: American Psychological Association, 1979.

GLATSTEIN, E. *Radiation Risks and Radiation Therapy*. Bethesda, Md.: National Institutes of Health, 1982.

GREINER, L., AND C. WEILER. "Early-Stage Breast Cancer: What Do Women

Know About Treatment Choices?" *American Journal of Nursing*, 83, no. 11 (November 1983): 1570.

HODGSON, T. A. "Social and Economic Implications of Cancer in the United States," *Annals of the New York Academy of Science*, no. 363 (1981): 189–204.

KRAYBILL, H. F., et al., eds. *NCI/EPA Collaborative Program on Environmental Carcinogenesis*. Bethesda, Md.: National Institutes of Health, 1982.

MEKHANN, C. F., M.D. *The Facts About Cancer: A Guide for Patients, Family and Friends*. Englewood Cliffs, N.J.: Prentice-Hall, 1981.

MEYEROWITZ, B. E., et al. "Quality of Life for Breast Cancer Patients Receiving Adjuvant Chemotherapy," *American Journal of Nursing*, 83, no. 2 (February 1983): 232–35.

MILLER, P. J. "Mastectomy: A Review of Psychosocial Research," *Health and Social Work*, 16, no. 2 (May 1981): 60–66.

MULLEN, B. D., AND K. A. MCGINN. *The Ostomy Book: Living Comfortably with Colostomies, Ileostomies and Urostomies*. Palo Alto, Calif.: Bull Publishing Co., 1980.

NELSON, N. "A Personal View of Occupational Cancer and Its Prevention," *Journal of the National Cancer Institute*, 67, no. 2 (August 1981): 227–31.

NEUHRING, E. M.; AND W. E. BARR. "Mastectomy: Impact on Patients and Families," *Health and Social Work*, 5, no. 1 (February 1980): 51–58.

Patient and Professional Education Materials for Ostomates: Selected Annotations. Bethesda, Md.: National Cancer Institute, 1981.

"Radiation Risks and Radiation Therapy." In *Medicine for the Layman*. Bethesda, Md.: National Institutes of Health, 1982.

REVENSON, T. A., et al. "Social Supports as Stress Buffers for Adult Cancer Patients," *Psychosomatic Medicine*, 45, no. 4 (August 1983): 321–31.

ROSENBAUM, E. H., AND I. R. ROSENBAUM. *A Comprehensive Guide for Cancer Patients and Their Families*. Palo Alto, Calif.: Bull Publishing Co., 1980.

SCHMALE, A. H., et al. "Well-Being of Cancer Survivors," *Psychosomatic Medicine*, 45, no. 2 (May 1983): 163–69.

SIEMIATYCKI, J., et al. "Discovering Carcinogens in the Occupational Environment: A Novel Epidemiological Approach," *Journal of the National Cancer Institute*, 66, no. 2 (February 1981): 217–25.

WELLISCH, D., et al. "Problems of the Homebound Cancer Patient," *Psychosomatic Medicine*, 45, no. 1 (March 1983): 11–21.

WILLETT, W. C. AND B. MACMAHON. "Diet and Cancer: An Overview," *New England Journal of Medicine*, 310, no. 11 (March 1984): 697–703.

YANCIK, R. *Perspectives on Prevention and Treatment of Cancer in the Elderly*. New York: Raven Press, 1983.

Chapter 4: The Dementias

Alzheimer's Guide for Practitioners. Washington, D.C.: National Institute on Aging, 1981.

ARONSON, M.; G. LEVIN; AND R. LIPKOWITZ. "Family Atmosphere and Alzheimer's Disease: Implications for Invention," *Gerontologist*, 21 (1981): 69–75.

ARONSON, M., AND R. LIPKOWITZ. "Senile Dementia, Alzheimer Type: The Family and the Health Care Delivery System" *Journal of the American Geriatrics Society*, 29, no. 12 (December 1981): 568–71.

BALL, M. J. "Alzheimer's Disease: A Challenging Enigma." *Archives of Pathology and Laboratory Medicine*, 106, no. 4 (April 1982): 157–62.

BECK, J. C., et al. "Dementia in the Elderly: The Silent Epidemic (Clinical Conference)," *Annals of Internal Medicine* 97, no. 2 (August 1982): 231–34.

BERESFORD, H. R., "Severe Neurological Impairment: Legal Aspects of Decisions to Reduce Care," *Annals of Neurology*, 15, no. 5 (May 1984): 409–14.

Choosing a Nursing Home for the Person with Intellectual Loss. Burke Rehabilitation Center, White Plains, N.Y.: n.d.

COONS, D. "Report to Families of the Study of Alzheimer's Disease: Subjective Experiences of Families," University of Michigan, Institute of Gerontology, 1983.

COYLE, J. T. "Alzheimer's Disease: A Disorder of Cortical Cholinergic Innervation," *Science*, 219 (1983): 1184–90.

DAHL, DAVID. "Diagnosis of Alzheimer's Disease," *Postgraduate Medicine*, 73, no. 4 (April 1983): 217–21.

The Dementias: Hope Through Research. Bethesda, Md.: National Institute of Neurological and Communicative Disorders and Stroke, 1981.

EISDORFER, C., AND D. COHEN. "Management of the Patient and Family Coping with Dementing Illness," *The Journal of Family Practice*, 12, no. 5: 831–37.

FISK, A. A. *A New Look at Senility: Its Causes, Diagnosis, Treatment, and Management.* Springfield, Ill.: Charles C. Thomas, 1981.

FISK, A. L. "Management of Alzheimer's Disease." *Postgraduate Medicine* 73, no. 4 (April 1983): 237–41.

"Alzheimer's Disease and Related Disorders," *Generations: Journal of the Western Gerontological Association*, Fall 1982, entire issue.

HAMSHER, K. "Mental Status Examination in Alzheimer's Disease: The Neuropsychologist's Role," *Postgraduate Medicine*, 73, no. 4 (April 1983): 225–28.

HEYMAN, A., et al. "Alzheimer's Disease: Genetic Aspects and Associated Clinical Disorders," *Annals of Neurology*, 14, no. 5 (1983): 507–15.

JURY, M., AND D. JURY. *Gramp.* New York: Grossman, 1976.

KANE, R., AND R. KANE. "Alternatives to Institutional Care for the Elderly." *The Gerontologist*, 20 (1980): 249–59.

KAPUST, L. R. "Living with Dementia: The Ongoing Funeral," *Social Work in Health Care*, 7, no. 4 (Summer 1982): 79–91.

KATZMAN, R. "Neurotransmitters and Aging," *Roche Seminars on Aging: The Scientific Aspects*, vol. 8, sec. 1.

KATZMAN, R., AND R. D. TERRY. *The Neurology of Aging.* Philadelphia: F. A. Davis, 1983.

KATZMAN, R.; R. D. TERRY; AND K. L. BICK, eds. *Alzheimer's Disease: Senile De-*

mentia and Related Disorders. Aging Series, vol. 7. New York: Raven Press, 1978.

KEYES, B., AND G. SZPAK. "Day Care for Alzheimer's," *Postgraduate Medicine, 73,* no. 4 (April 1983): 245–50.

KOKMEN, E. "Dementia-Alzheimer Type." *Mayo Clinic Proceedings,* 59 (1984): 35–42.

LAVARGA, D. "Group Treatment for Wives of Patients with Alzheimer's Disease," *Social Work in Health Care,* 5 (1979): 219–21.

LEVINE, N. B., et al. "Coping with Dementia," *Journal of the American Geriatrics Society,* 31, no. 1 (1983): 12–18.

MACE, N. L., AND P. V. RABINS. *The Thirty-six Hour Day: A Family Guide to Caring for Persons with Alzheimer's Disease, Related Dementing Illnesses, and Memory Loss in Later Life.* Baltimore: Johns Hopkins Press, 1982.

Managing the Person with Intellectual Loss at Home. White Plains, N.Y.: Burke Rehabilitation Center, 1980.

MORTIMER, J. A., AND L. M. SCHUMAN. *The Epidemiology of Dementia.* New York: Oxford University Press, 1981.

MORYCZ, R. H. "An Exploration of Senile Dementia and Family Burden," *Clinical Social Work Journal,* 8, no. 1 (Spring 1980): 16–27.

POWELL, L. S., AND K. COURTICE. *Alzheimer's Disease: A Guide for Families.* Reading, Mass.: Addison-Wesley, 1983.

RABINS, P. V.; N. L. MACE; AND M. J. LUKAS. "The Impact of Dementia on the Family," *Journal of the American Medical Association,* 248, no. 3 (1982): 333–35.

REISBERG, B., ed. *Alzheimer's Disease: The Standard Reference.* New York: The Free Press, 1984.

ROACH, M. "Another Name for Madness: A Family's Losing Battle with Alzheimer's Disease," *New York Times Magazine,* January 16, 1983, pp. 22–31.

SCHMIDT, G. "Mechanisms and Possible Causes of Alzheimer's Disease," *Postgraduate Medicine,* 73, no. 4 (April 1983): 206–13.

SELAN, B. H., AND S. SCHUENKE. "The Late Life Care Program: Helping Families Cope," *Health and Social Work,* 7, no. 3 (August 1982): 192–97.

SILVERSTONE, B., AND S. MILLER. "Isolation in the Aged: Individual Dynamics, Community and Family Involvement," *Journal of Geriatric Psychiatry,* 13 (1980): 27–47.

SOMERS, A. R. "Long-Term Care for the Elderly and Disabled." *New England Journal of Medicine,* 307, no. 4: 221–26.

TERRY, R. D., AND R. KATZMAN. "Senile Dementia of the Alzheimer's Type," *Annals of Neurology,* 14, no. 5 (November 1983): 497–506.

THOMAS, L. "On the Problem of Dementia." *Discover,* August 1981, pp. 34–37.

THORNTON, S. M., AND V. FRASER. *Understanding Senility: A Lady Person's Guide.* Potentials Development, 1982.

WELLS, C. E. "A Deluge of Dementia," *Psychosomatics,* 22, no. 10 (1981): 837–49.

————. "Diagnosis of Dementia: A Reassessment," *Psychosomatics*, 25, no. 3 (1984): 183–90.

ZARIT, S.; K. E. REEVER; AND J. BACH-PETERSON. "Relatives of the Impaired Elderly: Correlates of Feelings of Burden," *Gerontologist*, 20 (1980): 649–54.

Chapter 5: Diabetes

BENNETT, M. *The Peripatetic Diabetic*. New York: Hawthorn Books, 1969.

BIERMANN, J., and B. TOOHEY. *The Diabetic's Sports and Exercise Book*. Philadelphia: J. B. Lippincott, 1977.

The Diabetic's Total Health Book. Los Angeles: J. B. Tarcher, 1980.

Diabetic Forecast. American Diabetic Association, all issues.

DOLGER, H., AND B. SEEMAN. *How to Live with Diabetes*. 4th ed. New York: Schocken Books, 1978.

DUCAT, L., AND S. S. COHEN. *Diabetes*. New York: Harper & Row, 1983.

HAMBURG, B.; F. LIPSETT; G. E. INOFF; AND A. DRESH, eds. *Behavioral and Psychosocial Issues in Diabetes*. Washington, D.C.: GPO, 1977.

HANSEN, B., et al. "New Approaches to Therapy and Diagnosis of Diabetes," *Diabetologia*, 22 (1982): 61–67.

HAUSTER, S. T., AND D. POLLETS. "Psychological Aspects of Diabetes Mellitus: A Critical Review," *Diabetic Care*, 2, no. 2 (1979): 221–32.

JACOBSON, A. M., AND J. B. LEIBOVICH. "Psychological Issues in Diabetes Mellitus," *Psychosomatics*, 25, no. 1 (January 1984): 7–15.

KIVELOWITZ, T. *Diabetics: A Guide to Self-Management for Patients and Their Families*. Englewood Cliffs, N.J.: Prentice-Hall, 1981.

KRALL, L. P., ed. *Joslin's Diabetic Manual*. 11th ed. Philadelphia: Lea & Febiger, 1978.

National Diabetes Information Clearinghouse. *General Information About Diabetes: Selected Annotations*. Bethesda, Md.: NIH, August 1980.

PEDUSEN, J. *The Pregnant Diabetic and Her Newborn*. 2d ed. Baltimore: Williams & Wilkins, 1977.

PIRART, J. "Diabetes Mellitus and Its Degenerative Complications: A Prospective Study of 4,400 Patients Observed Between 1947–1973," *Diabetes Care*, 1, no. 3 (1978): 168–88.

PODOLSKY, S., ed. *Clinical Diabetes: Modern Management*. New York: Appleton-Century-Crofts, 1980.

PODOLSKY, S., AND B. EL-BEHERI. "The Principles of the Diabetic Diet," *Journal of Geriatrics*, 35, no. 12 (December 1980): 73–78.

REINSTEIN, L.; J. ASHLEY; AND K. HAAS MILLER. "Sexual Adjustment After Lower Extremity Amputation," *Archives of Physical Medicine and Rehabilitation*, vol. 59, November 1978.

SCHADE, D. S. "The Stress Factor," *Diabetes Forecast*, March–April 1982, pp. 18–21.

SIMS, D., ed. *The Positive Approach to Diabetes.* St. Louis: C. V. Mosby, 1980.

TATTERSALL, R. B. "Psychiatric Aspects of Diabetes: A Physician's View," *British Journal of Psychiatry,* 139 (December 1981): 485–93.

TEUTSCH, S. M. "Mortality Among Diabetic Patients Using Continuous Subcutaneous Insulin-Infusion Pumps," *New England Journal of Medicine,* 310, no. 6 (February 9, 1984): 361–68.

The Treatment and Control of Diabetics: A National Plan to Reduce Mortality and Morbidity. Report of the National Diabetes Advisory Board, November 1980.

WALTERS, J. "Coping With a Leg Amputation," *American Journal of Nursing,* July 1981, pp. 1347–52.

WHITEHOUSE, F. W., et al. "Outpatient Regulation of the Insulin-Requiring Person with Diabetes," *Journal of Chronic Disease,* 36, no. 6 (1983): 433–38.

WILKINSON, D. G. "Psychiatric Aspects of Diabetes Mellitus," *British Journal of Psychiatry,* 138 (January 1981): 1–9.

WISHNER, W. AND J. O'BRIEN. "Diabetes and the Family," *Medical Clinics of North America,* 62, no. 4 (1978): 849–56.

WRIGHT, A. D. "Therapeutic Progress—Review II: Control of Diabetes Mellitus," *Journal of Clinical and Hospital Pharmacy,* 6 (1981): 217–25.

LEVINE, S. E. "Nutritional Care of Patients with Renal Failure and Diabetes," *Journal of the American Dietary Association,* 81, no. 3: 261–67.

Chapter 6: The Epilepsies

ADAMS, R. D., AND M. VICTOR. *Principles of Neurology.* New York: McGraw-Hill, 1981.

BARRY, K. "The Health Education Needs of the Adult with Epilepsy," *Rehabilitation Nursing,* May–June 1982, pp. 30–33.

BENIAK, J. "Patient Education in Epilepsy," *Journal of Neurological Nursing* 14, no. 1 (February 1982): 19–22.

BLACK, R. B.; B. P. HERMANN; AND J. T. SHOPE, eds. *Nursing Management of Epilepsy.* Rockville, Md.: Aspen Publications, 1982.

BUCHANAN, N. "Treatment of Epilepsy: Whose Right Is It Anyway?" *British Medical Journal,* vol. 284, January 16, 1982.

Commission for the Control of Epilepsy and Its Consequences. *Plan for Nationwide Action on Epilepsy.* U.S. Department of Health, Education, and Welfare, Public Health Service, National Institutes of Health, DHEW Publication #(NIH) 78–276, 1978.

DELGARDO–ESCUETA, A. V.; D. M. TREIMAN; AND G. O. WALSH. "The Treatable Epilepsies," *New England Journal of Medicine,* 306 (June 1983): 1508–14, 1576–84.

DODRILL, C. B.; L. W. BATZEL; AND H. R. QUEISSER. "An Objective Method for the Assessment of Psychological and Social Problems Among Epileptics," *Epilepsia,* 21 (1980): 123–35.

EMERSON, R.; B. J. D'SOUZA; AND J. M. FREEMAN. "Stopping Medication in Children with Epilepsy," *New England Journal of Medicine*, 304, no. 19 (May 1981): 1125.

FALVO, D. R.; H. ALLEN; AND D. R. MAKI. "Psychosocial Aspects of Invisible Disability," *Rehabilitation Literature*, 43: nos. 1–2 (January/February 1982): 2–6.

FORD, C. A. "Epilepsy in Childhood." In T. S. Kerson et al., *Social Work in Health Settings: Practice in Context*. New York: Longmans, 1982, pp. 144–60.

GOLDENSOHN, E. S., AND A. V. WALTON. "A Little Counseling Goes a Long Way," *Consultant*, October 1982, pp. 43–48.

GROSS-SELBECK, G., AND H. DOOSE, eds. *Epilepsy: Problems of Marriage, Pregnancy, Genetic Counseling*. New York: Thieme-Stratton, 1981.

HEISLER, A. B., AND S. B. FRIEDMAN. "Social and Psychological Considerations in Chronic Disease: With Particular Reference to the Management of Seizure Disorders," Journal of Pediatric Psychology, 6, no. 3 (1981): 239–50.

HERMANN, B. P. *A Multidisciplinary Handbook of Epilepsy*. Springfield, Ill.: Charles C. Thomas, 1980.

HODGEMAN, C. H., et al. "Emotional Complications of Adolescent Grand Mal Epilepsy," *Journal of Pediatrics*, 95, no. 12 (1979): 309–12.

HOPKINS, A. *Epilepsy: The Facts*. New York: Oxford University Press, 1981.

JAN, J. E.; R. G. ZIEGLER; AND G. ERBA. *Does Your Child Have Epilepsy?* Baltimore: University Park Press, 1983.

LECHTENBERG, R. *Epilepsy and the Family*. Cambridge: Harvard University Press, 1984.

NELSON, K. B., AND J. H. ELLENBERG. "Maternal Seizure Disorder, Outcome of Pregnancy, and Neurologic Abnormalities in the Children," *Neurology*, 32 (November 1982): 1247–54.

PHILBERT, A., et al. "The Epileptic Mother and Her Child," *Epilepsia*, 23, no. 1 (February 1982): 85–99.

PINCUS, J., AND G. TUCKER. "Seizure Disorders." In Oxford University Press, *Behavioral Neurology*. 2d ed. New York: Oxford, 1978, pp. 3–57.

REYNOLDS, E. H., AND M. R. TRIMBLE, eds. *Epilepsy and Psychiatry*. London: Churchill Livingstone, 1981.

ROWLAND, L. P. *Merritt's Textbook of Neurology*. Philadelphia: Lea & Febiger, 1984.

SANDS, H., ed. Epilepsy: *A Handbook for the Mental Health Professional*. New York: Brunner/Mazel, 1982.

SCHEINER, A. P., AND I. F. ABRAMS, eds. *The Practical Management of the Developmentally Disabled Child*. St. Louis: C. V. Mosby, 1980.

SCHMIDT, D. *Adverse Effects of Antiepileptic Drugs*. New York: Raven Press, 1982.

SNYDER, M. "Effect of Relaxation on Psychosocial Functioning in Persons with Epilepsy," *Journal of Neurological Nursing*, 15, no. 4 (August 1983): 250–54.

SOLOMON, G. E., AND F. PLUM. *Clinical Management of Seizures*. Philadelphia: W. B. Saunders, 1983.

SUSUMU, S.; F. E. DREIFUSS; J. K. PENRY; D. D. KIRBY; AND Y. PALESCH. "Long-Term Follow-Up of Absence Seizures," *Neurology*, 33, no. 12 (December 1983): 1590–95.

TRIMBLE, M. R. "Personality Disturbances in Epilepsy," *Neurology*, 33, no. 10 (October 1983): 1332–34.

WADA, J. A., AND J. K. PENRY. *Advances in Epileptology: The 10th Epilepsy International Symposium.* New York: Raven Press, 1980.

WARD, A. A., et al. "Epilepsy." In W. Stolov and M. R. Clowers, eds., *Handbook of Severe Disability.* Washington, D.C.: U.S. Dept. of Education, 1981, pp. 155–67.

WOODBURY, D. M., et al. *Antiepileptic Drugs.* New York: Raven Press, 1982.

WOODWARD, E. S. "The Total Patient: Implications for Nursing Care of the Epileptic," *Journal of Neurosurgical Nursing*, 14, no. 4 (August 1982): 166–69.

WRIGHT, G. N. *Epilepsy Rehabilitation.* Boston: Little, Brown, 1975.

ZIEGLER, R. G. "Epilepsy: Individual Illness, Human Predicament and Family Dilemma," *Family Relations*, July 1982, pp. 435–44.

Chapter 7: Heart Disease

A Handbook of Heart Terms. Bethesda, Md.: U.S. Department of Health, Education, and Welfare, n.d.

American Heart Association. *Heartbook: A Guide to Prevention and Treatment of Cardiovascular Diseases.* New York: E. P. Dutton, 1980.

———. *Heart Facts: 1984.* Dallas: AHA's Office of Communications, 1984.

American Heart Association Cookbook. New York: David McKay, 1979.

BEDELL, S. E., et al. "Survival After Cardiopulmonary Resuscitation in the Hospital," *New England Journal of Medicine*, 309, no. 10 (September 8, 1983): 569–76.

BUELL, J. C., AND R. S. ELIOT. "Stress and Cardiovascular Disease," *Modern Concepts of Cardiovascular Disease*, 48, no. 1 (1979): 19–24.

BRAUNWALD, E. "Effects of Coronary-Artery Bypass Grafting on Survival," *New England Journal of Medicine*, 309, no. 19 (November 10, 1983): 1181–84.

CASS Principal Investigators. "Coronary-Artery Surgery Study (CASS): A Randomized Trial of Coronary-Artery Bypass Surgery: 'Quality of Life' in Randomized Subjects," *Circulation*, 68 (1983): 951–60.

"Coronary Bypass Surgery—Here To Stay," editorial in *The Lancet*, July 23, 1983, pp. 197–98.

COUSINS, N. *The Healing Heart: Antidotes to Panic and Helplessness.* New York: W. W. Norton, 1983.

CROOG, S. H., AND S. LEVINE. *The Heart Patient Recovers.* New York: Human Sciences Press, 1977.

———. *Life After a Heart Attack.* New York: Human Sciences Press, 1982.

DOEHRMAN, S. "Psycho-Social Aspects of Recovery for Coronary Heart Disease: A Review," *Social Science and Medicine*, 11 (1977): 199–218.

FISHER, A. *The Healthy Heart.* Alexandria, Va.: Time-Life Books, 1981.

HAVLIK, R. J., AND M. FEINLEIB, eds. *Proceedings of the Conference on the Decline in Coronary Heart Disease Mortality.* Washington, D.C.: U.S. Department of Health, Education, and Welfare, 1979.

HAYNES, S. G., AND M. FEINLEIB. "Women, Work and Coronary Heart Disease: Prospective Findings from the Framingham Heart Study," *American Journal of Public Health*, 70 (1980): 133–41.

HAYNES, S. G.; M. FEINLEIB; AND W. B. KANNEL. "The Relationship of Psychosocial Factors to Coronary Heart Disease," *American Journal of Epidemiology*, 111 (1980): 37–58.

"Heart Attacks," in *Medicine for the Layman.* U.S. Dept. of Health, Education, and Welfare, Public Health Service, National Institutes of Health. NIH Publication No. 79–1803, July 1979.

HOCHMAN, G. *Heart Bypass: What Every Patient Must Know.* New York: St. Martin's Press, 1982.

KANNEL, W. B., AND T. GORDON. *The Framingham Study: An Epidemiological Investigation of Cardiovascular Disease.* Washington, D.C.: Superintendent of Documents, 1974.

KULLER, L. "Risk Factor Reduction in Coronary Heart Disease." *Modern Concepts of Cardiovascular Disease*, 53, no. 2 (February 1984): 7–11.

LEAR, M. W. *Heartsounds.* New York: Simon & Schuster, 1980.

MOSS, A. L., et al. "Risk Stratification and Survival After Myocardial Infarction," *New England Journal of Medicine*, 306, no. 6 (August 11, 1983): 331–36.

RAZIN, A. M. "Psychosocial Intervention in Coronary-Artery Disease: A Review," *Psychosomatic Medicine*, 44, no. 4 (September 1982): 363–87.

RUBERMAN, W., et al. "Psychosocial Influences on Mortality After Myocardial Infarction," *New England Journal of Medicine*, 311, no. 9 (August 30, 1984): 552–39.

SANNE, H. *Readaptation After Myocaridal Infarction.* Monograph No. 1, International Exchange of Information in Rehabilitation, World Rehabilitation Fund, New York, 1979.

SPEEDLING, E. J., ed. *Heart Attack: The Family Response at Home and in the Hospital.* New York and London: Tavistock, 1982.

STALLONES, R. A. "The Rise and Fall of Ischemic Heart Disease," *Scientific American*, 243, no. 5 (November 1980): 53–59.

TAYLOR, C. B. "Behavioral Approaches to Hypertension." In J. M. Ferguson and C. B. Taylor, eds., *Comprehensive Handbook of Behavioral Medicine. Vol. 1.* New York: Spectrum, 1980, pp. 55–88.

TAYLOR, C. B., AND S. FORTMANN. "Essential Hypertension." *Psychosomatics*, 24, no. 5 (May 1983): 433–48.

WEISS, E. S., AND S. RUBENSTEIN. *Recovering from the Heart Attack Experience: Emotional Feelings, Medical Facts.* New York: Macmillan, 1981.

Chapter 8: Respiratory Disease

AGLE, D. P., AND G. L. BAUM. "Psychological Aspects of COPD," *Medical Clinics of North America*, 61 (1977): 749–58.

American Thoracic Society. "Pulmonary Rehabilitation," *American Review of Respiratory Disease*, 124 (November 1981): 1–3.

BECKER, A. B., et al. "The Bronchodilator Effects and Pharmokinetics of Caffeine in Asthma," *New England Journal of Medicine*, 310, no. 12 (March 22, 1984): 743–50.

BRECHER, R., AND E. BRECHER. *Breathing . . . What You Need to Know*. New York: American Lung Association, 1975.

BUTTS, J. R. "Pulmonary Rehabilitation Through Exercise and Education," *CVR*, December/January 1981, pp. 17–21; 60–61.

CRUVER, N., AND N. SOLLIDAY. "Fundamentals of Exercise Stress Testing for Lung Disease," *Respiratory Care*, 27, no. 9 (September 1982): 1150–57.

DAHMS, T. E., et al. "Passive Smoking: Effects on Bronchial Asthma," *Chest*, 80, no. 5 (November 1981): 530–34.

DETELS, R., et al. "The UCLA Population Studies of Chronic Obstructive Respiratory Disease," *American Review of Respiratory Disease*, 124, no. 6 (December 1981): 673–80.

FRITZ, G. K. "Childhood Asthma," *Psychosomatics*, 24, no. 11 (November 1983): 959–67.

HAAS, A., et al. *Pulmonary Therapy and Rehabilitation: Principles and Practices*. Baltimore: Williams & Wilkins, 1979.

Help Yourself to Better Breathing. New York: American Lung Association, 1982.

HODGKIN, J. E. "Exercise in the Pulmonary Patient." *Respiratory Care*, 27, no. 6 (June 1982): 671–73.

"Index of Risk for Obstructive Airways Disease," *American Review of Respiratory Disease*, 125, no. 2 (February 1982): 144–51.

KANDEL, G., AND A. ABERMAN. "Managing Exacerbations of COPD," *Respiratory Therapy*, November/December 1982, pp. 53–57.

KAUFFMAN, F., AND S. PERDRIZET. "Effect of Passive Smoking on Respiratory Function," *European Journal of Respiratory Disease*, 62, Supplement 113 (1981): 109–10.

KINSMAN, R. A., et al. "Levels of Psychological Experience in Asthma: General and Illness-Specific Concomitants of Panic-Fear Personality," *Journal of Clinical Psychology*, 36, no. 2 (April 1980): 552–61.

LERTZMAN, M. M., AND R. M. CHERNIAK. "Rehabilitation of Patients with Chronic Obstructive Pulmonary Disease," *American Review of Respiratory Disease*, 114 (1976): 1145–65.

MACDONELL, R. J. "The Pulmonary Rehabilitation Maze," *Respiratory Care*, 28, no. 2 (February 1983): 180–90.

MARTIN, A. J., et al. "Asthma from Childhood at Age 21: The Patient and His Disease," *British Medical Journal*, 284 (6313) (February 1982): 380–82.

National Heart, Lung and Blood Advisory Council. *Tenth Report (1982)*. NIH # 82–1127, 1982.

O'RYAN, J. A. "Essentials for a Comprehensive Pulmonary Rehabilitation Program," *Current Reviews in Respiratory Therapy*, 16, no. 2 (1980): 122–27.

PEARLE, J. L. "Smoking and Duration of Asbestos Exposure in the Production of Functional and Roentgenographic Abnormalities in Shipyard Workers," *Journal of Occupational Medicine*, 24, no. 1 (January 1982): 37–40.

PETTY, T. L. *Intensive and Rehabilitative Respiratory Care*. 3d ed. Philadelphia: Lea & Febiger, 1982.

PETTY, T. L., AND L. M. NETT. *Enjoying Life with Emphysema*. Philadelphia: Lea & Febiger, 1984.

ROSELLE, S., AND D'AMICO, F. J. "The Effect of Home Respiratory Therapy on Hospital Readmission Rates of Patients with Chronic Obstructive Pulmonary Disease," *Respiratory Care*, 27, no. 9 (October 1982): 1194–99.

ROSSER, R., et al. "Breathlessness and Psychiatric Morbidity in Chronic Bronchitis and Emphysema: A Study of Psychotherapeutic Management," *Psychological Medicine*, 13, no. 1 (February 1983): 93–110.

SCHUMAN, E., AND A. B. COHEN. "Effective Therapy for Chronic Bronchitis and Emphysema," *Geriatrics*, 37, no. 9 (September 1982): 74–76.

SCOGGIN, C. H., AND T. L. PETTY. *Clinical Strategies in Adult Asthma*. Philadelphia: Lea & Febiger, 1982.

SELECKY, P. A., ed. *Pulmonary Disease*. New York: John Wiley & Sons, 1982.

SJOBERG, E. L. "Nursing Diagnosis and the COPD Patient," *American Journal of Nursing*, 83 (February 1983): 245–48.

STORR, A. "Asthma: Disabilities and How To Live with Them," *The Lancet*, October 24, 1981, pp. 920–21.

U.S. Department of Health and Human Services. *Asthma and Allergies: An Optimistic Future*. Washington, D.C.: Public Health Service, NIH # 80–388, 1980.

———. *Chronic Obstructive Pulmonary Disease*. Washington, D.C.: Public Health Service, NIH # 832–020, 1983.

WEILL, H., ed. *Occupational Lung Diseases: Research Approaches and Methods*. New York: Marcel Decker, 1981.

WEISS, E. B., AND M. S. SEGAL, eds. *Bronchial Asthma: Mechanics and Therapeutics*. Boston: Little, Brown, 1976.

WILLIAMS, M. H. "Life-Threatening Asthma," *Archives of Internal Medicine*, 140 (1980): 1604.

Chapter 9: Stroke

ADLER, M. K., et al. "Stroke Rehabilitation: Is Age a Determinant?" *Journal of the American Geriatrics Society*, 28, no. 11 (November 1980): 499–503.

BACH-Y, R. A., ed. *Recovery of Function: Theoretical Consideration for Brain Rehabilitation*. Baltimore: University Park Press, 1980.

BRAY, G. P., AND G. S. CLARK. *A Stroke Family Guide and Resource.* Springfield, Ill.: Charles C. Thomas, 1984.

CHRISTIE, D. "Aftermath of Stroke: An Epidemiological Study in Melbourne, Australia," *Journal of Epidemiological Community Health,* 36, no. 2 (June 1982): 123–26.

COOPER, I. S. *Living with Chronic Neurologic Disease: A Handbook for Patient and Family.* New York: W. W. Norton, 1976.

DAHLBERG, C., AND J. JAFFE. *Stroke: A Doctor's Personal Story of His Recovery.* New York: W. W. Norton, 1977.

DEJONG, G., AND L. G. BRANCH. "Predicting the Stroke Patient's Ability to Live Independently," *Stroke,* 13, no. 5 (September–October 1982): 648–55.

Do It Yourself Again: Self-Help for the Stroke Patient. Dallas: American Heart Association, 1978.

DUCHARME, S. H., AND J. C. CUMMINS DUCHARME. "Sexual Adaptation," *Seminars in Neurology,* 3, no. 2 (June 1983): 135–40.

FOWLER, R. S. "Stroke and Cerebral Trauma: Psychosocial and Vocational Aspects." In W. C. Stolov and M. R. Clowers, eds., *Handbook of Severe Disability.* Washington: U.S. Department of Education, 1981, pp. 127–35.

GOODSTEIN, R. K. "Overview: Cerebrovascular Accident and the Hospitalized Elderly: A multidimensional Clinical Problem," *American Journal of Psychiatry,* 140 (1983): 141–47.

HEILMAN, K., AND E. VALENSTEIN. *Clinical Neuropsychology.* New York: Oxford University Press, 1979.

HELM-ESTABROOKS, N., AND M. L. ALBERT. "Rehabilitation of Speech and Language Disorders," *Seminars in Neurology,* 3, no. 2 (June 1983): 164–70.

JOHNSTONE, M. *Stroke Patients: Principles of Rehabilitation.* London and New York: Churchill, 1982.

LABI, M. L. C.; T. F. PHILLIPS; AND G. E. D. GRESHAM. "Psychosocial Disability in Physically Restored, Long-Term Stroke Survivors," *Archives of Physical Medicine and Rehabilitation,* 611 (1980): 561–65.

LIND, K. "A Synthesis of Studies on Stroke Rehabilitation," *Journal of Chronic Diseases,* 35, no. 2 (1982): 133–49.

LURIA, A. L. "The Functional Organization of the Brain," *Scientific American,* 222 (1970): 66–78.

MESULAM, M. M. "A Cortical Network for Directed Attention and Unilateral Neglect," *Annals of Neurology,* 10, no. 4 (October 1981): 309–25.

POSER, C. M., AND R. G. FELDMAN, eds. "Rehabilitation of the Neurologically Impaired," *Seminars in Neurology,* vol. 3, no. 2, June 1983, entire issue.

POSNER, J. D., et al. "Stroke in the Elderly," *Journal of American Geriatrics Society,* 32, no. 2 (February 1984): 95–102.

PRESCOTT, R. J.; W. M. GARRAWAY; AND A. J. AKHTAR. "Predicting Functional Outcome Following Acute Stroke Using a Standard Clinical Examination," *Stroke,* 13, no. 5 (September–October 1982): 641–47.

RADERSTORF, M., et al. "A Young Stroke Patient with Severe Aphasia Returns to War: A Team Approach," *Journal of Rehabilitation,* 50, no. 1 (January 1984): 23–26.

ROBINSON, R. G., AND T. R. PRICE. "Post-Stroke Depressive Disorders: A Follow-up Study of 103 Patients," *Stroke*, 13, no. 5 (September–October 1982): 635–41.

ROGERS, E. J. "Goals in Hemiplegia Care," *Journal of the American Geriatrics Society*, 28, no. 11 (November 1, 1980): 497–98.

ROWLAND, L. P. *Merritt's Textbook of Neurology*. 7th ed. Philadelphia: Lea & Febiger, 1984.

RUSKIN, A. P. "Understanding Stroke and Its Rehabilitation," *Current Concepts of Cerebrovascular Disease*, 17, no. 6 (November–December 1982): 27–32.

SCHWARTZ, D. "Catastrophic Illness: How It Feels," *Geriatric Nursing*, September–October 1982, pp. 303–6.

SESSLER, G. J. *Stroke*. Englewood Cliffs, N.J.: Prentice-Hall, 1981.

SMITH, D. S., et al. "Remedial Therapy After Stroke: A Randomized Controlled Trial," *British Medical Journal*, 282 (1981): 517–20.

SRARR, F. *Stroke Patients: Personal Narrative*. New York: Vantage, 1984.

STARR, L. B., et al. "The Social Functioning Exam: An Assessment for Stroke Patients," *Social Work Research and Abstracts*, 18, no. 4 (Winter 1982): 28–33.

Strike Back at Stroke. Dallas: American Heart Association, 1982.

TAYLOR, MARTHA L. *Understanding Aphasia: A Guide for Family and Friends*. New York: New York University Institute of Rehabilitation Medicine, 1977.

TOOLE, J. F. *Cerebrovascular Disorders*. 3d ed. New York: Raven Press, 1984.

———. *Diagnosis and Management of Stroke*. Dallas: American Heart Association, 1979.

"Up and Around: A Booklet to Aid the Stroke Patient in Activities of Daily Living." Dallas: American Heart Association, n.d.

WEINFELD, F. D. *The National Survey of Stroke*. Bethesda, Md.: National Institute of Neurological and Communicative Diseases and Stroke, 1983.

Chapter 10: Substance Abuse

ABELSON, A.; P. M. FISHBURNE; AND I. CISIN. *National Survey on Drug Abuse: 1977*. Rockville, Md.: National Institute on Drug Abuse, 1977.

ADLER, I., AND D. B. KENDEL. "Cross-Cultural Perspectives on Developmental Stages in Adolescent Drug Use," *Journal of Studies on Alcohol*, 42 (1981): 701–15.

Al-Anon Family Headquarters. *Al-Anon Faces Alchoholism*. Cornwall, N.Y.: Cornwall Press, 1965.

Alcohol and Health. Fifth Special Report to the U.S. Congress. Rockville, Md.: National Institute on Alcohol Abuse and Alcoholism, 1983.

Alcoholics Anonymous. New York: Alcoholics Anonymous World Services, 1955.

BRECHER, EDWARD M., AND THE EDITORS OF *Consumer Reports*. *Licit and Illicit Drugs*. Boston: Little, Brown, 1972.

BURGIN, J. E. *Guidebook for the Family with Alcohol Problems*. Center City, Minn.: Hazelden, 1982.

CORRIGON, E. M. *Alcoholic Women in Treatment.* New York: Oxford University Press, 1980.

COTTON, N. S. "The Familial Incidence of Alcoholism," *Journal of Studies on Alcohol,* 40 (1979): 89–115.

"Depression and Alcoholism." *American Journal of Psychiatry,* Special issue, vol. 136, no. 4B, April 1979.

Drug Abuse Council. *The Facts About "Drug Abuse."* New York: Free Press, 1980.

Drugs of Abuse. Washington, D.C.: Government Printing Office, 1979.

"Drug Abuse in Selected Metropolitan Areas: Reports on Trends and Lifestyles." Forecasting Branch, Division of Data and Information Development, National Institute on Drug Abuse, Rockville, Md., 1982.

First Statistical Compendium on Alcohol and Health. Rockville, Md.: National Institute on Alcohol Abuse and Alcoholism, 1981.

GLYNN, J., ed. *Drugs and the Family.* Rockville, Md.: National Institute on Drug Abuse, Research Issue 29, 1981.

GRINSPOON, LESTER. *Marijuana Reconsidered.* Cambridge, Mass.: Harvard University Press, 1982.

HAWKINS, R. O., JR. "Adolescent Alcohol Abuse: A Review," *Journal of Developmental and Behavioral Pediatrics,* 3, no. 2 (June 1982): 83–7.

HILL, SHIRLEY Y. "Alcohol and Brain Damage: Cause or Association," *American Journal of Public Health,* 73, no. 5 (May 1983): 487–89.

HOYUMPA, A. M., JR., et al. "Major Drug Interactions: Effect of Liver Disease, Alcohol, and Malnutrition," *Bulletin of Narcotics,* 33 (1982): 113–49

KALANT, O. J., ed. *Alcohol and Drug Problems in Women.* New York: Plenum Press, 1980.

KELLER, MARK, ed. *International Bibliography of Studies on Alcohol.* New Brunswick, N.J.: Rutgers Center of Alcohol Studies, 1980.

LENDER, M. E., AND J. K. MARTIN. *Drinking in America: A History.* New York: Free Press, 1982.

McINTOSH, I.D. "Alcohol-Related Disabilities in General Hospital Patients: A Critical Assessment of the Evidence," *International Journal of Addiction,* 17, no. 4 (May 1982): 609–39.

NELSON, J. E.; H. W. PEARSON; M. SAYERS; AND T. GLYNN. *Guide to Drug Abuse Research Terminology.* Rockville, Md.: National Institute on Drug Abuse, Research Issues 26, 1982.

NICHOLI, ARMAND M. "The Nontherapeutic Use of Psychoactive Drugs," *New England Journal of Medicine,* 308, no. 16 (April 21, 1983): 925–33.

Occupational Alcoholism: A Review of Research Issues. Research Monograph 8, National Institute on Alcohol Abuse and Alcoholism. Washington, D.C.: GPO, 1982.

Occupations and Alcoholism: 1982. Alcohol and Health Research Monograph 8. Rockville, Md.: National Institute on Alcohol Abuse and Alcoholism, 1982.

ORME, T. C., et al. "Alcoholism and Child Abuse: A Review," *Journal of Studies on Alcohol,* 42, no. 3 (March 1981): 273–87.

PATTISON, E. M., AND E. KAUFMAN, ed. *Encyclopedic Handbook of Alcoholism.* New York: Gardner Press, 1982.

PATTISON, E. M.; M. B. SOBELL; AND L. C. SOBELL. *Emerging Concepts of Alcohol Dependence.* New York: Springer, 1977.

PETERSEN, R. C., AND R. C. STILLMAN. *Phencyclidine (PCP) Abuse: An Appraisal.* Rockville, Md.: National Institute on Drug Abuse, 1978.

ROSS, H. L. *Deterring the Drinking Driver: Legal Policy and Social Control.* New York: Lexington Books, 1983.

SCHNOLL, S. H. *Alcohol and Other Substance Abuse in Adolescents in Addiction Research and Treatment: Converging Trends.* New York: Pergamon, 1979.

SELLERS, E. M., et al. "Drug Therapy: Drugs to Decrease Alcohol Consumption," *New England Journal of Medicine,* 305, no. 21 (19 November 1981): 1255–62.

SMART, R. G., et al. "A Review of Trends in Alcohol and Cannabis Use Among Young People," *Bulletin of Narcotics,* 33, no. 4 (1981): 77–90.

Special Populations. Alcohol and Health Research Monograph 4. Rockville, Md.: National Institute on Alcohol Abuse and Alcoholism, 1982.

STRACHAN, J. G. *Alcoholism: Tractable Disease.* Center City, Minn.: Hazelden, 1982.

TUCKER, J. A., et al. "Alcohol's Effects on Human Emotions: A Review of the Stimulation/Depression Hypothesis," *International Journal of Addiction,* 17, no. 2 (January 1982): 155–80.

WEGSCHEIDER, SHARON. *Another Chance: Hope and Health for the Alcoholic Family.* Palo Alto, Calif.: Science and Behavior Books, 1981.

WEIL, A., AND W. ROSEN. *Chocolate to Morphine: Understanding Mind Active Drugs.* Boston: Houghton-Mifflin, 1983.

WISEMAN, J. P. *Stations of the Lost: The Treatment of Skid Row Alcoholics.* Englewood Cliffs, N.J.: Prentice-Hall, 1970.

Index